Connected Health in Smart Cities

T0093730

Abdulmotaleb El Saddik • M. Shamim Hossain •
Burak Kantarci
Editors

Connected Health in Smart Cities

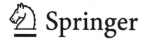

Editors
Abdulmotaleb El Saddik
School of Electrical Engineering and
Computer Science
University of Ottawa
Ottawa, ON
Canada

M. Shamim Hossain
Computer and Information Sciences
King Saud University
Riyadh, Saudi Arabia

Burak Kantarci
School of Electrical Engineering and
Computer Science
University of Ottawa
Ottawa, ON
Canada

ISBN 978-3-030-27846-5   ISBN 978-3-030-27844-1   (eBook)
https://doi.org/10.1007/978-3-030-27844-1

This Springer imprint is published by the registered company Springer Nature Switzerland AG.
The registered company address is: Gewerbestrasse 11, 6330 Cham, Switzerland

Preface

The book *Connected Health in Smart Cities* seeks to provide an opportunity for researchers, academics, and practitioners to explore the relationship between connected health techniques, theoretical foundations, essential services, and recent advances of solutions to problems, which may arise in a variety of problem domains of connected health in a smart city context. This book can serve as a repository of significant reference material.

This book aims to report the theoretical foundations, fundamental applications, and the latest advances in various aspects of connected services in health, more specifically the state-of-the-art approaches, methodologies, and systems in the design, development, deployment, and innovative use of multisensory systems, platforms, tools, and technologies for health management for the success of smart cities ecosystem.

The title of each of the book chapters is self-explanatory and a good hint to what is being covered. The overview of each chapter is as follows:

Chapter "Image Recognition-Based Tool for Food Recording and Analysis: FoodLog"—Maintaining food consumption and habits and analyzing food records is indispensable for the well-being of the citizen in a smart city context. To this end, FoodLog, a smart phone-based image recognition tool, is used for food recording and analysis from digital food image through image recognition or searching. FoodLog's application can be used for the management of food-related data of the athletes or sports activities. This chapter also has better insights related to improved health for healthy diet selection to control various diseases.

Chapter "A Gesture Based Interface for Remote Surgery"—At present, specially equipped vehicles or air-lifting to nearest hospitals/clinics is not affordable for the citizens in emergency cases or inadequate for areas with a large population that is remote from emergency surgical services. These vehicles can only serve a few patients or citizens every day. In this situation, there is a need for remote surgical services by skilled surgeons. Considering the above facts, this chapter discusses the application of gesture-based interactive user interfaces in performing remote endovascular surgery. The conducted experiments in the chapter demonstrate the feasibility of the approach and also the accuracy of the robotic controller at the base of the catheter, before it enters an artery.

Chapter "Deep Learning in Smart Health: Methodologies, Applications, Challenges"—Today, deep learning is one of the emerging theoretical foundations of connected health that can support healthcare professionals to find out the hidden opportunities in healthcare data and its pattern to assist doctors in order to have better analysis for improved health care for the citizens of smart cities. Keeping the above benefits in mind, this chapter presents very good insights of how deep learning techniques can be used for smart health data analysis, processing, and prediction. It also discusses about the emerging applications of deep learning techniques in smart health from cancer diagnosis to health status predictions.

Chapter "Emotional States Detection Approaches Based on Physiological Signals for Healthcare Applications: A Review"—Emotional health is one important consideration for improving citizens' quality of life and well-being in the smart cities. With these issues in mind, this chapter discusses existing emotional state approaches using machine and/or deep learning techniques, the most commonly used physiological signals in these approaches, and existing physiological databases for emotion recognition and highlights the challenges and future research directions in this field. It also discusses about how to incorporate accurate emotional state detection wearable applications (e.g., patient monitoring, stress detection, fitness monitoring, wellness monitoring, and assisted living for elderly people) within the smart cities so that it can aid to alleviate mental disorders, stress problems, or mental health.

Chapter "Toward Uniform Smart Healthcare Ecosystems: A Survey on Prospects, Security, and Privacy Considerations"—Security and privacy consideration is of paramount importance in the connected healthcare applications for the citizens' safety and well-being in smart cities. To this end, this chapter explores the latest trends in connected healthcare applications along with enabling technologies (e.g., sensing, communication, and data processing) and solutions (e.g., low-power short-range communication, machine learning, and deep learning) that might be driving forces in future smart health care. It reports the latest cyber-attacks and threats, which could be major vulnerabilities and weaknesses of the future smart healthcare ecosystem. It concludes with the proposed solutions and their associated advantages and disadvantages of each solution and analyzes their contribution to the overall security as an integral part of the connected healthcare system.

Chapter "Biofeedback in Healthcare: State of the Art and Meta Review"—This chapter begins by discussing the scope of utilizing biofeedback technology in smart healthcare systems. It presents a brief history of biofeedback technology and highlights the sensory technology in biofeedback systems by presenting the different types of sensors and their features. Recent research of biofeedback-based healthcare systems will be explored by presenting a range of applications in different fields. A set of challenges/issues that affect the deployment of biofeedback in healthcare systems will be discussed.

Chapter "Health 4.0: Digital Twin for Health and Well-Being"—With the advances in wearable computing, smart living, and communication technologies, personalized healthcare technology has entered a new era of healthcare industry to provide personalized proactive and preventive care in real time without being in close proximity. Digital Twins is an emerging technology to revolutionize healthcare and clinical processes. A digital twin virtualizes a hospital to have more personalized care. This chapter gives an overview of the existing literature and aims to provide an overview of existing literature on digital twins for personal health and well-being—key terminologies, key technologies, key applications, and the key gaps.

Chapter "Incorporating Artificial Intelligence into Medical Cyber Physical Systems: A Survey"—The emerging Medical Cyber-Physical Systems (MCPS) can revolutionize our connected healthcare system with high-quality, efficient, and continuous medical care for citizens of smart cities by providing remote patient healthcare monitoring, accelerate the development of new drugs or treatments, and improve the quality of life for patients who are suffering from different medical conditions, among other various applications. This chapter starts with the general description of the MCPS components and then discusses (1) how multisensory sensor devices and body sensor networks can assist in healthcare data acquisition, aggregation, and preprocessing and (2) how machine intelligence algorithms process the medical data from the previous steps to facilitate monitoring through connected healthcare systems and make self-directed decisions without much involvement of healthcare staff in a secure way to preserve the privacy of the citizens of smart cities.

Chapter "Health Promotion Technology and the Aging Population"—One of the important aspects for the success of connected health is the use of emerging healthcare technologies, which are of paramount importance in connected health services to the aging population in cities to improve the quality of care. To this end, this chapter provides an overview of assisted technologies and a survey of how the technology can be used to affect the elderly population to integrate healthier habits into their lives. The variety of accessible technologies allows individuals to use them in conjunction for their desired outcomes.

Chapter "Technologies for Motion Measurements in Connected Health Scenario"—The proactive and efficient care is one of the utmost requirements for connected health or technology-enabled care (TEC) in smart cities. For such care, smart sensing technology-based wearable solutions are essential for human motion tracking, rehabilitation, and remote healthcare monitoring. In such a context, this chapter presents an unobtrusive sensing solution (e.g., the Internet of Things (IoT)-enabled sensing) based on key enabling technologies with the aim of providing human motion measurement accompanied by motion measurement-related research and open issues. Finally, it demonstrates how the human motion measurements in motion tracking can contribute to the remote health monitoring system based on IoT and publish/subscribe communication paradigm.

Chapter "Healthcare Systems: An Overview of the Most Important Aspects of Current and Future m-Health Applications"—With the increasing number of aging population and the widespread use of mobile devices and communication technologies, citizens in smart cities would like to access the connected health service from anywhere at any time. In this respect, the mobile health care (m-healthcare) can provide affordable care for people in a convenient, accessible, and cost-effective manner. This chapter reports an overview of a generic m-Health application along with its main functionalities and components. The use of a standardized method for the treatment of a massive amount of patient data is necessary to integrate all the collected information resulting from the development of m-Health devices, services, and applications. To this end, this chapter discusses about the requirements of a standardization in healthcare, which is supported by related international and European healthcare projects.

Chapter "Deep Learning for EEG Motor Imagery-Based Cognitive Healthcare"— Owing to the massive amounts of complex healthcare data being produced in environments, such as smart cities, deep learning and cognitive capability are necessary to the idea of connected health. Deep learning-based cognitive systems can help various stakeholders, such as medical experts, healthcare professionals, and patients to develop insights into medical data that can help improve health care and provide a better quality of life to smart city residents. Hence, this chapter leverages deep learning techniques for understanding MI EEG data. The improvement in classification accuracy for motor imagery can help impart cognitive intelligence to machines and enable smart city residents to control the environment through sensors attached to their heads. This chapter proposes novel techniques for cross-subject accuracy and achieves outstanding improvement that can usher in new concepts about these complex brain signals.

The target audience of this book includes researchers, research students, and health practitioners in digital health. The book is also of interest to researchers and industrial practitioners in healthcare industry and smart city. We would like to express our great appreciation to all the contributors, including the authors, reviewers, and Springer staff, for their kind support and considerable efforts in bringing this book to reality.

We hope that the chapters from this book will serve as a repository of significant reference material and contribute to the roadmap of emerging use of services, techniques, and technologies for connected healthcare in smart cities.

Ottawa, ON, Canada   Abdulmotaleb El Saddik
Riyadh, Saudi Arabia   M. Shamim Hossain
Ottawa, ON, Canada   Burak Kantarci

Contents

Image Recognition-Based Tool for Food Recording and Analysis: FoodLog

Kiyoharu Aizawa

Abstract While maintaining a food record is an essential means of health management, there has long been a reliance on conventional methods, such as entering text into record sheets, in the health medicine field. Food recording is a time-consuming activity; hence, there is a need for innovation using information technology. We have developed the smartphone application "FoodLog," as a new framework for food recording. This application uses digital pictures and is supported by image recognition and searches. It is available for general release. In this paper, we present an overview of this framework, the data statistics obtained using FoodLog, and the future prospects of this application.

Keywords Food recognition · Image processing · Text search · Visual search

1 Food Recording Tool Using Analysis: FoodLog

We have developed and constructed a system, known as FoodLog, as a technical platform to record and utilize daily consumption data using multimedia information [1]. Although there are many tools to record details of the food consumed daily, the vast majority of these involve the input and output of text. Although there is much effort required for input, the records generated cannot be intuitively understood with just a single glance. The greatest distinguishing characteristic of FoodLog from existing tools is that it supports image recognition and searches through image-based recordings. Additionally, an important advantage of images is that the records can be perused and grasped with just a single glance. Initially, this was developed as a web-based system; now, this system has also been developed as a smartphone application [2, 3]. The functionality has gradually been expanded. The smartphone version released in 2013 supported image searches; since June 2016, an

K. Aizawa (✉)
Department of Information and Communication Engineering, The Faculty of Engineering, University of Tokyo, Tokyo, Japan
e-mail: aizawa@hal.t.u-tokyo.ac.jp

© Springer Nature Switzerland AG 2020
A. El Saddik et al. (eds.), *Connected Health in Smart Cities*,
https://doi.org/10.1007/978-3-030-27844-1_1

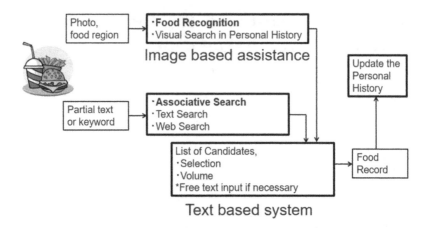

Fig. 1 Outline of FoodLog supported by food recognition and search

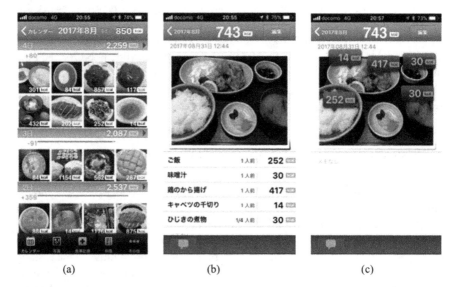

(a)   (b)   (c)

Fig. 2 Screenshots of FoodLog app. (**a**) Diary view, (**b**) food records, and (**c**) energy view

update supports image recognition as a method of record entry (image recognition is currently limited to the iPhone version).

An overview of the current functionality is shown in Fig. 1. A representative screenshot of the application's functionality is shown in Fig. 2. This framework supports record input based on image recognition and searches; notably, keywords are input with text only when image support is insufficient, significantly reducing the effort required to input data. The typical input procedures performed are described as follows:

1. The user photographs the food.

2. On inputting the record, the user starts up the FoodLog app. The FoodLog application automatically distinguishes between various images and presents the food photos from the album. Indeed, it is also possible to manually select the images from the album.
3. The users specify the food area in which they would like to record the presented food photo.
4. Automatic recognition of the food occurs, and the top 20 food items are presented in terms of probability. Additionally, an image search is conducted simultaneously on the individual history, and the top 20 consumed food items are presented in descending order of similarity.
5. If there is a desired item in the presented list, it is selected and the quantity is specified. This step completes the recording.
6. If a food item close to the desired item is included in the presented list (for example, a hamburger instead of a cheeseburger), an associative search is performed; then, the presented list is updated, and if the desired item appears, that item is selected and the quantity is specified. These steps complete the recording.
7. In case the desired item has still not appeared in the list, you can enter a keyword and update the candidate list; also, at the location of the desired item, this entered information is selected and the quantity specified. These steps complete the recording.
8. In case the target food item cannot be found with image or text search, you can describe the food name in free text as a newly appearing item; once this information is entered, it will be available for future searches.

It is not necessary to perform steps 1 and 2 at the same time. It is my personal practice to first take the picture and enter the record later. The photo is an essential mnemonic while inputting the record at a later time.

In case of the app screenshot shown in Fig. 2, (a), (b), and (c) show a list of the food records in calendar format, the record content of the individual food pictures, and a format in which just the calories are superimposed on the images. Furthermore, Fig. 3(a) and (b) shows the food area specified on the screen when entering the food records and a display of the recognition results, respectively. In the published version, this includes the detailed nutritional values of approximately 2000 foods that are typically found in Japan; of these details, only the calories are displayed. Datasets, with detailed nutritional values can, where necessary, be switched to those with high variation. At present, there are approximately 400 food items that have a high number of record registrations that can be detected. The number of food items detected can be easily increased through data quantity, without affecting the performance of the recognizer device. Using associative searches, this app searches a total of about 2000 typical foods based on similarity of food name, nutritional value, or recipe [4].

FoodLog is used by Diabetics [5]; notably, this app is under investigation at Tokyo University as a self-diagnostics tool for diabetes. It is also being used in the application Gluco Note, which Tokyo University is also evaluating [6].

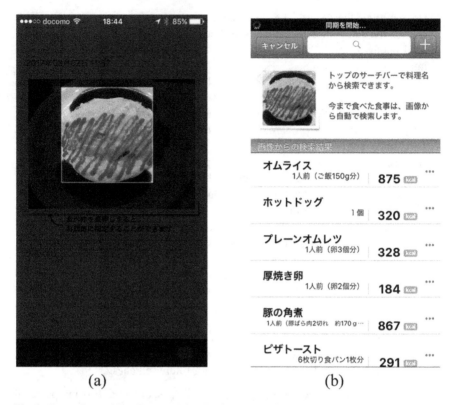

(a)   (b)

Fig. 3 Screenshots of FoodLog app. (**a**) Food area specified on the screen and (**b**) the list of candidates by image recognition

2 Trends Visible from FoodLog Data: (1) Frequent Foods

Since the implementation of the FoodLog application in 2013, more than 200,000 users have uploaded at least one photo, and 6 million food items have been recorded so far. The variation in food names registered by the users themselves has greatly exceeded expectations, evidenced by the fact the number of unique food names has exceeded 250,000 items.

Owing to the fact that there is a wide variety of food names registered by all users, it is necessary to summarize these appropriately to produce meaningful statistics. For example, we want to consider "yogurt" and "plain yogurt" as the same food item. To achieve this, we had to perform normalization processing on the recorded names using compression representation [7]. Specifically, (1) the respective foods are broken down into vocabulary words, (2) food names are selected from similar vocabulary words, a vocabulary graph is generated, and (3) representative food names are set based on the collections of shortest path vocabulary words.

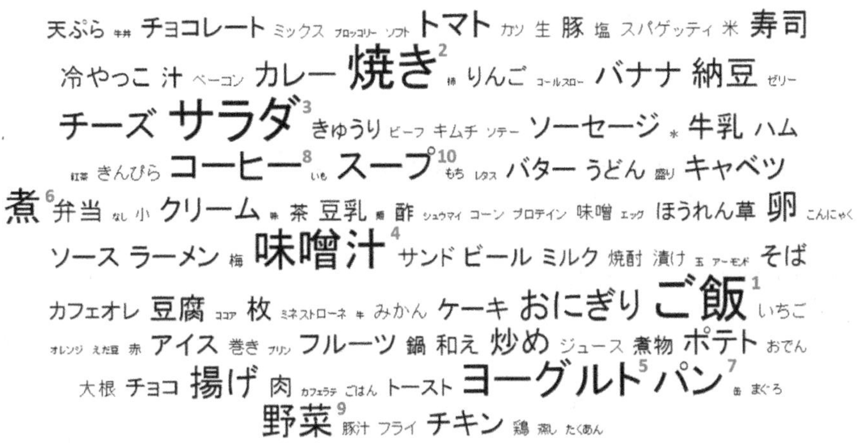

天ぷら 牛丼 チョコレート ミックス ブロッコリー ソフト トマト カツ 生 豚 塩 スパゲッティ 米 寿司
冷やっこ 汁 ベーコン カレー 焼き りんご コールスロー バナナ 納豆 ゼリー
チーズ サラダ きゅうり ビーフ キムチ ソテー ソーセージ 牛乳 ハム
きんぴら コーヒー スープ もち レタス バター うどん 盛り キャベツ
煮 弁当 なし 小 クリーム 茶 豆乳 酢 シュウマイ コーン プロテイン 味噌 エッグ ほうれん草 卵 こんにゃく
ソース ラーメン 梅 味噌汁 サンド ビール ミルク 焼酎 漬け アーモンド そば
カフェオレ 豆腐 ココア 枚 ミネストローネ みかん ケーキ おにぎり ご飯 いちご
オレンジ えだ豆 赤 アイス 巻き プリン フルーツ 鍋 和え 炒め ジュース 煮物 ポテト おでん
大根 チョコ 揚げ 肉 カフェラテ ごはん トースト ヨーグルト パン 缶 まぐろ
野菜 豚汁 フライ チキン 鶏 蒸し たくあん

Fig. 4 Top 100 frequent food records of all users of FoodLog

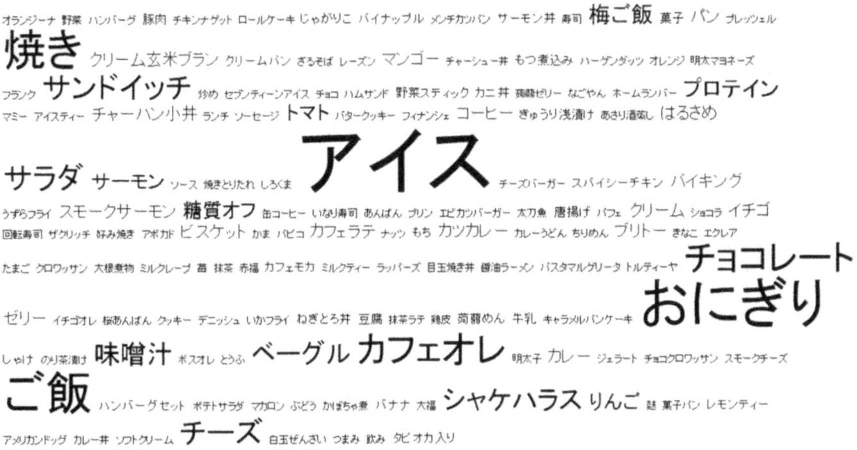

オランジーナ 野菜 ハンバーグ 豚肉 チキンナゲット ロールケーキ じゃがりこ パイナップル メンチカツパン サーモン丼 寿司 梅ご飯 菓子 パン プレッツェル
焼き クリーム玄米ブラン クリームパン ざるそば レーズン マンゴー チャーシュー丼 もつ煮込み ハーゲンダッツ オレンジ 明太マヨネーズ
フランク サンドイッチ 炒め セブンティーンアイス チョコ ハムサンド 野菜スティック カニ 珈琲ゼリー なごやん ホームランバー プロテイン
マミー アイスティー チャーハン 小丼 ランチ ソーセージ トマト バタークッキー フィナンシェ コーヒー きゅうり浅漬け あさり酒蒸し はるさめ
サラダ サーモン ソース 焼きとりたれ しろくま アイス チーズバーガー スパイシーチキン バイキング
うずらフライ スモークサーモン 糖質オフ 缶コーヒー いなり寿司 あんぱん プリン エビカツバーガー 太刀魚 唐揚げ パフェ クリーム ショコラ イチゴ
回転寿司 ザクリッチ 好み焼き アボカド ビスケット かま パピコ カフェラテ ナッツ もち カツカレー カレーうどん ちりめん ブリトー きなこ エクレア
たまご クロワッサン 大根煮物 ミルクレープ 苗 抹茶 赤福 カフェモカ ミルクティー ラッパーズ 目玉焼き丼 醤油ラーメン バスタマルゲリータ トルティーヤ チョコレート
ゼリー イチゴオレ 桜あんぱん クッキー デニッシュ いかフライ ねぎとろ丼 豆腐 抹茶ラテ 鶏皮 葛餡めん 牛乳 キャラメルパンケーキ おにぎり
しゃけ のり茶漬け 味噌汁 ボスオレ とうふ ベーグル カフェオレ 明太子 カレー ジェラート チョコクロワッサン スモークチーズ
ご飯 ハンバーグセット ポテトサラダ マカロン ぶどう かぼちゃ煮 バナナ 大福 シャケハラス りんご 某子パン レモンティー
アメリカンドッグ カレー丼 ソフトクリーム チーズ 白玉ぜんざい つまみ 飲み タピオカ入り

Fig. 5 Top 100 frequent food records of a particular user for its 6 weeks

We analyzed data trends using the first year of data (~1 million items) generated by the FoodLog application. The representative food names that appear frequently among the users are shown in Fig. 4. The frequently occurring items for all users are food names that are very familiar to all users. At the top of the list, names such as "baked" and "boiled" appear; however, because baked items and boiled items are overcompressed in the automatic processing for the normalization process, names of the cooking methods also appear.

In contrast to this, the same processing performed in relation to 6 weeks of data for a particular user is shown in Fig. 5, and this displays the order of frequency of records for just a single user. It is highly evident that this is very different to the trend for all users, which is very interesting. These food trends for individual users can be intuitively grasped.

3 Trends Visible from FoodLog Data: (2) Food Frequency Temporal Changes

The amount of food records greatly depends on the degree to which the user likes food. Food itself is also greatly influenced by seasonal factors and specific events. Additionally, consumption of newly emerging food items may increase as a result of mass media advertising.

We attempted to investigate changes in food frequency over time using the records recorded by FoodLog. Using the record frequency of food in FoodLog as an indicator, we used the ratio of the number of people that recorded a specific food item among all people who recorded consumption for that day. For reference purposes, we also investigated changes over time using search words on Google (Google Trend). Although Google Trend can intuitively grasp social concerns, the granularity of food is coarse; hence, while looking at the top 500 items in terms of frequency in FoodLog, only ~300 of these could be surveyed. Among these 300, there will always be words included that are not necessarily limited to food; thus, there is no certainty that they are expressing a particular interest in food. However, from ~300 items, frequency changes in 42 of the food names demonstrated a strong correlation (≥ 0.7) between FoodLog and Google Trend. From these, we selected items of particular interest and demonstrated fluctuations over 3 years, as shown in Fig. 6. Each of these was normalized to a maximum value of 1 within the period.

For all four examples in Fig. 6, trends of interest in terms of frequency trends in FoodLog records or Google search terms are extremely similar. Figure 6(a) and (b) are examples in which the frequency trends change considerably depending on the season or events. (a) Yudofu (boiled bean curd) appears frequently during winter, while (b) fried chicken peaks appear only during Christmas. In contrast to this, natto (fermented bean curd) in Fig. 6(c) is a food eaten daily, and its consumption, for both indices, gently increases over the period of approximately 3 years. (d) Chicken salad only became well known at the end of 2013, and from that point on exhibited a rapidly increasing trend for both indices. The fact that is interesting about (c) and (d) is that they are both health-oriented food items. In this manner, compared to Google, FoodLog, despite having a significantly small user base, is a tool that can be used

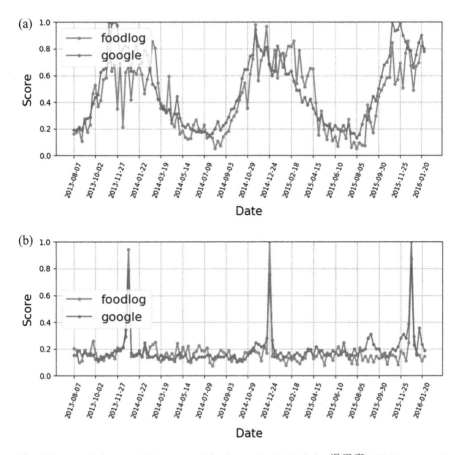

Fig. 6 Temporal changes of frequency of food records. (**a**) Yudofu (湯豆腐): Highly seasonal changes. (**b**) Fried chicken: Highly event-dependent changes. (**c**) Natto (納豆): Growing trend of a dairy food. (**d**) Salad Chicken: Growing trend of newly appearing food. It started widely selling in November 2013 at Seven Eleven Stores

to look at food-related fluctuations in detailed categories. Among these, items that relate to the interests of all users match with similar information from Google to a significantly higher degree.

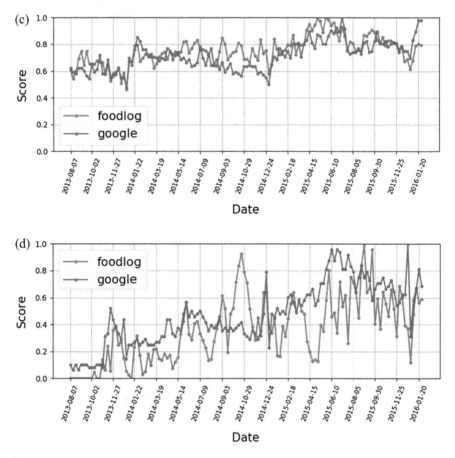

Fig. 6 (continued)

4   Conclusion

In this chapter, we presented an overview of our research and development of FoodLog as a tool to record information concerning food consumption in which the use of images is maximized. Additionally, from an analysis of the recorded data, we introduced examples of visualized food trends, both overall and individual, and changes over time for the frequency of food consumption over long periods.

As a tool, FoodLog is still in the developmental stage and we would like it to be increasingly convenient. For example, it would be useful if it could create a record by just inserting the picture, without the need to specify the food area. In actual fact, great efforts are being made in research and development for this purpose, and many innovations are planned for the interface in the next version of FoodLog.

The trends seen from the data in this paper, as demonstrated in the two examples, show its importance not only as a tool for recording but also as a platform for analyzing food records. Food surveys, which traditionally have taken months from data collection to publication, can be produced in real time through the use of FoodLog. Additionally, based on data from a large number of users, we are addressing the task of estimating records over a long period based on only few days' data for a particular user [8]. In addition, for FoodLog's application in the fields of self-management for health and dietary purposes, its functionality is also being expanded for the management of food-related data and information from other activities of sports athletes.

References

1. K. Aizawa, M. Ogawa, FoodLog: Multimedia tool for healthcare applications. IEEE Multi Media **22**(2), 4–9 (2015)
2. FoodLog. http://app.foodlog.jp/
3. K. Aizawa, K. Maeda, M. Ogawa, Y. Sato, M. Kasamatsu, K. Waki, H. Takimoto, Comparative study of the routine daily usability of FoodLog: A smartphone-based food recording tool assisted by image retrieval. J. Diabetes Sci. Technol. **8**, 203–208 (2014)
4. S. Amano, S. Horiguchi, K. Aizawa, K. Maeda, M. Ogawa, Food search based on user feedback to assist image-based food recording systems, in *ACM Multimedia Workshop on Multimedia Assisted Dietary Management (MADiMa)*, (2016), pp. 71–75
5. K. Waki, K. Aizawa, S. Kato, H. Fujita, H. Lee, H. Kobayashi, M. Ogawa, K. Mouri, T. Kadowaki, K. Ohe, DialBetics with a multimedia food recording tool, FoodLog: Smartphone-based self-management for type 2 diabetes. J. Diabetes Sci. Technol. **9**(3), 534–540 (2015)
6. GlucoNote. http://uhi.umin.jp/gluconote/ (2016)
7. S. Amano, K. Aizawa, M. Ogawa, Food category representatives: Extracting categories from meal names in food recordings and recipe data, in *IEEE International Conference on Multimedia Big Data, At Beijing, China*, (2015), pp. 48–55
8. A. Tsubakida, S. Amano, K. Aizawa, M. Ogawa, Prediction of individual eating habits using short-term food recording, in *International Joint Conference on Artificial Intelligence (IJCAI) Workshop CEA* (2017), pp. 45–48

A Gesture-Based Interface for Remote Surgery

Irene Cheng, Richard Moreau, Nathaniel Rossol, Arnaud Leleve, Patrick Lermusiux, Antoine Millon, and Anup Basu

Abstract There has been a great deal of research activity in computer- and robot-assisted surgeries in recent years. Some of the advances have included robotic hip surgery, image-guided endoscopic surgery, and the use of intra-operative MRI to assist in neurosurgery. However, most of the work in the literature assumes that all of the expert surgeons are physically present close to the location of a surgery. A new direction that is now worth investigating is assisting in performing surgeries remotely. As a first step in this direction, this chapter presents a system that can detect movement of hands and fingers, and thereby detect gestures, which can be used to control a catheter remotely. Our development is aimed at performing remote endovascular surgery by controlling the movement of a catheter through blood vessels. Our hand movement detection is facilitated by sensors, like LEAP, which can track the position of fingertips and the palm. In order to make the system robust to occlusions, we have improved the implementation by optimally integrating the input from two different sensors. Following this step, we identify high-level gestures, like push and turn, to enable remote catheter movements. To simulate a realistic environment we have fabricated a flexible endovascular mold, and also a phantom of the abdominal region with the endovascular mold integrated inside. A mechanical device that can remotely control a catheter based on movement primitives extracted from gestures has been built. Experimental results are shown demonstrating the accuracy of the system.

I. Cheng · N. Rossol · A. Basu (✉)
Department of Computing Science, University of Alberta, Edmonton, AB, Canada
e-mail: locheng@ualberta.ca; nrossol@ualberta.ca; basu@ualberta.ca

R. Moreau · A. Leleve
Ampere Lab, INSA, Lyon, France
e-mail: rmoreau@insa-lyon.fr; leleve@insa-lyon.fr

P. Lermusiux · A. Millon
CHU Hospital, Lyon, France
e-mail: patrick.lermusiaux@chu-lyon.fr

© Springer Nature Switzerland AG 2020
A. El Saddik et al. (eds.), *Connected Health in Smart Cities*,
https://doi.org/10.1007/978-3-030-27844-1_2

Keywords Gesture recognition · Remote control of catheter · Endovascular
surgery

1 Introduction

Despite the increasing popularity of computer- and robot-assisted surgeries, there
is still a need for remotely performing surgical tasks. At present, it is difficult to
perform surgeries in remote locations. Very often patients in emergency situations
need to be driven long distances in specially equipped vehicles or airlifted to
nearest hospitals. These emergency transportations are not only very expensive
but are also very demanding on fragile patients resulting in a negative effect on
their chance of survival. Also, these special transportations are far from guaranteed.
For example, the STARS air ambulance in Alberta, Canada, needs to hold several
fundraising lotteries every year to support their operating costs. Furthermore, the
air ambulance can only serve a few clients every day. While an ad hoc solution
like this is somewhat functional for a sparsely populated region with low demand,
it is completely inadequate for areas with large population that are remote from
emergency surgical services. According to a report from the Fraser Institute entitled
"The Effect of Wait Times on Mortality in Canada," over a 16 -year period surgical
wait times have led to over 44,000 deaths in an advanced country like Canada
with a relatively small population. This fact can give us some insight into the very
positive effect remote surgeries can have at a global level, if skilled surgeons could
collaborate from around the world.

With the above discussion in mind, in this chapter we discuss the application of
gesture-based interactive user interfaces in surgery. This new technology, which will
provide touch-free environments for interaction with 3D medical data, will improve
both the ease of use and efficiency of a number of medical devices and procedures.
Despite the large increase in popularity of touch-based devices, such as the iPad
and other tablet computers, in recent years, interaction with these devices remains
limited to physically touching the screen. There are many scenarios, particularly
in healthcare, where the ability to control a device through touch-free mechanisms
offers a significant advantage. During medical scans and procedures, for example,
a touch-free user interface will help (1) decrease the risk of spreading infection
by reducing the need for the device operator to touch potentially contaminated
surfaces; (2) eliminate the need for an extra assistant to help view and interact with
image data; (3) improve ergonomic conditions for a medical technician by removing
the need to concurrently use one hand for a medical probe and the other to operate
a computer keyboard; and (4) give surgeons the ability to leave a surgical room and
still be able to interact with a surgical procedure without touching any contaminated
surface.

A specific application area is Endovascular surgery, which is a type of Minimally
Invasive Surgery (MIS), designed to access target regions of the human body
through blood vessels [1, 2]. While endovascular surgery is being increasingly

deployed to replace classical surgery for improving recovery time and patient safety, there are still challenges to sustain a safe environment for patients as well as doctors. Ongoing research aims at reducing surgery time, and minimizing exposure to radiation. Currently, medical personnel require heavy cumbersome protective clothing which, nevertheless, can cover only part of the body. The ability to perform a surgery while keeping some distance from sources of radiation will improve the safety of surgeons and medical staff. In addition, the ability to interact with medical devices through gestures will increase patient safety by reducing the potential for contamination.

Several studies have examined active endoscopes and the effective control of catheters [3–5]; while the impact of stiffness of surgical manipulators was discussed in [6]. However, how to control a catheter using only gestures has not been addressed before.

Endovascular surgery has become a very important part of the therapeutic arsenal for the treatment of vascular diseases, such as abdominal aortic aneurysms [7]. These techniques are part of mini-invasive surgery and related to a decreased immediate postoperative morbidity and mortality. Yet, all these benefits are balanced by an additional cost and several challenges still remain.

Endovascular surgery exposes the patient and medical staff to a significant amount of radiation during the procedure [8]. Repetitive exposures to radiation increase the risk of cancer [9] and other diseases, such as cataract and skin injuries [10]. Thus, the ability to keep the surgeon and the staff distant from radiations without any loss of efficiency during the procedure is highly desirable in future endovascular surgeries.

Avoiding contact between the surgeon and the patient also reduces the risk of per-operative contamination. Stent-graft [11] infections are rare but associated with high morbidity and mortality rates [12]. Aortic stent-graft infections require, in most of the cases, the surgical explantation of the stent-graft [13].

From another perspective, gesture-based interactive user interfaces for surgery could be used for training of junior surgeons. The role of simulators in medical training is becoming more and more important [14–16]. Using such simulators, junior surgeons would be able to reproduce preoperative gestures during a surgical simulation, improve their skills before performing surgery on real patients, and have their learning evaluated through objective metrics.

2 Materials and Methods Used in Our System

There are various steps involved in our overall system to access the feasibility of using gestures to conduct or assist remotely in a surgery. These include:

- Extracting blood vessels from CT and identifying arteries
- Planning a path to follow during endovascular surgery
- Detecting hand movements and interpreting gestures; and
- Robotically controlling a catheter based on gestures performed remotely.

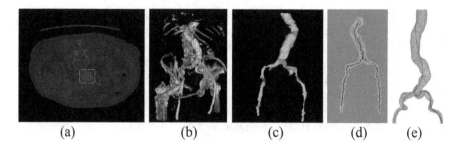

Fig. 1 Various steps in endovascular surgical planning: (**a**) A low contrast CT slice in axial view with the aorta inside the rectangle; (**b**) artery neighborhood detected using the OSIRIX software; (**c**) 3D segmentation using initialization of livewires followed by using the Turtleseg software; (**d**) medial axis generated inside the artery 3D model; and (**e**) artery phantom: with optimal path chosen by a surgeon for catheter navigation

The novelty in this work is in the last two areas mentioned above. However, we will briefly outline some of our work in the first area as well. We extracted the blood vessel and the medial axis (the curve in the middle that is equidistant from all sides) using several segmentation techniques. We used a new scale-space skeletonization algorithm for robust 3D medial axis extraction. Our algorithm is adaptive and can adjust the scale so that both narrow and wide regions of a blood vessel can be processed accurately. Figure 1 describes some of the methods related to preprocessing the medical image data that have been developed by us over the past few years. These include enhancing segmentation algorithms to extract blood vessels and arteries; skeletonization to find the path close to the center of the blood vessels; and designing and fabricating a phantom representing the actual arteries in a CT scan to allow surgical training. Details on some of these procedures are available in our earlier publication in [17, 18].

Endovascular surgery has become a very important part of the therapeutic arsenal for the treatment of vascular diseases, such as abdominal aortic aneurysms [7]. These techniques are part of mini-invasive surgery and related to a decreased immediate postoperative morbidity and mortality. Yet, all these benefits are balanced by an additional cost and several challenges still remain.

Endovascular surgery exposes the patient and medical staff to a significant amount of radiation during the procedure [8]. Repetitive exposures to radiation increase the risk of cancer [9] and other diseases, such as cataract and skin injuries [10]. Thus, the ability to keep the surgeon and the staff distant from radiations without any loss of efficiency during the procedure is highly desirable in future endovascular surgeries.

Avoiding contact between the surgeon and the patient also reduces the risk of per-operative contamination. Stent-graft [11] infections are rare but associated with high morbidity and mortality rates [12]. Aortic stent-graft infections require, in most of the cases, the surgical explantation of the stent-graft [13].

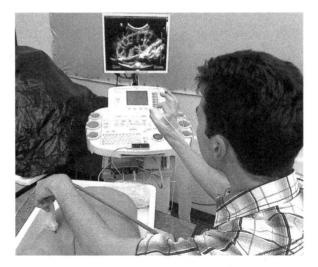

Fig. 2 A hand gesture tracked interface for controlling an ultrasound workstation

From another perspective, gesture-based interactive user interfaces for surgery could be used for training of junior surgeons. The role of simulators in medical training is becoming more and more important [14–16]. Using such simulators, junior surgeons would be able to reproduce preoperative gestures during a surgical simulation, improve their skills before performing surgery on real patients, and have their learning evaluated through objective metrics.

Figure 2 shows our work on detecting gestures being used for controlling the user interface of an ultrasound workstation. In the system we developed, the hand gestures that can be used to adjust the gain, brightness, zoom, and other parameters on the display shown in the figure without the fingers touching the screen.

Our hand gesture detection system uses the LEAP motion sensor. However, there are several challenges in situations with high occlusion. Many skeletal hand pose estimation techniques follow particle-filter approaches, which can get trapped in a local minimum due to inadequate visible data to resolve ambiguity. Incorrect pose may be identified as long as the hand pose remains static. Traditional approaches like the Kalman Filter [5] may not be adequate because the distribution of noise is similar for correct vs. incorrect detection scenarios [20]. Also, for fast movements of the fingers, tracking angular velocities of the fingers to predict future positions may not work.

We address the issues raised by occlusion using multiple sensors that are strategically placed with different viewing angles. We process the skeleton information provided by the Leap motion sensor instead of depth maps. The skeleton information consists of a collection of points with lines, representing a simplified version of the human skeleton of the hand. This type of data is easier to process than 3D depth information that may be available from other sensors, because of the limited amount of data that needs to be considered. Alternative strategies were considered to

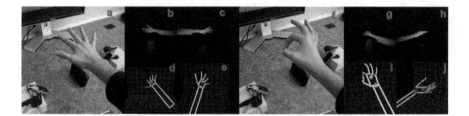

Fig. 3 Summary of our recent work in [19]. Using multiple sensors, we can reduce the effect of occlusion. For example, for the pair of images on the left, both of the sensors can detect the open hand pose. However, for the pair of images on the right, one sensor detects the pinch pose while the other incorrectly detects an open hand. Intelligently combining the results from the two sensors, it is possible to correctly detect the pinch gesture on the right

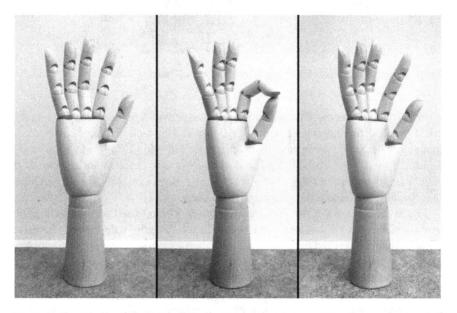

Fig. 4 Various hand poses used to compare performance against ground truth

determine the best way of combining (or fusing) data from multiple sensors. Figure 3 shows some results of our approach implemented in real time.

To determine the accuracy of our approach, we used a flexible hand phantom as shown in Fig. 4. Various alternative approaches were compared, including (1) Single Sensor, (2) Averaging of Multiple Sensors, (3) Sensor Confidence, (4) Weighted Fusion, and (5) Our Intelligent Fusion Approach. These results are shown in Fig. 5. It can be seen that our results are closest to the best possible if a person already knows which sensor to use.

Following the recording of gestures, we need to control the movement of a catheter potentially at a location that is distant from where the gestures were captured and analyzed. There are at least two scenarios where this approach is

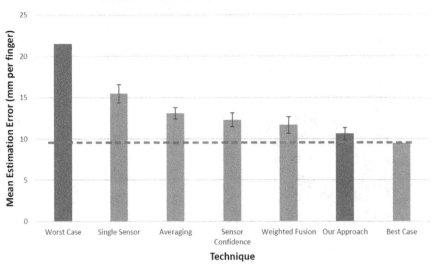

Fig. 5 Comparison of various approaches for hand pose estimation

very valuable. First, creating some distance between a surgeon and a patient in an operating room would reduce, if not eliminate, surgeons being exposed to radiation from intra-operative X-rays during surgery. At present, surgeons need to wear protective clothing with lead barriers to reduce radiation exposure. This type of clothing is heavy and uncomfortable, and still does not eliminate exposure to the face, arms, and legs. The second utility of our approach lies in surgeons being available to perform an emergency surgery even from a remote location. This will support greater access to patients who are unable to travel to a limited number of specialized urban centers that have surgical facility available.

We designed and built an electromechanical system for precise computerized control of a catheter. Our device consists of a motorized XZ Table that can move in two directions, coupled with two conveyor belts. The velocities of the two conveyors can be controlled through a computer or if necessary by a remote joystick. The guidewire is placed in between the two conveyor belts. The XZ Table is connected to one of the conveyors, while the other conveyor is fixed. By moving the two conveyors, we can move the guidewire backward or forward, while rotations of the guidewire can be realized through radial movements of the XZ Table. Figure 6 shows the composition of the electromechanical system built by us for controlling a catheter.

In order to determine the precision of our system we built an artery phantom. The phantom was designed by segmenting the arteries of an actual patient from the CT scans captured before a surgery. Figure 7 demonstrates our system. On the left, the mechanical system and the joystick are shown. On the right, the artery phantom is shown connected to the mechanical system. Inside the artery phantom, the catheter being controlled electronically can be seen.

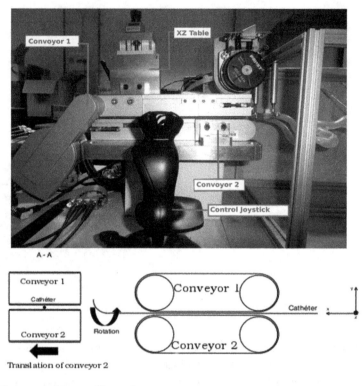

Fig. 6 Our system for controlling catheter movements

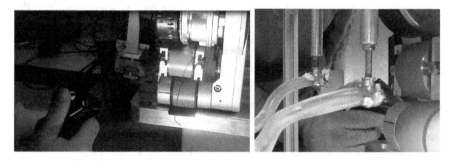

Fig. 7 Moving a catheter electronically into an artery phantom

3   Results in a Simulated Environment

We have already conducted experiments to verify our proposed methodology. Hand gestures were recorded and processed at the University of Alberta, Canada, using the Leap motion sensor. From these recordings, the primitives of the hand gestures were automatically extracted. Finally, these primitives were transmitted to Lyon,

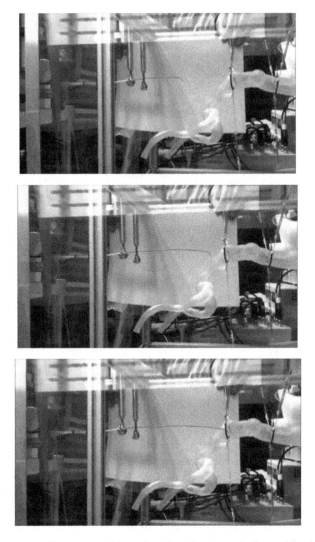

Fig. 8 Various stages of movement of the catheter based on remotely detected hand gestures

France, where they were used to remotely control a catheter. Figure 8 shows the position of the catheter at various stages of the process. Part of the endovascular phantom is not tied up in Fig. 8 so that the catheter can be seen more clearly.

Figure 9 compares the expected trajectory of the catheter with its actual trajectory. The blue line is based on Gesture Detection and the red line is based on the actual trajectory. The position was measured at the output of the robotic controller.

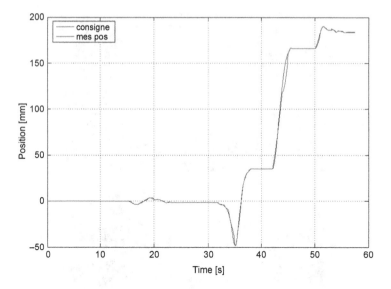

Fig. 9 Comparison of expected trajectory and actual trajectory of a catheter

4   Discussion

The current experiments verify the feasibility of our approach and also the accuracy of the robotic controller at the base of the catheter, before it enters an artery. However, the accuracy of the position and orientation, relative to the desired ones, at the tip of the catheter are still unknown. Additional errors can be encountered at the tip of a catheter resulting from unexpected bending and twisting. To correct for such distortions, we need to incorporate tracking methodologies at the tip; this could be done through visual (camera) feedback for testing the accuracy in a simulation. In the long term, we will also measure the accuracy of magnetic trackers in getting position and orientation feedback at the tip of a catheter. We also plan to conduct tests on laboratory animals to determine the feasibility of the approach in a real surgery.

5   Conclusion and Future Work

Despite significant achievements in computer- and robot-assisted surgery in recent years, limited advancements have been made in remotely conducting surgeries. In addition, the use of gestures rather than complex robotic tools to acquire input during conducting a surgery has been rarely considered. Taking these observations into account, we proposed a new direction of gesture-based interfaces for remote surgery. The description in this chapter outline preliminary work demonstrating the feasibility of the approach in performing remote endovascular surgery. However, there are many hurdles to overcome to realize a prototype even for this specific application. Some of the future tasks to build a functional prototype include obtaining accurate location and orientation information on the tip of a catheter inside blood vessels using magnetic sensors; providing feedback to a remote surgeon possibly through haptic and tactile means; and graphical interfaces preferably with light wearable glasses to allow more mobility.

Acknowledgements The financial support from Alberta Innovates and INSA, Lyon, France in conducting this research is gratefully acknowledged.

References

1. S. Guo, H. Kondo, J. Wang, J. Guo, T. Tamiya, A new catheter operating system for medical applications. Proceedings IEEE International Conference on Complex Medical Engineering, Beijing, China, 2007, pp. 82–86
2. L.W. Klein et al., The catheterization laboratory and interventional vascular suite of the future: Anticipating innovations in design and function. Catheter Cardiovasc. Interv. **77**, 447–455 (2011)
3. V. De Sars et al., A practical approach to the design and control of active endoscopes. Mechatronics **20**(2), 251–264 (2009)
4. M. Simi, G. Sardi, P. Valdastri, A. Menciassi, P. Dario, Magnetic levitation camera robot for endoscopic surgery. IEEE International Conference on Robotics and Automation, Shanghai, China, 2011, pp. 5279–5284
5. J. Hao, J. Zhao, M. Li, Spatial continuity incorporated multi-attribute fuzzy clustering algorithm for blood vessels segmentation. Science China Inf. Sci. **53**, 752–759 (2010)
6. M. Mahvash, P. Dupont, Stiffness control of surgical manipulators. IEEE Trans. Robotics **27**(2), 334–345 (2011)
7. B. Lindbald, Commentary on 'impact of shaggy aorta in patients with abdominal aortic aneurysm following open or endovascular aneurysm repair. Eur. J. Vasc. Endovasc. Surg. **52**(5), 620 (Nov. 2016)
8. S. Monastiriotis, M. Comito, N. Labropoulos, Radiation exposure in endovascular repair of abdominal and thoracic aortic aneurysms. J. Vasc. Surg. **62**(3), 753–761 (Sep 2015)
9. S. Yoshinaga, K. Mabuchi, A.J. Sigurdson, M.M. Doody, E. Ron, Cancer risks among radiologists and radiologic technologists: Review of epidemiologic studies. Radiology **233**, 313–321 (2004)
10. T.R. Koenig, D. Wolff, F.A. Mettler, L.K. Wagner, Skin injuries from fluoroscopically guided procedures. Am. J. Roentgenol. **177**, 3–20 (July 2001)
11. W.K. Wong et al., Endovascular stent graft repair is an effective and safe alternative therapy for arteriovenous graft Pseudoaneurysms. Eur. J. Vasc. Endovasc. Surg. **52**(5), 682–688 (November 2016)
12. M.R. Smeds, A.A. Duncan, M.P. Harlander-Locke, P.F. Lawrence, S. Lyden, J. Fatima, M.K. Eskandari, Treatment and outcomes of aortic Endograft infection. J. Vasc. Surg. **63**(2), 332–340 (February 2016)
13. X. Chaufour, J. Gaudric, Y. Goueffic, R.H. Khodja, P. Feugier, S. Malikov, G. Beraud, J.-B. Ricco, A multicenter experience with infected abdominal aortic Endograft explantation. J. Vasc. Surg. **65**(2), 372–380 (2017)
14. R. Aggarwal et al., Virtual reality simulation training can improve inexperienced surgeons' endovascular skills. Eur. J. Vasc. Endovasc. Surg. **31**(6), 588–593 (2006)

15. A. Saratzis, T. Calderbank, D. Sidloff, M.J. Bown, R.S. Davies, Role of simulation in endovascular aneurysm repair (EVAR) training: A preliminary study. Eur. J. Vasc. Endovasc. Surg. **53**(2), 193–198 (2017)

16. S. Sinceri, M. Carbone, M. Marconi, A. Moglia, M. Ferrari, V. Ferrari, Basic endovascular skills trainer: A surgical simulator for the training of novice practitioners of endovascular procedures. Conf. Proc. IEEE Eng. Med. Biol. Soc. **2015**, 5102–5105 (2015)

17. L. Shi, I. Cheng, A. Basu, Anatomy preserving 3D model decomposition based on robust skeleton-surface node correspondence. IEEE International Conference on Multimedia and Expo, 6 p 2011

18. I. Cheng, A. Firouzmanesh, A. Leleve, R. Shen, R. Moreau, V. Brizzi, M.-T. Pham, P. Lermusiaux, T. Redarce, A. Basu, *Enhanced Segmentation and Skeletonization for Endovascular Surgical Planning* (SPIE Medical Imaging, San Diego, February 2012), p. 7

19. N. Rossol, I. Cheng, A. Basu, A multisensor technique for gesture recognition through intelligent skeletal pose analysis. IEEE Trans. Human Mach. Syst. **46**(3), 350–359 (2016)

20. J. D. Hoelscher, MS Thesis, *Development of a Robust, Accurate Ultrasonic Tracking System for Image Guided Surgery*, Southern Illinois University Carbondale, 2008

Deep Learning in Smart Health: Methodologies, Applications, Challenges

Murat Simsek, Alex Adim Obinikpo, and Burak Kantarci

Abstract The advent of artificial intelligence methodologies pave the way towards smarter healthcare by exploiting new concepts such as deep learning. This chapter presents an overview of deep learning techniques that are applied to smart health-care. Deep learning techniques are frequently applied to smart health to enable AI-based recent technological development to healthcare. Furthermore, the chapter also introduces challenges and opportunities in deep learning particularly in the healthcare domain.

Keywords Predictive analytics · Deep learning · Smart health · Medical imaging

1 Introduction

Urban and regional planning is an aspect of human endeavor that has expanded as man improves in knowledge and understanding. This expansion has seen tremendous improvement in the way and manner humans move about within and outside their immediate vicinity. This success was no doubt assisted by tools used for proper town planning of which maps and other location positioning services are part of. The need to constantly get the best within our community and outside our community has led to the improvement of the tools used for location positioning and other factors that contribute to a better-planned city [32]. This constant improvement

M. Simsek
School of Electrical Engineering and Computer Science, University of Ottawa, Ottawa, ON, Canada

Department of Astronautical Engineering, Istanbul Technical University, Istanbul, Turkey
e-mail: msimsek@uottawa.ca

A. A. Obinikpo · B. Kantarci (✉)
School of Electrical Engineering and Computer Science, University of Ottawa, Ottawa, ON, Canada
e-mail: aobin064@uottawa.ca; Burak.Kantarci@uottawa.ca

© Springer Nature Switzerland AG 2020
A. El Saddik et al. (eds.), *Connected Health in Smart Cities*,
https://doi.org/10.1007/978-3-030-27844-1_3

was helped and continuously being helped by improved technological output. Digitalization of our cities is seeing daily improvement with the aid of powerful devices embedded with sensors for data acquisition, environmental monitoring, digital transportation, health improvement, easy access to amenities and facilities, and overall service provision for everyone within the city. A digital city is more often than not called a smart city. A smart city has various components which are all interlinked with improved technology and the need to provide quality services to its citizenry [15]. One of this components is smart health.

Smart health is the use of high technological devices for improved and quality health delivery. In other words, it contains the use of smart devices, electronic health monitoring gadgets, web services all connected(or not) to a data hub where positive inferences could be made about an individual's health status or a community's health status. The ubiquitousness of smart health has made its development a welcome change; this coupled with the ever-growing production of technological tools has seen the demand for smart health applications go up in recent years. As an example, an individual could check his or her blood pressure with his or her mobile devices thanks to the embedded sensors and applications found on these devices [7]; it is also possible to check the weather or climate readings of an area within a city and to know which part of the city to avoid if the weather is not suitable for your health [41]; a medical professional can check his or her patients health condition using the application both of them share with the purpose of advising the patients should any emergency occurs and so on. These examples are just a few of the many advantages smart health has to offer and with the increase in technological advancements, better devices are being produced to cope with the demands of the smart health industry. These devices not only serve as health tools but they also serve as good data acquisition tools, in which case the generated data could be processed and useful inference can be made in the long run. This also makes Smart Health applications integral parts of smart cities development. However, for smart health to be a successful element within a smart city, it ought to be able to measure up to the level of growth when compared to other aspects of a smart city. In other words, smart health needs to advance with technology just like the other components of a smart city. For this to work, processing of a smart health dataset would require proper and improved techniques; this is somewhat becoming a research hurdle as the datasets are generated by different devices with various operating capabilities thus leading to datasets with varying output type and format. The question now becomes; how do we process these datasets effectively and efficiently considering the volume and format of these generated data in order to achieve the goals of smart health? To provide answers to this question and others like it, different methods were developed and proposed by various data scientists. These methods would further metamorphous into much broader techniques, the most popular of them being machine learning.

Machine learning (ML) is the ability of a machine to learn from inputs with the goal of producing powerful algorithms for decision making. With advancing technologies, comes different learning ways by which a machine learns. This learning evolution has led to the development of more sophisticated tools like deep learning, extreme learning, etc. These tools have proven to be better to keep up with the aspect of new technological developments than conventional machine learning techniques. In fact, deep learning (one of the new tools) has a wide range of applications in smart health, specifically bioinformatics [36], medical imaging [18], disease prediction and analysis [40] to mention but a few. In the next section, we will talk about the improvement of the deep learning that is the next generation of machine learning.

2 Evolution of Deep Learning

The dataset generated by devices requires some form of processing for it to be useful. This processing was done using techniques that include the conventional machine learning algorithms. There two major types of machine learning algorithms; Supervised learning algorithm, where an input data with labeled responses are fed to the machine and the machine predicts the output (Support vector machines, decision trees, etc.); and unsupervised learning algorithms, which groups the input data into different classes or clusters based on certain characteristics (for example, K-means, DBScan, etc.). Machine learning algorithms use the features within a dataset to teach the machine how to identify patterns or specific characters like handwriting and speech [38]. The usefulness of machine learning algorithms in certain fields, for example, health care [51], computer vision [25], and so on [6], made them the "go to" tools for data processing and analysis. However, due to the increase in volume of datasets and the unstructured nature of data, these machine learning algorithms tend to face limitations in achieving the desired results. These and many other shortcomings lead to the development of a more computationally intensive and powerful learning technique called deep learning.

Deep learning algorithms have been described as a set of algorithms that think like the human brain [45]. A deep learning algorithm divides the dataset into layers and learn each layer, one by one, more like a "Divide and conquer" approach to problem solving. Deep learning techniques are gaining relevance as the year goes by due to the ease in which deep learning algorithms tackle problems in relative shorter time while consuming less memory. The development of deep learning was a gradual process borne out of the need to develop a machine that can deliver faster and work with high level of dimensions. This urge was given a boost when in 1958, Rosenblatt invented "perceptron." Hence, the first Artificial Neural Network (ANN) emerged and more development was begun [43]. The goal is to model the machine to think like the human brain and learn on its own. ANNs were used to do tasks that ordinarily could have been difficult for the computer without certain defined rules. However, as the year went by, improvements were needed to help the early invention keep up with the changing trend in computation. One of these improvements was introduced by Ivakhnenko [24] where he developed an algorithm for supervised deep feed-forward network; in this algorithm, layers grow incrementally, then trained using regression analysis and trimmed using validation sets to give effective output. Then in 1970, Linnainmaa developed the back propagation technique which is considered as the backbone of deep learning. Fukushima [17] while building his deep neocognition architecture introduced and added weights to convolutional neural networks. This created a gradient-based deep learning algorithms. All these were done in order to find a better way to train multiple layered network. To further expand on previous stated techniques, LeCun et al. [29], combined the back Propagation (BP) algorithm with a deep neural network in his research on hand written zip code recognition which proved successful. This further led to other useful ways to properly train a multilayered perceptron and further develop deep learning algorithm as seen in [3, 11, 19, 20, 46]. These historical developments of deep learning can be summed up into two major characteristics of deep learning. The first characteristic is the ability to discover hidden structures within large datasets using the back propagation algorithm which tells a machine how it should handle its parameters used in the computation of a layer and its successor. This argument sometimes lead to deep learning been termed as an example of representation learning. Another characteristic is deep learning adjust to unforeseen circumstances even if it has no knowledge of the rule governing such problems before hand. This is a necessary characteristic since the machine cannot be trained with loose data. Loose data occurs when proper problem description cannot be delivered to the machine thus leading to inadequate data that could have helped the machine make meaningful inference.

Deep learning is an effective tool in all fields through these two properties, especially healthcare. The diverse applications of deep learning in healthcare have evolved over the years and would be discussed in details in subsequent sections of this chapter. However, deep learning methods in healthcare mainly discussed in the following section.

3 Deep Learning-Based Methods

The following subsections will mention about the various type of deep learning methods that are mostly applied on smart health technologies. Fundamental notations which are required to understand mathematical relations in the remaining part of the section can be seen in Table 1, which has been adopted from [39].

3.1 Deep Feed-Forward Networks

Deep feed-forward primarily aims to approximate a function $f*$ by defining a mapping $y = f(x, \theta)$ which learns the value of θ in order to get a best approximation. To get the final value of y, several iterations are done within the layers. A typical feed-forward neural network consists of three fundamental layers. The input layer and the output layer should equal to the dimension of the input

Table 1 Basic notations used in the chapter

Notations	Definition
x	Samples
y	Outputs
v	Visible vector
h	Hidden vector
q	State vector
W	Matrix of weight vectors
M	Total number of units for the hidden layer
w_{ij}	Weights vector between hidden unit h_j and visible unit v_i
t_i	Signals
a_{ik}	Mixing weights
S_j	Binary state of a vector
s_i^q	Binary state assigned to unit i by state vector q
Z	Partition factor
b_j	Biased weights for the j-th hidden units
a_i	Biased weights for the i-th visible units
z_i	Total i-th inputs
v_i	Visible unit i
w_{kj}^2	Weight vector from the k-th unit in the hidden Layer 2 to the j-th output unit
w_{ji}^1	Weight vector from the j-th unit in the hidden Layer 1 to the i-th output unit
W_{ji}^1	Matrix of weights from the j-th unit in the hidden Layer 1 to the i-th output unit
$E(q)$	Energy of a state vector v
σ	Activation function
$P_r(q)$	Probability of a state vector q
$E(v, h)$	Energy function with respect to visible and hidden units
$pdf(v, h)$	Probability distribution with respect to visible and hidden units
$(A(n(t|m)))$	Entropy of the posterior

space and output space of the model. The hidden layer can be single or multiple according to the complexity of the model. Training process is required to ensure that $f(x)$ matches $f*$. In this case every sample in x has an accompanying attribute in $y \approx f * (x)$. In order to get the better approximations of $f * (x)$, the algorithm develops and uses the hidden layers. The hidden layers are the iterative computations which are done before the final result is sent to the output layer.

Mathematically, a basic feed-forward network with single hidden layer can be described in Eq. (1). Let $y_1, \ldots, y_k, ..y_M$ be M outputs for N dimensional input x and H_1 the number of neurons in the single hidden layer, then general output y_k could be given as follows:

$$y_k(x, w) = \sigma \left(\sum_{k=1}^{M} w_{kj}^{(2)} \sum_{j=1}^{H_1} \sigma_j \left(\sum_{i=1}^{N} w_{ji}^{(1)} x_i \right) + w_{j0}^{(1)} \right) + w_{k0}^{(2)} \tag{1}$$

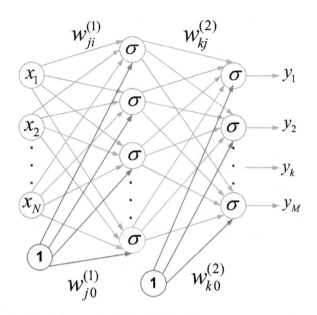

Fig. 1 Basic feed-forward network with single hidden layer

where $w_{kj}^{(2)}$ and $w_{k0}^{(2)}$ are weights associated with output layer; $w_{ji}^{(1)}$ and $w_{j0}^{(1)}$ are weights associated with hidden layer. Nonlinear modeling can be possible through nonlinear activation function σ.

Deep feed-forward network in Fig. 2 has more hidden layer than basic feed-forward network in Fig. 1. Number of hidden layer H can be shown in Fig. 2. The more hidden layer provides more processing capability for Deep Networks.

3.2 Linear Factor Models

Given a latent variable h and a real variable x, and if

$$h \approx p(h) \tag{2}$$

Then we can define a linear model as Eq. (3).

$$x = wp(h) + b + noise \tag{3}$$

where $p(h)$ is a factorial distribution, b is the bias, and w is the weight, and the noise is independent over all dimensions and Gaussian dependent.

Equation (3) is the base linear factor model where other forms will be derived from as we will see in later subsections.

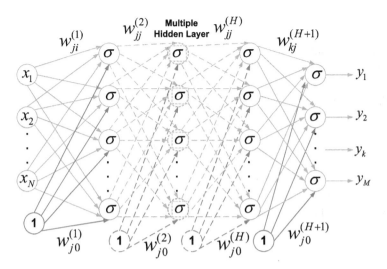

Fig. 2 Deep feed-forward network with H number of hidden layers

3.2.1 Probabilistic Principal Component Analysis (PCA)

The first variant of the linear factor model is the PCA. In order to utilize Eq. (3), the PCA allows the noise variation to occur when approximating the latent variable h before the real valued variable x is observed. That is,

$$h \approx N(h; 0, I) \tag{4}$$

With variables x_i assumed to be conditionally independent with respect to h, we get the following:

$$x \approx N(x; b, WW^T + \psi) \tag{5}$$

In this case, x is a multivariate normal random variable, ψ is the covariant matrix given as $\psi = diag(\sigma^2)$. We can define σ^2 as per-variable variance and it is represented in vector form $[\sigma_1^2 + \sigma_2^2 + \ldots + \sigma_n^2]^T$. Substituting this into Eq. (4) and adjusting the initial model equation (5), we obtain

$$x \approx N(x; b, WW^T + \sigma^2 I) \tag{6}$$

Equation (6) is the model for the PCA and $WW^T + \sigma^2 I$ is the covariance of the variable x. Decomposing Eq. (6) further gives

$$x = Wh + b + \sigma z \tag{7}$$

where $z \approx N(z; 0, \sigma I)$ is the introduced Gaussian noise.

3.2.2 Independent Component Analysis (ICA)

The second variant of linear factor models is the ICA. The ICA divides observed signals into many independent non-Gaussian parts, then fuse them to become the observed/input data.

Suppose, we have T signal divided into $T = (t_1, \ldots, t_n)^T$ and a random vector x given as $x = (x_1, \ldots, x_m)^T$, then the input data can be of the form

$$x_i = a_{i,1}t_1 + \ldots + a_{i,k}t_k + \ldots + a_{i,n}t_n \tag{8}$$

where $a_{i,k}$ is the mixing weights.

Now, if we let $x_1, x_2, \ldots, x_m$ be the set of binary variables from m monitors with a corresponding $y_1, y_2, \ldots, y_n$ of n sources, then we have

$$x_i = \vee_{j=1}^{n}(g_{ij} \wedge y_i), i = 1, 2, \ldots, m \tag{9}$$

where $\vee$ is Boolean "OR" and $\wedge$ is Boolean "AND." Equation (9) is called the binary ICA model and the monitors and sources are in binary form.

3.3 Autoencoder

An autoencoder [22, 49] is a fully connected neural network which consists of three layers such as input, hidden, and output. The autoencoder can be decoupled into two separate parts: an encoder $h = f(x)$ and a decoder $r = g(h)$, both sharing the layer which is often referred to as base vector as depicted in Fig. 3. If the autoencoder successfully learns to place $g(f(x)) = x$ everywhere, then it becomes irrelevant

Fig. 3 Autoencoder network

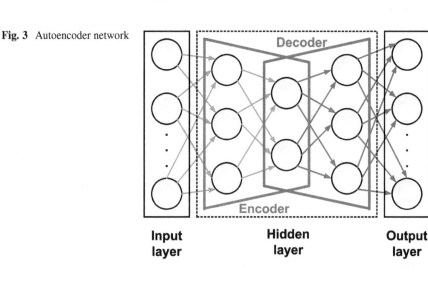

Input layer   Hidden layer   Output layer

because autoencoders are usually made just to be able to copy the original a bit but not perfectly. They are viable tools for dimensionality reduction, feature learning, and generative modeling.

There are various types of autoencoders which will be described briefly:

- Undercomplete Autoencoders: have a smaller dimension for hidden layer compared to the input layer. This helps to obtain important features from the data. Objective function in Eq. (10) minimizes the loss function by penalizing the $g(f(x))$ for being different from the input x. Objective is to minimize the loss function by penalizing the $g(f(x))$ for being different from the input x.

$$L = |x - g(f(x))| \qquad (10)$$

where L is the loss function.
- Regularized Autoencoders: This kind of autoencoder trains any type of architecture by choosing the code dimension and other properties based on the complex nature of the dataset to be modeled [4]. The regularized autoencoder uses a loss function most times to give the model a leeway in exploiting other encoder properties rather than limiting itself to just the ability to copy inputs to outputs.
- Sparse Autoencoders: have hidden neurons greater than input neurons. Sparsity constraint is introduced on the hidden layer which is to prevent output layer exactly copy to input data. They can still discover important features from the data. The sparse autoencoder's training requirement involves the imposition of a sparsity penalty $\Omega(h)$ on the hidden layer h, together with the reconstruction error equation (11).

$$L = |x - g(f(x))| + \Omega(h) \qquad (11)$$

Again, sparse autoencoders are sometimes used to learn features during a classification task.
- Denoising Autoencoder: is a stochastic autoencoder as a stochastic corruption process to set some of the inputs to zero [49]. Denoising refers to intentionally adding noise to the input before providing it to the network. Denoising autoencoders minimizes the loss function equation (12) between the output node and the corrupted input $\tilde{x}$ which is obtained by adding noise to the input.

$$L = |\tilde{x} - g(f(x))| \qquad (12)$$

- Contractive Autoencoders: is another regularization technique like sparse autoencoders and denoising autoencoders. It can be considered to have a robust learned representation which is less sensitive to small variation in the data. Robustness of the data representation is ensured by applying Frobenius norm of the Jacobian matrix as a penalty to the loss function [42]. This penalty for the hidden layer is calculated with respect to input. Once penalty term in Eq. (11) is changed by Eq. (13), then Eq. (14) is used as Frobenius norm in Eq. (13). Hence, loss function can be obtained by changing the Eq. (11).

$$\Omega(h) = \lambda \left\| J_f(x) \right\|_F^2 \tag{13}$$

$$\left\| J_f(x) \right\|_F^2 = \sum_{ij} \left(\frac{a h_j(x)}{\partial x_i} \right)^2 \tag{14}$$

In this case, the penalty $\Omega(h)$ is called the Frobenius norm.

The contractive autoencoders are trained to discourage any form of perturbation of their input values, so they try to map the neighborhood of input values into a much smaller neighborhood of output values.

3.4 Convolutional Neural Network (CNN)

Convolutional Neural Net is a more powerful deep learning technique to improve the performance for current visual recognition tasks [1, 12]. CNN's structure can be determined in terms of the size, quality, and type of dataset. They are neural networks that use mathematical convolutions besides general matrix multiplications. CNNs consist of multiple receptive layers that process portions of the input image. The outputs of CNNs are arranged in such a way that it creates some form of overlapping in the input area, in order to obtain a higher-resolution representation of the original image. The same procedure is run for every layer that is present in the network. Moreover, the goal of CNNs is to learn data-specific kernels instead of predefined kernels.

3.4.1 CNN Architecture

CNNs will utilize a series of convolutions and pooling operations during which the features are detected. The fully connected layers will work as a classifier using these extracted features. All operations in CNN are summarizes in Fig. 4. It is worthy to note that though, any CNN might have a few amount of convolutional layers coupled with pooling layers, it is optional for it to have fully connected layers.

- Convolutional Layer: Convolution is one of the main building blocks of CNNs. The convolution is used for the mathematical combination of two functions and the result is a function as well. The convolution is executed by sliding the filter over the input. A matrix multiplication is performed for every location and sums the result onto the feature map. The convolutional layer has a $m \times m \times r$ input image, where m is the height and width of the image and r is the number of channels. It has k filters (or kernels) and size of each is $n \times n \times q$. n in this case, is smaller than the image dimension. q could either be the same as the amount

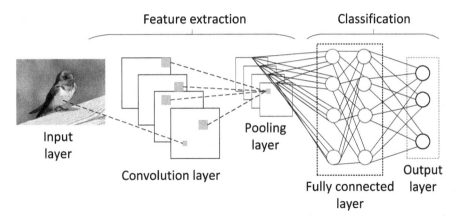

Fig. 4 Architecture of a CNN

of channels r or it might be smaller for every kernel. The filters' size leads to connected structures where each structure is linked with the image to constitute k feature maps of size $m - n + 1$.

- Pooling Layer: After a convolution layer, a pooling layer is commonly added between CNN layers. The main function of pooling layer is to reduce the dimensionality to satisfy lower the number of parameters and computation in the network. Hence, the training time is reduced and it can be possible to control overfitting. Pooling layer sub-samples their input by applying a maximum operation to the result produced by each filter or kernel. One major property of pooling is to generate a fixed size output matrix that is required for classification. The most favorite pooling is max pooling, which takes the maximum value in each window.

- Fully Connected Layer: After the convolution and pooling layers, the last part is required to be fully connected regular Neural Network to classify input images. Neurons in a fully connected layer are connected to the activation functions in the previous layer.

3.5 Deep Belief Network (DBN)

The DBN consists of stochastic binary unit layers where each connected layers have some weight. The DBN has multiple layers of latent variables that is connected between layers [21, 23]. Though with these connections amongst layers, there exists no visible connections amongst units that are within a particular layer. Again, the DBN learns to do a new construction of its inputs, and thereafter train them for classification tasks. One important feature of the DBN is that, they are learned one particular layer per time using the greedy scheme. The DBN has the following properties:

- When learning the generative weights, a layer by layer approach is used which determines how each variable in a layer depends on variables in another layer that is above it.
- After learning each latent variable, their values are inferred using a single pass which begins with an observed data in the least layer.

Furthermore, suppose, we have the visible units v, the hidden units, h that are conditionally independent, the weights W, that is learned by a restricted Boltzmann machine, then the probability of generating a visible vector v, is

$$p(v) = \sum_h p(h\backslash W)p(v\backslash h, W) \tag{15}$$

where $p(h\backslash W)$ is the prior distribution over hidden vectors and $p(v\backslash h, W)$ is the posterior distribution over visible vectors.

In one sense, if a DBN has just one hidden layer, it is called a restricted Boltzmann machine (RBM). In this case using a constructive divergence method, we can train the first RBM which subsequently leads to the training of DBN after certain number of iterations.

3.6 Boltzmann Machine (BM)

BM is a symmetrically connected network of neuron-like units (Fig. 5) that make binary stochastic decisions [2]. The learning algorithms of BMs allow them to fully discover useful and important features that portrays complex regularities in datasets. BMs are mostly used to solve search and learning problems.

To get a better understanding, assume a unit i has an opportunity to always update its binary state at any given time; it computes its total input as seen in Eq. (16), below.

$$z_i = b_i + \sum_j s_j w_{ij} \tag{16}$$

where w_{ij} refers to the connection weight between units i, j, and s_j is 1 if j is on or 0 when j is off. The probability that unit i comes on is given as

$$P_r(s_i = 1) = \frac{1}{1 + e^{-z_i}} \tag{17}$$

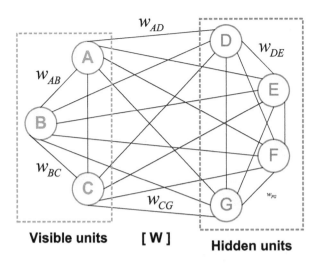

Fig. 5 Boltzmann network

Now, if each unit is updated sequentially, the network in the probability of a state vector v can be obtained in Boltzmann distribution as follows:

$$P_r(q) = \frac{e^{-E(q)}}{\sum_u e^{-E(u)}} \tag{18}$$

where $E(q)$ is the energy of state vector q and defined as

$$E(q) = -\sum_i s_i^q b_i - \sum_{i<j} s_i^q s_j^q w_{ij} \tag{19}$$

where s_i^q refers to the binary state assigned to unit i by state vector q.

Should any of these connections weights be selected in a way that the energies of each state vectors represent their costs, then we can view the stochastic nature of a BM as a means of exiting from an inappropriate local optima while it continues its search for low-cost solutions.

When learning a BM, it can be done with the hidden units or without them. There are special cases or types of BM, out of which two are highlighted below.

Mean Field Boltzmann Machines. This kind of BM uses mean field units which possesses deterministic values between 0 and 1, and they are used to compute the main value for a unit's state based on the current states of the other units.

High-order Boltzmann machines. In this type, the structure and the rule for learning encourage the use of energy functions that are complicated.

3.7   Restricted Boltzmann Machines (RBM)

In an RBM, there exists layers of visible and hidden units with intraconnections within these layers (that is, no hidden-hidden nor visible-visible connections) [22, 28].

With the hidden units (h) being independent conditionally on the visible (v) vector, the unbiased samples from $\langle s_i s_j \rangle_{data}$ can be obtained in one single step. In order to take samples from $\langle s_i s_j \rangle_{model}$ requires a number of iterations with alternating activities between updating the hidden units and the visible units in parallel times [44].

Mathematically, the energy function of an RBM with hidden and visible units consisting of $W = (w_{ij})$ (where W is the matrix of weights) associated with the connection between hidden unit h_j and visible unit v_i, can be written as

$$E(v, h) = -\sum_i a_i v_i - \sum_j b_j h_j - \sum_i \sum_j v_i w_{i,j} h_j \qquad (20)$$

with a probability distribution of

$$pdf(v, h) = \frac{1}{Z} e^{-E(v,h)} \qquad (21)$$

After learning is finished for one hidden layer, the activity vectors of the hidden units can be treated as "data" to train another RBM. This particular computation can be repeated as many times as possible in order to learn as many hidden layers as needed. After learning many hidden layers, the entire network can be seen as a single but multi-layered generative model where additional hidden layers contribute to the improvement of the lower bound (Fig. 6).

Learning hidden layers one at a time has been seen as a very efficient way to learn and understand deep neural networks that possess multiple hidden layers with quite a number of weights. The learning might be unsupervised but the highest features are generally useful for classification purposes.

3.8   Variational Autoencoders (VAE)

These autoencoders use learned approximations to make inference. They are trained mainly using gradient-based methods. To obtain a sample from an already built model, the VAE chooses a sample t from the distribution $p_{model}(t)$ and runs it through a generator network $g(t)$. After which, the random variable m is chosen randomly from the distribution $p_{model}(m; g(t)) = p_{model}(m|t)$. While training is

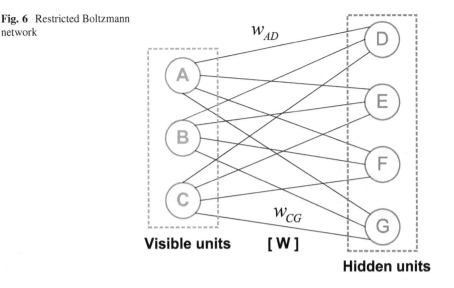

Fig. 6 Restricted Boltzmann network

Visible units [W]

Hidden units

going on, the generated approximate inference network $n(l)$ is used to derive t while $p_{model}(m|t)$ becomes the encoder of the network. In other words a VAE could be trained properly if the variational lower bound $D(n)$ that is associated with the random variable m is maximized such that

$$D(n) = E_{t \approx n(t|m)} log p_{model}(t, m) + A(n(t|m)) \qquad (22)$$

where $A(n(t|m))$ refers to the entropy of the posterior.

If n is a Gaussian distribution with an additive noise added to its predicted mean value, then a maximum entropy value would increase the value of the standard deviation of the noise. Another way of saying this is, the entropy value allows the variational posterior to place a steep probability mass function on a number of t items which would have produced m rather than reducing it to just a point estimate of the most probable value.

While some approaches to VAE infer the value of n through an optimization algorithm, the main goal however is to train any parametric encoder to produce parameters of n. Thus, if t is a continuous variable, then carrying out a back propagation on the samples of m will give a gradient with respect to the encoder(θ).

One important feature with the VAE is that it is very possible to train a combined parametric encoder and generator network function, thus giving the model the ability to learn a predictable coordinate system which the encoder captures.

3.9 Auto-Regressive (AR) Model

An auto-regressive (AR) model is utilized to predict future characteristics based on past values. AR is also used for forecasting when there is some correlation between values in a time series and the values [27, 35]. Since AR requires past data to model the behavior, the name auto-regressive is related to "self." The process is very similar to a linear regression of the data in the current series opposing one or more past values in the series.

The AR process is a stochastic process, which has degrees of uncertainty or randomness built in. The randomness means that AR might be able to predict future trends accurately in terms of past data, but this accuracy is never going to get %100. Generally, the process can be close enough to the desired response. AR models are also called conditional models or Markov models.

An $AR(p)$ model is an auto-regressive model where specific lagged values of y_t are used as predictor variables. The value for "p" is called the order. $AR(1)$ indicates the first-order auto-regressive process. The response in a first-order AR process at some point in time t is related only to time delayed response. The high order AR process is related to the corresponding time delayed response data. $AR(p)$ model formulation is given as follows:

$$y_t = \delta + \varphi_1 y_{t-1} + \varphi_2 y_{t-2} + \ldots + \varphi_p y_{t-p} + A_t \tag{23}$$

where A_t is white noise and φ indicates constant values. Moreover y_{t-1} indicates the first-order time delayed response.

δ in (24) is seen in (23).

$$\delta = \left(1 - \sum_{i=1}^{p} \phi_i\right) \mu \tag{24}$$

where μ is the process mean.

3.10 Nonlinear Auto-Regressive (NAR) Neural Networks

Nonlinear auto-regressive (NAR) neural networks are mostly suitable for prediction and forecasting [14, 16]. The output of NAR neural network is generated by regarding different ordered delayed outputs. Hence previous output data are used for prediction of the future output. Nonlinear activation functions provide a nonlinear relationship between time delayed data and the current time output. The structure of NAR neural network can be seen in Fig. 7.

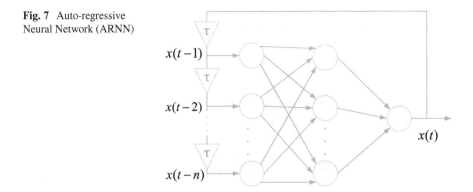

Fig. 7 Auto-regressive Neural Network (ARNN)

4 Applications

Health care systems are being revolutionized due to rapid growth in technology. The applications of various technological innovations have contributed immensely to the growth of quality healthcare delivery. As stated in Sect. 1, the growth of smart health can be attributed to the ever-growing ecosystem in the technological space. And as this growth increases, comes the burden of specialization in terms of proper algorithms for problem solving; ability to synchronize the data acquired with the intended technique for data analysis; how and when to use a particular technique; what techniques should be used for effective results, amongst many others. These are some of the many problems plaguing the smart health industry. However intimidating these problems might seem, research has been conducted to provide up-to-date solutions to these problems. Most research was conducted according to various themes in the industry which includes but not limited to data acquisition, data processing, data analytics, and learning techniques. That said, for any meaningful progress to be made, there is always a base case. The base case for smart health care is a 2-prong one: data acquisition and data analytics. Data acquisition can occur in various forms with different output format. This often leads to data heterogeneity when various devices are used to acquire data for experimental purposes. The format of the acquired data determines what kind of techniques that would be used for analytics. Deep learning, one of the tools used for data analytics has proven to be an effective tool due to its accuracy, runtime, and usage with almost any kind of data. Deep learning can make classify, cluster, and predict possible by getting signals, or structures in datasets. When deep network is trained, it can be used for prediction about the data. The prediction error of it can be measured regarding with the training set. What's more is that deep learning has a range of applications in the smart health industry. In this section of the chapter, we shall be looking at a few applications of deep learning techniques in smart health. These applications shall be discussed based on three health categories; bioinformatics, medical imaging, and predictive analytics.

4.1 BioInformatics

Bioinformatics is one area in the health industry that has been receiving lots of attention in recent years. This is not far-fetched since the health industry is currently experiencing massive digitization and the utilization of this massive technological growth is evident. Deep learning techniques are being used widely in the bioinformatics area of health care. Specific cases are summarized as follows. Understanding protein structures is a key research topic in the medical area. This is due to the fact that protein structures are key components in the understanding of the functions of proteins. The authors in [36] proposed a deep learning technique called sparse autoencoder for sequence-based determination of the distance between two neighboring $c\alpha$ atoms represented by the angles between $C\alpha_{i-1} - C\alpha_i - C\alpha_{i+1}$ (θ) and $C\alpha_i - C\alpha i + 1$ (τ). They believed that accurate predictions of these angles can appropriately give a more accurate distance. Also, the predicted α and τ values could be used to construct local structures with good accuracies. In the same vein, the authors in [5] show that DNA- and RNA- binding proteins sequence specificities can be derived from experimental data. They called this approach "DeepMind." This method uses the convolutional neural network for training the acquired data and then used back propagation to compute the derivative of all parameters that are in the model. The result obtained from Deepmind was better than other methods used in this particular application area. Also, Lee and Yoon [30] used a deep learning-based technique-restricted Boltzmann machines to predict protein secondary structure. The demand for protein secondary structure predictions is on the increase in the protein discovery sphere of bioinformatics. The authors generated multiple layers for the intended network from a dataset of 1230 protein chains, used the RBM for training, analysis, and prediction. The outcome of the prediction was evaluated using the SOV scoring functions. Their proposed method generated a result of 80.7% accuracy when tested with an independent test dataset. In their work, Leung et al. [31] used deep neural network to create a model that can predict splicing patterns in individual tissues as well as individual differences found in splicing patterns across tissues. Zhang et al. [52] with a view to model the structural binding for RNA-binding proteins used a deep learning framework. The developed learning framework constructed a representation for the specificities of the RNA-binding proteins and also predict new binding sites within the RNA being studied. Motivated by the need to accurately recognize gene expressions, the authors in [9] used D-GEXT (feed-forward neural network-based technique) to determine the expressions of certain target genes. The result from this experiment showed that D-GEX outperforms other methods by 6.57%. Aside gene classifications and expressions, deep learning is also being used in cancer research. Specifically, to enhance diagnosis of cancer, Fakoor et al. [13] proposed a method that is based on two deep learning techniques (principal component analysis and autoencoder). Their proposed method was able to detect and classify cancer types accurately from different cancer datasets. In similar vein, Danaee et al. [10] used the stacked denoising autoencoder for feature extraction and classification of cancer types from high dimensional gene expression dataset with a view to accurately detect cancer. Again, a deep learning-based model was proposed by Wei et al. [50] for breast cancer image classification. The deep learning technique used for this research was convolutional neural network where class and sub-class labels of breast cancer are labeled in such a way that the distance between features in breast cancer images are restricted within a certain threshold. This method produced a classification accuracy of 97%. Similarly, Liu et al. [34] developed "XmasNet" a convolutional neural networks-based classification technique for prostate cancer identification.

4.2 Medical Imaging

While deep learning has a presence in bioinformatics, its presence is also found in medical imaging. Over the years, scientist and health care professionals have been seeking for new ways to process and analyze medical images properly and in a timely manner. And since deep learning surfaced, various deep learning-based techniques have been developed. These techniques have produced results that have outperformed the traditional image processing techniques. A case specific example is the use of deep learning algorithm for the detection of melanoma (a deadly form of skin cancer). In order to detect this tumor, the algorithm learns more about the features of the disease from a dataset containing medical images and makes appropriate predictions. Similarly, Li et al. [33] developed a method based on deep learning (CNN) for the detection of mitotic cells from pathological slides. This is done by first creating a deep segmentation of the mitosis region and there after designing a deep detection network for the localization of the mitosis region. The results from this showed a better F-score when compared to other methods. Aside tumor detection, deep learning is also being used to track tumor growth and development by generating probability heat maps which provides various information on the shape, size, density, and location of tumors [47]. In [48], the authors used deep learning-based technique called the stacked autoencoder to identify and categorize organs in MRI images from unlabeled and unstructured dataset. This they did with the hope of developing a working technique for organ identification within abnormal datasets. This technique achieved an accuracy of 96%. In order to be able to detect diabetic retinopathy early, Gulshan et al. [18] developed a deep learning algorithm that detects diabetic retinopathy early using images in the retinal fundus photographs. The deep learning algorithm used was the CNN and it had an accuracy of 97% in detecting this deadly case of diabetes. For brain lesion segmentation, Kamnitsas et al. [26] proposed a CNN-based technique to overcome earlier computational burden experienced during brain lesion segmentation; this technique is 11 layers deep and has proven to be an effective scheme when run on the MRI dataset of patients with brain injuries and brain tumors. Using non-medical image database, the CNN was used to identify various types of pathologies present in chest X-ray images; the idea was to use the algorithm/result to prove that deep learning could be applied to databases that are all non-medical and still produce useful results and this experiment yielded a 93% accuracy [8].

4.3   Predictive Analytics

Predictive analytics is the use of past data coupled with some computations or analytical tools to predict an event. In the medical case, it is the use of a medical history or health care history to predict the outcome of an event. Predictive analytics has been an ongoing activity in recent years as successful prediction can help avoid adverse health condition of a patient or help reduce the effect of an outbreak. Various techniques have been employed in predictive analytics, of which deep learning is one of them. Some of the applications of deep learning in this aspect of health care are highlighted in the following sentences. Miotto et al. [37] proposed a method called Deep Patient, which used denoising autoencoder for deep feature learning and EHR data extraction with the view to properly facilitate clinical prediction of patients' health status. In similar vein, Pham et al. [40] developed DeepCare whose sole purpose is to read medical records and make predictions of future health outcomes. DeepCare uses long short-term memory for this purpose. Both Deep Patient and DeepCare showed a high performance rate with regard to disease predictions.

Table 2 shows a summary of the major applications of deep learning and their associated techniques.

Table 2 A summary of deep learning applications in smart health

Smart health theme		Deep learning technique used
Bioinformatics	Protein Structure prediction	Sparse autoencoder [36]
		CNN [5]
		RBM [30]
	Gene expression	DNN [31, 52]
		Feed-forward network [9]
	Cancer detection and identification	PCA,Autoencoder [13]
		Denoising autoencoder [10]
		CNN [34, 50]
Medical imaging	Tumor detection	CNN [33, 47]
	Brain lesion	CNN [26]
	Organ Identification	Stacked Autoencoder [18, 48]
Predictive analytics	Patients health prediction	Denoising autoencoder [37, 40]
		Auto-regressive NN [16]

5 Challenges in Deep Learning

Deep learning algorithms require huge amount of data to enable them perform excellently. The more perfection you want; the more data you will need to feed to the machine to enable the algorithms produce models that are powerful enough for your needs. This is mostly the bane of deep learning. And with big data comes the huge amounts of parameters required to get the deep learning algorithm properly tuned. In most cases, this huge amount of data is not available and whenever they are, it is mostly not enough as such, researchers are expected to augment the learning process through approximation.

Another challenge is the issue of overfitting. This is usually common in neural networks where there is a huge difference in the error that occurs when training a dataset and that which occur when a new dataset is introduced. This is an issue since the reason a model is being trained is to be able to perform well when it is used on a new dataset rather than the one it was developed with.

Again, deep learning usually requires huge resource deployments for it to perform excellently well. That is, the more powerful your computing resources are, the more likely you are to get a more effective result from the deep learning algorithm. Aside computing resources, you would also require a huge amount of storage capabilities to train models effectively. Also, deep learning algorithm requires more time to train a dataset than the usual machine learning techniques.

Furthermore, deep learning algorithms are problem specific. That is, when a model is trained for a particular problem, it is usually difficult to tweak it for another kind of problem. This lack of flexibility is an issue because, it would lead to a waste of time to retrain and redevelop a new model for a seemingly similar problem.

6 Conclusion

Deep learning is proving to be an emerging and usable technique in smart health processing and applications. Even with its challenges, its use has been widely accepted in smart health.In the beginning of this chapter, we discussed briefly the emergence of smart city and its links to smart health. We also talked about the link between smart health and machine learning in the introductory section of this chapter. The recent transition from machine learning to deep learning was also discussed in Sect. 2, where we briefly highlighted the deep learning development timeline and evolution. Then, we introduced the basic deep learning techniques (feed-forward networks, autoencoders, linear factor models, convolutional neural networks) that are been used in smart health along with their major formulations. Furthermore, we highlighted the applications of deep learning techniques in smart health from cancer diagnosis to health status predictions. These applications were divided along the lines of bioinformatics, medical imaging, and predictive analytics. Lastly, the challenges of deep learning were discussed in the last section of this chapter.

References

1. A.H. Abdulnabi, G. Wang, J. Lu, K. Jia, Multi-task CNN model for attribute prediction. IEEE Trans. Multimedia **17**(11), 1949–1959 (2015)
2. D.H. Ackley, G.E. Hinton, T.J. Sejnowski, A learning algorithm for Boltzmann machines. Cogn. Sci. **9**(1), 147–169 (1985)
3. I.N. Aizenberg, N.N. Aizenberg, G.A. Krivosheev, Multi-valued and universal binary neurons: learning algorithms, application to image processing and recognition. Lecture Notes Comput. Sci. **1715**(4), 306–316 (1999)
4. G. Alain, Y. Bengio, S. Rifai, Regularized auto-encoders estimate local statistics, in *Proc. CoRR* (2012), pp. 1–17
5. B. Alipanahi, A. Delong, M.T. Weirauch, B.J. Frey, Predicting the sequence specificities of DNA- and RNA-binding proteins by deep learning. Nat. Biotechnol. **33**(8), 831 (2015)
6. E. Alpaydin, *Introduction to Machine Learning* (MIT Press, Cambridge, 2014)
7. M.M. Baig, H. Gholamhosseini, Smart health monitoring systems: an overview of design and modeling. J. Med. Syst. **37**(2), 9898 (2013)
8. Y. Bar, I. Diamant, L. Wolf, H. Greenspan, Deep learning with non-medical training used for chest pathology identification, in *SPIE Medical Imaging*, vol. 9414 (2015), pp. 94140V-1–94140V-7
9. Y. Chen, Y. Li, R. Narayan, A. Subramanian, X. Xie, Gene expression inference with deep learning. Bioinformatics **32**(12), 1832–1839 (2016)
10. P. Danaee, R. Ghaeini, D.A. Hendrix, A deep learning approach for cancer detection and relevant gene identification, in *Pacific Symposium on Biocomputing* (World Scientific, Singapore, 2017), pp. 219–229
11. A. De Carvalho, M.C. Fairhurst, D.L. Bisset, An integrated Boolean neural network for pattern classification. Pattern Recogn. Lett. **15**(8), 807–813 (1994)
12. L. Deng, O. Abdelhamid, D. Yu, A deep convolutional neural network using heterogeneous pooling for trading acoustic invariance with phonetic confusion, in *IEEE International Conference on Acoustics, Speech, and Signal Processing (ICASSP)* (2013), pp. 6669–6673
13. R. Fakoor, F. Ladhak, A. Nazi, M. Huber, Using deep learning to enhance cancer diagnosis and classification, in *Proceedings of the International Conference on Machine Learning*, vol. 28 (2013)
14. R. Fan, F.-L. Zhang, M. Zhang, R.R. Martin, Robust tracking-by-detection using a selection and completion mechanism. Comput. Visual Media **3**(3), 285–294 (2017)
15. M. Finger, M. Razaghi, Conceptualizing "smart cities". Informatik-Spektrum **40**(1), 6–13 (2017)
16. M. Frandes, B. Timar, D. Lungeanu, A risk based neural network approach for predictive modeling of blood glucose dynamics. Stud. Health Technol. Inform. **228**, 577–581 (2016)
17. K. Fukushima, Neocognitron: a self-organizing neural network model for a mechanism of pattern recognition unaffected by shift in position. Biol. Cybern. **36**(4), 193–202 (1980)
18. V. Gulshan, L. Peng, M. Coram, M.C. Stumpe, D. Wu, A. Narayanaswamy, S. Venugopalan, K. Widner, T. Madams, J. Cuadros, et al., Development and validation of a deep learning algorithm for detection of diabetic retinopathy in retinal fundus photographs. JAMA **316**(22), 2402–2410 (2016)
19. G.E. Hinton, Learning multiple layers of representation. Trends Cogn. Sci. **11**(10), 428 (2007)
20. G.E. Hinton, P. Dayan, B.J. Frey, R.M. Neal, The "wake-sleep" algorithm for unsupervised neural networks. Science **268**(5214), 1158 (1995)
21. G.E. Hinton, S. Osindero, Y.-W. Teh, A fast learning algorithm for deep belief nets. Neural Comput. **18**(7), 1527–1554 (2006)
22. G.E. Hinton, R.R. Salakhutdinov, Reducing the dimensionality of data with neural networks. Science **313**(5786), 504–507 (2006)

23. G. Huang, H. Lee, E. Learnedmiller, Learning hierarchical representations for face verification with convolutional deep belief networks, in *2012 IEEE Conference on Computer Vision and Pattern Recognition* (2012), pp. 2518–2525

24. A.G. Ivakhnenko, V.G. Lapa, Cybernetic predicting devices. Transdex (1966)

25. M.I. Jordan, T.M. Mitchell, Machine learning: trends, perspectives, and prospects. Science **349**(6245), 255–260 (2015)

26. K. Kamnitsas, C. Ledig, V.F.J. Newcombe, J.P. Simpson, A.D. Kane, D.K. Menon, D. Rueckert, B. Glocker, Efficient Multi-Scale 3D CNN with fully connected CRF for accurate brain lesion segmentation. Med. Image Anal. **36**, 61–78 (2017)

27. Y. Kim, J.W. Chong, K.H. Chon, J. Kim, Wavelet-based AR–SVM for health monitoring of smart structures. Smart Mater. Struct. **22**(1), 015003 (2012)

28. H. Larochelle, Y. Bengio, Classification using discriminative restricted Boltzmann machines, in *International Conference* (2008), pp. 536–543

29. Y. Lecun, B. Boser, J.S. Denker, D. Henderson, R.E. Howard, W. Hubbard, L.D. Jackel, Backpropagation applied to handwritten zip code recognition. Neural Comput. **1**(4), 541–551 (2014)

30. T. Lee, S. Yoon, Boosted categorical restricted Boltzmann machine for computational prediction of splice junctions, in *International Conference on Machine Learning* (2015), pp. 2483–2492

31. M.K.K. Leung, H.Y. Xiong, L.J. Lee, B.J. Frey, Deep learning of the tissue-regulated splicing code. Bioinformatics **30**(12), i121–i129 (2014)

32. J.M. Levy, *Contemporary Urban Planning* (Taylor & Francis, London, 2016)

33. C. Li, X. Wang, W. Liu, L.J. Latecki, DeepMitosis: mitosis detection via deep detection, verification and segmentation networks. Med. Image Anal. (2018)

34. S. Liu, H. Zheng, Y. Feng, W. Li, Prostate cancer diagnosis using deep learning with 3D multiparametric MRI, in *Medical Imaging 2017: Computer-Aided Diagnosis*, vol. 10134 (International Society for Optics and Photonics, Bellingham, 2017), page 1013428

35. F.S. Lu, S. Hou, K. Baltrusaitis, M. Shah, J. Leskovec, R. Sosic, J. Hawkins, J. Brownstein, G. Conidi, J. Gunn, J. Gray, A. Zink, M. Santillana, Accurate influenza monitoring and forecasting using novel internet data streams: a case study in the Boston Metropolis. JMIR Public Health Surveill. **4**(1), e4 (2018)

36. J. Lyons, A. Dehzangi, R. Heffernan, A. Sharma, K. Paliwal, A. Sattar, Y. Zhou, Y. Yang, Predicting backbone cα angles and dihedrals from protein sequences by stacked sparse auto-encoder deep neural network. J. Comput. Chem. **35**(28), 2040–2046 (2014)

37. R. Miotto, L. Li, B.A. Kidd, J.T. Dudley, Deep patient: an unsupervised representation to predict the future of patients from the electronic health records. Sci. Rep. **6**(1), 26094 (2016)

38. M. Mohri, A. Rostamizadeh, A. Talwalkar, *Foundations of Machine Learning* (MIT Press, Cambridge, 2012)

39. A. Obinikpo, B. Kantarci, Big sensed data meets deep learning for smarter health care in smart cities. J. Sens. Actuator Netw. **6**(4), 22 (2017)

40. T. Pham, T. Tran, D. Phung, S. Venkatesh, DeepCare: a deep dynamic memory model for predictive medicine, in *Advances in Knowledge Discovery and Data Mining. PAKDD 2016*, ed. by J. Bailey, L. Khan, T. Washio, G. Dobbie, J. Huang, R. Wang. Lecture Notes in Computer Science, vol. 9652 (Springer, Cham, 2016)

41. S. Poslad, *Ubiquitous Computing: Smart Devices, Environments and Interactions* (Wiley, New York, 2011)

42. S. Rifai, Y. Bengio, Y. Dauphin, P. Vincent, A generative process for sampling contractive auto-encoders (2012). Preprint arXiv:1206.6434

43. F. Rosenblatt, The perceptron: a probabilistic model for information storage and organization in the brain. Psychol. Rev. **65**(6), 386 (1958)

44. R. Salakhutdinov, A. Mnih, G. Hinton, Restricted Boltzmann machines for collaborative filtering, in *International Conference on Machine Learning* (2007), pp. 791–798

45. J. Schmidhuber, Deep learning in neural networks: an overview. Neural Netw. **61**, 85–117 (2014)

46. J. Schmidhuber, Learning complex, extended sequences using the principle of history compression. Neural Comput. **4**(2), 234–242 (2014)
47. M. Shah, C. Rubadue, D. Suster, D. Wang, Deep learning assessment of tumor proliferation in breast cancer histological images (2016). Preprint arXiv:1610.03467
48. H.-C.C. Shin, M.R. Orton, D.J. Collins, S.J. Doran, M.O. Leach, Stacked autoencoders for unsupervised feature learning and multiple organ detection in a pilot study using 4D patient data. IEEE Trans. Pattern Anal. Mach. Intell. **35**(8), 1930–1943 (2013)
49. P. Vincent, H. Larochelle, I. Lajoie, Y. Bengio, P.-A. Manzagol, Stacked denoising autoencoders: learning useful representations in a deep network with a local denoising criterion. J. Mach. Learn. Res. **11**(Dec), 3371–3408 (2010)
50. B. Wei, Z. Han, X. He, Y. Yin, Deep learning model based breast cancer histopathological image classification, in *2017 IEEE 2nd International Conference on Cloud Computing and Big Data Analysis (ICCCBDA)* (IEEE, Piscataway, 2017), pp. 348–353
51. M.N. Wernick, Y. Yang, J.G. Brankov, G. Yourganov, S.C. Strother, Machine learning in medical imaging. IEEE Signal Process. Mag. **27**(4), 25–38 (2010)
52. S. Zhang, J. Zhou, H. Hu, H. Gong, L. Chen, C. Cheng, J. Zeng, A deep learning framework for modeling structural features of RNA-binding protein targets. Nucleic Acids Res. **44**(4), e32 (2015)

Emotional States Detection Approaches Based on Physiological Signals for Healthcare Applications: A Review

Diana Patricia Tobón Vallejo and Abdulmotaleb El Saddik

Abstract Mood disorders, anxiety, depression, and stress affect people's quality of life and increase the vulnerability to diseases and infections. Depression, e.g., can carry undesirable consequences such as death. Hence, emotional states detection approaches using wearable technology are gaining interest in the last few years. Emerging wearable devices allow monitoring different physiological signals in order to extract useful information about people's health status and provide feedback about their health condition. Wearable applications include e.g., patient monitoring, stress detection, fitness monitoring, wellness monitoring, and assisted living for elderly people, to name a few. This increased interests in wearable applications have allowed the development of new approaches to assist people in everyday activities and emergencies that can be incorporated into the smart city concept. Accurate emotional state detection approaches will allow an effective assistance, thus improving people's quality of life and well-being. With these issues in mind, this chapter discusses existing emotional states' approaches using machine and/or deep learning techniques, the most commonly used physiological signals in these approaches, existing physiological databases for emotion recognition, and highlights challenges and future research directions in this field.

Keywords Affective recognition · Deep learning · Emotional states · Emotions · Machine learning · Physiological signals · Quality of life · Smart city · Well-being

D. Tobón Vallejo
Universidad de Medellin, Medellin, Colombia

A. El Saddik (✉)
Multimedia Communications Research Laboratory, University of Ottawa, Ottawa, ON, Canada
e-mail: elsaddik@uottawa.ca

© Springer Nature Switzerland AG 2020
A. El Saddik et al. (eds.), *Connected Health in Smart Cities*,
https://doi.org/10.1007/978-3-030-27844-1_4

47

1 Introduction

Negative emotional states changes affect physical health. They can be originated by several conditions such as depression, stress, mood disorders, drug addiction, and anxiety, thus affecting people's quality of life and well-being. Healthcare applications can aid to alleviate these consequences providing feedback for therapies, treatments, and prevention by means of monitoring, detecting, and analyzing physiological and emotional state information about people's health status [1]. Burgeoning technologies and applications allow these healthcare applications to occur. Internet of Things (IoT) incorporated within the smart city concept allows that "the things" (i.e., sensors and actuators) can interact between them and send physiological information in real time for complete health assistance. Thus, citizens can be monitored in their everyday activities in order to assist them with health situations. The big picture of this application is depicted in Fig. 1. The user will wear biomedical sensors to monitor physiological signals. That information will be sent to a central device (or server) to be processed and analyzed. Then, the results of this analysis will provide information about actions or treatments to take in order to improve the citizen's health condition.

The use of wearable technology has been increasing in the last few years. The global analyst firm, CCS insight Ltd, indicates that the wearable market is

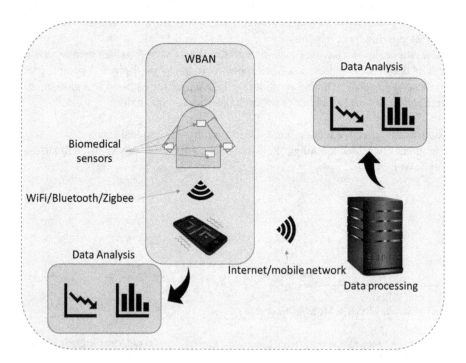

Fig. 1 Envisioned proposed application

increasing from 84 million units in 2015 to 245 million units in 2019. This is due to the so-called quantified-self applications, where users are interested in monitoring their physiological signals by themselves without requiring a health practitioner, unless there is an emergency about a disease condition [2]. Consequently, wearable technology applications can contribute to reducing healthcare costs and providing quality healthcare services.

On the other hand, according to the World Health Organization (WHO), the population aged over 60 years will increase from 12% in 2015 to 22% in 2050, thus pressing for effective and accurate wearable-based applications for senior people. Hence, cost-saving healthcare applications where elderly people can be safe, independent, and move freely are required [3]. Thereby, assisted living applications will allow independency and a healthier lifestyle. This can be achieved not only for elderly people but also for people suffering from diseases, stress [4], requiring treatments, or therapies, as well as those looking for improving their well-being [5]. Stress, e.g., has been identified as a risk factor for depression, anxiety, gastroesophageal reflux, hypertension, and coronary disease [6]. Healthcare applications can aid to control and reduce health problems related to high levels of stress. In [7], e.g., a platform was proposed to assist learners in stressful educational activities. Changes in physiological signals associated with stress are detected to further recommend learners to relax through ambient sensors. The learners perceive recommended actions in terms of light, sound, or vibration at a relaxation breath rate in order to maximize learning engagement. Consequently, learners' physiological states are controlled by regulating breathing. Another example of stress detection is presented in [8]. Emotional state detection was performed for drivers suffering from tiredness and stress. Four emotional states such as concentration, tension, tiredness, and relaxation are identified in real-world driving situations. These emotional states are identified using a body sensor network (WBSN) to be integrated into a vehicular onboard unit, where emergency messages are transmitted to other vehicles, emergency services, or roadside units in order to avoid fatal accidents.

Emotional states are connected to physical health. Hence, the importance of measuring emotional state changes. This has been a field of interest for the affective computing research. Emotional states are detected using hardware and software technologies [6]. The main goal is to design innovative human interaction models, where the human and the system can interact in a natural manner through multi-modal human communication [9]. Affective computing has two main branches such as detection and recognition, and simulation of emotional states in computers [6]. Emotional states can be recognized through physiological sensors since emotions induce physiological changes (e.g., heartbeat and respiration increase with fear [1]). Hence, emotional states detection systems can help users to enhance their experience, motivate toward a certain goal, and model human behaviors [10].

The terms affect and emotion have been used in affective computing interchange-ably [11]. Psychologists describe affect as the experience of emotion [12] in terms of discrete categories (in a language daily life [9]) of basic emotions such as happiness, sadness, fear, anger, disgust, and surprise [1]. Researchers in [13, 14] studied this basic emotions description, where it is indicated that humans perceive emotions in

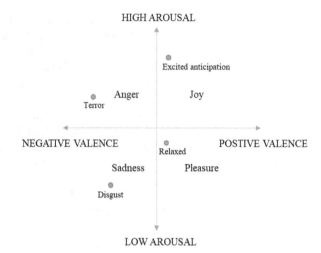

Fig. 2 Two-dimensional model comprising arousal and valence [17]

the same way that facial expressions. Other emotions such as frustration and stress have been studied in [6]. Human behavior is influenced by physiological changes due to emotional states. These physiological changes are divided into categories such as arousal and valence [6, 15]. Arousal is linked to the autonomic nervous system (ANS) and allows the evaluation of valence through physiological sensors. Discrete emotion recognition systems are based on a representation in 2D dimension [9, 16], where it is simplified in classifications such as two class (positive vs. negative and active vs. passive) as depicted in Fig. 2 [17]. Thus, the 2D dimension corresponds to evaluation and activation, which reflect the main characteristics of emotion. The evaluation dimension measures human feelings from positive to negative (i.e., valence). The activation dimension, in turn, measures if humans take actions under an emotional state from active to passive (i.e., arousal) [9]. A 3D model was suggested in [18], where attention–rejection was additionally added to the 2D model as shown in Fig. 3. These tendencies have been associated with stance dimension (e.g., fear associated with the action of flight, and anger associated with the action of fight [17]).

In [19], it was reported that positive emotions help to recover from aftermath caused by negative emotions, thus supporting the theory that negative emotions induce the organism to escape from homeostasis, while positive emotions bring the organism to return to homeostatic levels [17]. Thus, ANS activity provides reliable indications about emotional state changes [20]. It allows exploring the correlation between mood disorders and neurobiological and psychophysiological factors [21]. Researches have shown how ANS changes according to valence and arousal. Those are the two main dimensions of the affect model known as circumplex model of affect (CMA) [22]. Some approaches have provided evidence that the accuracy of arousal discrimination is higher than valence discrimination. The reason could

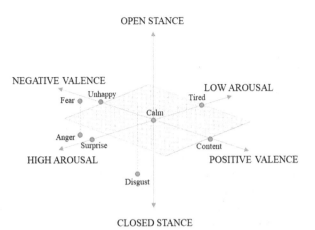

Fig. 3 Three-dimensional model comprising arousal, valence, and stance [17]

be that arousal corresponds to discharge in ANS activities and can be measured directly (e.g., from sweat gland and blood pressure). Valence, in turn, requires cross-correlated ANS reaction analysis [17].

Machine and/or deep learning (DL) approaches can contribute to scenarios where human interpretation is difficult, and facilitate the diagnosis or health issues detection by reducing the uncertainty in the process of decision [23]. These approaches will allow the integration of several physiological signals that monitor people's health status for the emotional detection task. The information collected by the sensors is sent to a server to be processed and analyzed. As a result, users will obtain a feedback about their health status based on the outcomes from the emotional state detection approach. Those outcomes are used to guide the users to take actions in order to improve their well-being and quality of life, as well as to detect emergency events that need assistance from a health practitioner. Given the importance of emotional states detection in improving well-being, this chapter pretends to give an overview about existing machine and/or DL approaches for emotional state detection using physiological signals and highlights current challenges and possible research directions in this field. Therefore, questions that arise are (1) Which approaches are used to detect people' emotional states using physiological signals? (2) Are the existing approaches able to detect correctly people's emotional states to improve their quality of life and well-being?

The rest of this chapter is organized as follows: Sect. 2 presents the most commonly used physiological signals for the emotional state detection task, Sect. 3 summarizes some existing machine and/or DL approaches for emotional state detection, Sect. 4 surveys available emotional state detection databases, and Sect. 5 discusses the challenges and futures research directions in this field.

2   Used Physiological Signals for Emotional State Detection

Existing low-cost wearable biological sensors in the market allow detecting physiological signal changes induced by emotions [1]. These sensors give the possibility
to monitor humans' emotions anywhere at any time in order to detect biological
patterns that reflect emotional states changes [11]. They can be integrated in
everyday activities in watches, T-shirts, and shoes [24], and are able to monitor
different conditions in healthcare applications [25, 26]. A combination of several
biological sensors (i.e., multimodal approach) has presented better performance
for emotion recognition than only one biological sensor (i.e., unimodal approach)
[7]. That combination aids to alleviate the uncertainty in the raw signals [11]. The
importance of physiological signal monitoring lies in the central and autonomic
nervous system (ANS) is responsible for several reactions of emotions and regulates
stress and anxiety [27]. Consequently, many of these reactions can be observed
by analyzing the physiological signals' behavior. Typical employed physiological
signals for emotional state recognition are explained to follow and summarized in
Table 1.

- **Electroencephalogram (EEG):** This signal corresponds to the brain activity
  measured by electrodes on the scalp. It shows the voltage fluctuations resulting
  from the ionic current within the neurons. The EEG signals are divided into
  four frequency rhythms. Delta waves corresponding to frequencies below 4 Hz
  that have the highest amplitude (about 250–325 μV) and slowest rhythms.
  Theta waves that are between 4 Hz and 8 Hz with greater amplitudes. Alpha
  waves are between 8 and 12 Hz resulting from relaxed and alerted stages.
  Finally, Beta waves are between 14 and 32 Hz or 50 Hz corresponding to
  high-frequency rhythms and low voltage [28]. Ongoing brain activity can be
  recorded to find the EEG relation with emotional states [29]. It allows monitoring
  of different emotional states since physiological manifestations are produced
  due to ANS stimulation. For example, stress response that is originated in the
  amygdala, is then communicated with the hypothalamus, which further initiates
  the ANS response [30]. Hence, the induced potentials between the amygdala and
  hypothalamus are recorded at the scalp [31]. EEG features are used to classify
  emotional dimensions such as arousal, valence, and dominance (i.e., stance) [11].
  Two types of neural activity are attention and meditation. Attention is related
  to an increase in Beta waves and indicates alertness [8]. Meditation, in turn,
  is related to increases in Alpha waves and indicates relaxation. Studies have
  shown that positive emotions such as joy, happiness, and interest are associated
  with the left frontal area. Negative emotions such as sadness, fear, and disgust
  are associated with the right frontal region [32]. However, EEG signals are
  highly contaminated with muscle artifacts generated by muscle contractions, thus
  imposing the use of effective EEG denoising techniques.
- **Electromyogram (EMG):** This signal measures the electrical activity of muscle's motor units that are controlled by the nervous system. The signals are collected either on the surface or intramuscular. Surface EMG signals are recorded

Table 1 Summary of used physiological signals for the emotional state detection task

Physiological signal	Abbreviation	Body measure	Measured emotion	Limitation
Electroencephalogram	EEG	Brain activity	Stress, joy, happiness, interest, sadness, fear, disgust	Muscle artifacts
Electromyogram	EMG	Electrical activity of muscle	Reflect negative valence emotions	Presence of artifacts and EMG complex pattern
Electrocardiogram	ECG	Heart activity	Stress, depression, fear, sadness, anger, happiness, surprise, disgust, joy, amusement	Affected by movement, respiration, muscle artifacts
Electrodermal activity	EDA, GSR, SC	Changes in the skin conductance, sweat gland activity (finger or wrist)	Engagement, excitement, stress, calmness, boredom, disengagement	Noise, artifacts
Photoplethysmography	PPG	Change of blood's volume in the tissues over time	Same as ECG since heart rate can be detected	Motion artifact
Respiration	RESP	Breathing capture	Stress	Artifacts by body movement
Skin temperature	ST	Corporal temperature	Positive and negative emotions (valence)	Artifacts by body movement

using non-invasive electrodes. Intramuscular EMG signals, in turn, use invasive sensors. Surface EMG measurements are preferred in healthcare applications. These EMG measurements permit to understand the human body's behaviors under pathological and normal conditions [33]. In the emotion recognition field, this signal has been used to reflect negative valence emotions [11, 34]. However, the signal analysis is difficult due to artifacts and the EMG complex pattern. Those artifacts come from electronic equipment and physiological factors.

- **Electrocardiogram (ECG):** This signal shows the heart activity waveform. It is one of the most commonly measured physiological signals in wireless body area networks (WBANs) and wearable applications. According to the Heart and Stroke Foundation, it is a powerful tool that helps clinicians to diagnose, detect, and monitor heart diseases. Beyond diagnosis, ECG signals have been used in applications such as stress detection, athlete endurance, remote patient monitoring, patient rehabilitation, biofeedback, assisted living, biometrics, fitness, depression states detection, performance, and wellness monitoring [2]. Heart rate variability (HRV) is a noninvasive assessment of the ANS in healthy and patients with cardiac diseases [35]. The ANS is composed of the sympathetic (prepares the body for action and maintains homeostasis) and parasympathetic (vagal) systems (stimulates the body for relaxation). The heart rhythm changes according to the ANS activity. The parasympathetic nervous system is associated with mental states and physical well-being. Positive emotions are associated with the increase in the vagal activity, while decreasing in the vagal activity is associated with mortality, anxiety, cardiovascular disease [36], and depression [37]. Existing studies have shown the relationship between ECG and emotional states. For example, in [38] it was reported that emotions such as fear, sadness, and anger produce higher heart rate (HR) than happiness, surprise, and disgust. In [39], decreased HRV was associated with happiness, while an increased HRV was associated with joy and amusement. In addition, stress states can be monitored examining the ANS activity by analyzing the HR. A stressful situation induces an increase in the HR. Thus, it allows monitoring how fast the body responds to stress, how long the stress response lasts, and how fast the parasympathetic system can act to reduce the stress [6]. Conventionally, 12 electrodes are connected to the body to measure the ECG signal. Nevertheless, Lead I configuration is the most used in affective computing systems, which only requires two electrodes [11, 40].

- **Electrodermal activity (EDA):** This signal is commonly also known as Galvanic Skin Response (GSR) and Skin Conductance (SC). It shows changes in SC at the surface while an activity is monitored. The SC is based on sweat gland activity [6]. It is usually measured at the finger and not always requires gel for conductivity [6]. It is one powerful measure of the ANS neural pathway since it is controlled directly by the sympathetic branch. An EDA sensor placed on fingers has been used to identify emotional changes produced by affective sounds in [5]. Higher EDA reactions have been found compared to neutral stimuli in response to valence stimuli [20]. Other studies have depicted EDA responses generated by emotional arousal [41, 42]. Higher levels of EDA are associated with higher levels of arousal and indicate a user more engaged, excited, or stressed. Lower levels of EDA, in turn, are related to calmness, boredom, or disengagement and indicate lower levels of arousal [8]. In addition, some research works have shown measurements at the wrist to be highly correlated to the finger. This helps to improve wearability in healthcare applications [43, 44]. Stress detection approaches use skin measurements since they provide an easy setup. High-stress situations activate the gland causing resistance to current flow and affecting the skin conductivity. In [17], it was found that SC is linearly correlated with arousal changes while listening to music.
- **Photoplethysmography (PPG):** This signal measures the change of blood's volume in the tissues over time. The skin is illuminated through a pulse oximeter

to measure the light absorption. A light-emitting diode (LED) is radiated toward the skin and received the reflected light from the photodetector [45]. The PPG signal periodicity is similar to the ECG due to blood goes to the capillary vessels at every beat of heart [45]. Thus, the heart rate can be estimated from PPG signals. The physiological analysis of PPG signals is known that is the result of the interaction between autonomic, respiratory, and cardiovascular systems [46]. The PPG measurement technique is also used to measure blood volume pressure (BVP), thus allowing the detection of the two phases of cardiac cycle, i.e., systole and diastole. In every heartbeat, the blood is pushed from the ventricles to the aorta. This produces a pressure wave that travels from the heart to the peripherals vessels. That flow depends on arterial properties such as elasticity, stiffness, or thickness. Since the blood pressure depends on the arterial properties, it can give information about the status of the cardiovascular system [47].

- **Respiration (RESP):** The signal can be measured using noninvasive sensors such as piezoelectric sensors, linear variable differential transformers, strain gauges, and respiratory inductive plethysmographs to capture breathing [48]. The piezoelectric sensor, e.g., composed of a crystal that when compressed or stretched, it generates a voltage [49]. The respiration signal can be affected by nervous system, cardiovascular system, and excretory system, thus providing an indication of failure of those systems [48]. The respiration rate reflects arousal [11, 50] and its activity can be an indication of stress. Physical stress results in ventilation as a response to the ANS activity [50]. In the hyperventilation process, more CO_2 leaves the body causing reductions in O_2 delivery. These lead to physiological alterations that have been usually sensed from ECG and EEG directly [6].
- **Skin temperature (ST):** It carries information about the autonomic nervous system. The sympathetic system activation will conduct to vasoconstriction in the extremities, which will produce lower extremity temperatures [51]. Several studies have reported changes in the skin temperature with the emotion. For example, in [11] was reported that skin temperature has valence information. In addition, higher skin temperatures for low-intensity negative emotions were reported in [52] compared to low-intensity positive emotions.

Several approaches for emotional states detection based on physiological signal monitoring have been proposed. A platform for helping learners to control stress was developed in [7]. Physiological signals such as temperature, SC, and ECG were collected to identify users' needs. Feedback messages are generated in order to guide the user to relax using ambient sensors (e.g., light, sound, and vibration). Thus, the platform guides the learner to breathe slowly when high levels of stress are detected. EDA signals were used in [53] to quantify the sympathetic activation in bipolar patients, thus supporting the hypothesis about a relationship between pathological mood states and autonomic dysfunctions. SC and EMG were found to be linearly correlated with arousal change in [17]. In addition, it was found that ECG and RESP features are dominant for valence differentiation. Inter beat interval (IBI) HRV metric was studied to predict workload in [54], where IBI measures the variability between consecutive R waves in the ECG in milliseconds. In [55], emotional states were modeled as a combination of arousal and valence according to the circumplex model. It was reported that affective sounds produce emotional states changes reflected in the ANS dynamics. Therefore, although physiological signals are highly affected by noise and artifacts due to user's movement and present difficulty to allow extracting emotional patterns, they are less affected by environmental noise and permit to analyze the user's state in real time. One advantage is that physiological signals are not caused by unnatural emotions or social masking [56] (e.g., smile during negative emotional state). In addition, information can be continuous gather from users, which is convenient for the so-called poker face users that "hide" their emotional state. In this specific case, audiovisual recording systems cannot detect the emotional changes [17].

3 Machine and/or DL Approaches for Emotion Recognition Based on Physiological Signals

This section presents a summary of the machine and/or DL approaches for emotional states recognition using physiological signals. Several machine learning methods such as support vector machines (SVM), neural networks (NN), linear discriminant analysis (LDA), quadratic discriminant analysis (QDA) classifiers, k-nearest neighbors (kNN), decision trees, hidden Markov models, and Fisher linear projection have been employed [1, 10]. On the other hand, DL is a burgeoning technique based on artificial neural networks (ANN) and is a potent machine learning tool for artificial intelligence (AI). Convolutional Neural Networks (CNNs) have impacted the field of health informatics [23]. They have been used for object recognition in images, as well as for facial expression recognition [57]. Deep Neural Networks (DNNs) are able to learn novel features and patterns in supervised and unsupervised ways [23]. Perceptron is a proposed NN for binary classification and inspired in how the biological neuron works. It consists of an input layer connected to an output node as depicted in Fig. 4. This connection emulates a biochemical process (i.e., information processed by the brain through interconnected neurons) through and activation or transfer function and few weights. Thus, the perceptron learns to classify patterns separable linearly by changing the weights [23]. Representative approaches that use machine and/or DL techniques using physiological signals are described next and summarized in Table 2.

EEG signals have been commonly used in affective computing applications. For example, emotional states recognition during music listening was presented in [29]. SVM was employed to classify emotional states such as joy, anger, sadness, and pleasure. An averaged classification accuracy of 82.29 $\pm$ 3.06% was found. Feature extraction methods for emotion recognition is explored in [62]. The authors compare available feature extraction methods using machine-learning techniques for feature selection. QDA with diagonal covariance estimates was used. Experimental

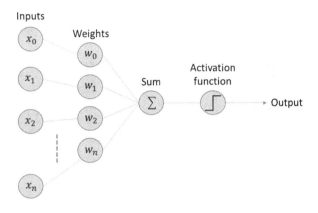

Fig. 4 Representation of a perceptron for binary classification

results showed that multivariable feature selection techniques performed slightly better compared to univariate methods. Feature extraction methods such as Higher Order Crossings (HOC), Higher Order Spectra (HOS), and Hilbert-Huang Spectrum (HHS) outperformed the common power spectral bands. In addition, it was reported preference locations over parietal and center-parietal lobes. EEG was employed for music preference such as "like" and "dislike" in [68]. The authors evaluated four classifiers in the complete dataset (user-independent), i.e., k-NN, SVM, QAD, and Mahalanobis. An accuracy of 86.52 ± 0.76% was achieved using k-NN classifier and HHS-based feature vectors. Beta and gamma bands showed to contain emotional arousal information. Multilayer perceptron (MLP) and SVM were evaluated for EEG-based emotion recognition in [29]. The implemented MLP has an input layer, a hidden layer with a sigmoid function (neural excitation), and an output layer (i.e., four neurons corresponding to joy, anger, sadness, and pleasure) as depicted in Fig. 5. The number of neurons in the input and hidden layer varied according to the used feature type, which were derived from electrodes located near the frontal and the parietal lobes. The backpropagation algorithm was used within the network layers to adjust the weight coefficients. MLP obtained a classification accuracy of 81.52% compared to 82.29% using SVM.

Even though EEG signals carry relevant emotional states information, other physiological signals have been collected along with EEG to better characterize users' emotions. For example, physiological signals such as EEG, ECG, EDA, and RESP were collected in [8] to detect emotions in real time such as concentrated, tension, tired, and relaxed. The authors propose an architecture to detect emotions using body sensor networks (BSN) and logistic regression. The proposed architecture can be communicated from a vehicle to emergency services, and vehicular ad hoc networks (VANETs) in order to improve the driver's experience and prevent car accidents. A kappa index of 0.5455 and a level of agreement of 0.7186 were found. Pictures from the International Affective Picture System (IAPS) are used in [63] to discriminate among pleasant, unpleasant, high arousal or low arousal, by collecting

Table 2 Summary of representative emotional states recognition approaches using physiological signals

References	Physiological signals	Stimulus	Emotional states	Approaches	Performance
[20]	EDA	IADS	Arousal and valence	k-NN	Arousal: 77.33% Valence: 84%
[10]	HR, EDA	IAPS, IADS	Regret and rejoice	CART	Rejoice: 67% Regret: 61%
[58]	ECG, EMG, EDA	Interaction with an intelligent tutoring system (AutoTutor)	Boredom, confusion, curiosity, delight, flow, engagement, surprise, and neutral	k-NN LBNC	Kappa = 0.42, F1 = 0.82 Kappa = 0.34, F1 = 0.70
[8]	EEG, EDA	Drive in two types of conditions and self-reports	Concentrated, tension, tired, and relaxed	Logistic regression	Kappa = 0.5455
[29]	EEG	Oscar's film Soundtracks	Joy, anger, sadness, and pleasure	SVM	Average accuracy: 82.29 ± 3.06%
[59]	EEG, EDA, BVP, RESP, and ST	Tetris game	Boredom, engagement, and anxiety	QDA, LDA	Accuracy after fusion: 63%
[60]	HR, EDA, PPG	Popular film website	Amusement, anger, grief, and fear	Random forests	Overall accuracy: 74%
[17]	EMG, ECG, EDA, RESP	Musical induction method	Positive/high arousal, negative/high arousal, negative/low arousal, and positive/low arousal	Emotion-specific multilevel dichotomous classification (EMDC)	Overall CCR: 95%
[61]	EDA, HR	Six tests using a robot	Arousal and valence	NN	Accuracies between 73% and 82%
[62]	EEG	IAPS	Happy, curious, angry, sad, and quiet	QDA	Accuracy ranges from 25% to 47.5%
[54]	HR	Four workload situations	Mental, physical, and temporal demands; own performance; effort; and frustration	Fuzzy-based model	$R^2 = 0.7144$

Ref	Signals	Stimuli	Emotional states	Classifier	Results
[63]	EEG, EDA	IAPS	Pleasant, unpleasant, high arousal or low arousal	C4.5 decision tree	Average accuracy: 77.68%
[64]	EDA, EMG, PPG	Audio-video clips from YouTube	Positive or negative valence	Gaussian process classifiers	Accuracy between 80% and 90%
[55]	ECG	IADS	Arousal and valence	QDC	Arousal: 84.26% Valence: 84.72%
[65]	RESP	Film clips/slide films	Love, sadness, joy, anger, and fear	PNN	Accuracy: 88%
[66]	HR, EDA, and ST	Trait scale State–Trait Anxiety Inventory (T-STAI)	Non-agitated state, transitional state, and agitated state	Proposed SVM architecture	Accuracy: 91.4%
[67]	ECG, EDA, and RESP	IAPS	Arousal and valence	QDC	Accuracy > 90%
[68]	EEG	Musical excerpts	Like and dislike	k-NN	Accuracy: $86.52 \pm 0.76\%$
[69]	EMG, BVP, and EDA	IAPS	Arousal, valence, and dominance	ANN	Classification rate: 70.1%
[56]	EDA, ECG, ST, and PPG	Rated audio–visual film clips	Sadness, fear, surprise, and stress	SVM	Accuracy: 100%
[21]	ECG	Pictures	Depressive and euthymic status	MLP	Euthymia: 99.56% Depression: 99.98%
[57]	EDA and BVP	Video game	Relaxation, anxiety, excitement, and fun	CNN	Accuracies between 70% and 75%

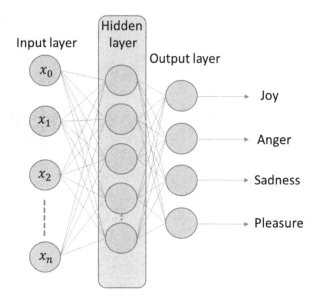

Fig. 5 Multilayer perceptron implemented in [29] for emotion recognition

EEG signals along with EDA signals. A data mining approach was combined with a distance-based classification algorithm named Mahalanobis metric. C4.5 decision tree algorithm was employed to differentiate valence dimension. After, the gender and valence information are input to the Mahalanobis distance classifier to divide the data into high and low arousal. The success recognition average rate was 77.68% to discriminate the four emotional states. Game difficulty is adapted according to player's emotion in [59]. EEG signals, questionnaire responses, and peripheral signals (i.e., EDA, BVP, RESP, and ST) of players playing Tetris at three different levels are collected such as (1) boredom (low pleasure, low pressure, low arousal, and low motivation; (2) engagement (higher arousal, higher pleasure, higher motivation, and higher amusement); and (3) anxiety (high arousal, high pressure, and low pleasure). LDA and QDA were employed in this study. Experimental results showed an accuracy of 63% after fusing the EEG and peripheral signals, thus showing the importance of adapting the game according to player's emotions to preserve the player's engagement.

ECG is a primary signal for feature extraction in the emotional recognition field. By quantifying emotions, actions can be taken in order to improve the coordination of the ANS system, thus potentially helping to improve people's quality of life. Several approaches have been proposed based on ECG signals features. Emotional states elicited by affective sounds are analyzed through the cardiovascular dynamics in [55]. Emotions are classified into four different levels of arousal (intensity) and two levels of valence (unpleasant and pleasant). HRV features are extracted and the Leave One Subject Out (LOSO) procedure was applied to the training set, whereas quadratic discriminant classifier (QDC) was applied to the test set. The study suggested that ANS measures such as mean HRV, standard deviation (std), root mean squared (RMSSD), triangular index, spectral measures, and Lagged Poincare plots (LPP) are the most reliable HRV metrics to identify emotional states induced by affective sounds. Experimental results showed an accuracy of 84.72% for valence dimension and 84.26% for arousal dimension. A fuzzy-based model technique using the HR is proposed in [54] to remove uncertainties from the modeling problem. To this end, a finite-mixture model was used to analyze the uncertainties in order to adapt a workload model to the physiological conditions of a subject. Thus, the fuzzy-based tool can be used in real-world scenarios in the presence of uncertainties. Four workload situations were evaluated: (1) manual mode with open workplace; (2) manual mode with glove box; (3) partial automation mode; and (4) full automation mode. The method achieved an accuracy of $R^2 = 0.7144$ compared to $R^2 = 0.4627$ with a Bayesian regularization NN. Depressive states for bipolar patients were characterized using an MLP in [21]. HRV assessment was used to characterize the status of bipolar patients. Relevant pictures were used for emotional stimuli. Linear and nonlinear features were estimated to further be used as inputs of an MLP in order to discriminate between depressive and euthymic states. The MLP was trained using a supervised learning method. In the training phase, the artificial function of the artificial neurons is calculated for each data record. The backpropagation algorithm is employed to the resulting error between inputs and outputs to adapt the weight of a generic neuron. The MLP has a response (i.e., Boolean vector) that represents the activation function of an output neuron. The implemented MLP has three layers such as input (i.e., seven neurons), hidden (i.e., five neurons), and output layers (i.e., two neurons, each of them corresponding to the two classes to recognize). Experimental results showed an accuracy of 99.56% for euthymia and 99.98% for depression states.

Skin responses such as sweating, vasomotor, and piloerection are responses induced by emotional states. Hence, EDA signals reflect activity within the sympathetic system of the ANS and measures changes in sympathetic arousal associated with emotion and attention [44, 58, 70]. A framework based on EDA recordings and clustering algorithms is proposed in [20] to discern arousal and valence levels. Affective sounds from the International Affective Digitized Sound System (IADS) database are used for emotion stimuli. Three levels of arousal (i.e., neutral, low, medium, and high) and two levels of valence (i.e., positive and negative) were evaluated. The authors employed a multivariate pattern recognition analysis followed by LOSO and k-NN classifier. The experimental results showed a recognition accuracy of 84% for valence and 77.33% for arousal. EDA signals have been analyzed along HR to classify arousal (excited-bored) and valence (happy-unhappy) states in [61]. It was found that both signals are predictive of arousal states, while HR is predictive of valence. The objective of this study was to develop a computational algorithm for patient emotional classification using nursing robots in medical service. Wavelet analysis was used to effectively extract features from the physiological signals. A machine learning algorithm using NN structures was developed to classify patient emotional states in real time during the interaction with the robot. The classification accuracies result for arousal and valence are between 73 and 82%. Another approach using these two signals is presented in [10]. A comparison between Classification and Regression Tree (CART), C4.5 classification, and random forest classification algorithms was performed to predict emotions of regret and rejoice in a financial decision context. These changes have been observed when traders experience loss, or are regretted about their decision. Three methods, namely, binary (i.e., regret or rejoice), tristate (i.e., only regret, only rejoice, or blended), and tetra state blended (i.e., only regret, only rejoice, both, neither emotion) were compared to detect emotions using the HR and EDA. The authors were interested in comparing accuracies across different types of decision trees since they are better suited for real-time analysis (less computationally compared to SVMs). Tenfold cross validation was used to prevent overfitting and for pruning the decision trees. The comparison using 100 features set showed 67% accuracy for binary rejoice, 44% for a tristate, and 45% for a tetra state blended models with highest accuracies achieved by CART. These results were replicated using only three proposed delta features based on the triphasic cardiac form such as the difference between the maxima and minima in the anticipatory–parasympathetic, anticipatory–sympathetic, and parasympathetic–sympathetic phases. Emotional states such as amusement, anger, grief, and fear were analyzed in [60] for several subjects that watch individually the same film. A multivariant correlation method (i.e., random matrix theory) is applied before feature extraction to detect common patterns using HR, EDA, the first derivate of EDA, and fingertip oxygen saturation (OXY). After correlation analysis, local scaling dimension (LSD) is applied to characterize the physiological changes. After, conventional affective features and the LSD affective physiological features are applied to a random forest to discriminate the different emotional states plus a baseline state. It was obtained an overall correct rate of 74% for classifying amusement, anger, grief, fear, and the baseline.

Existing solutions have used EDA and ECG signals along other physiological signals. For example, in [58], the authors addressed the efficacy of emotion detection using several classification techniques on three physiological signals such as ECG, EMG, and EDA, as well as their combinations. A number of classification approaches and feature selection techniques using naturalistic emotion physiological dataset were evaluated. Eight emotion states such as boredom, confusion, curiosity, delight, flow/engagement, surprise, and neutral were evaluated. The experimental results showed a better emotion recognition performance for k-NN (kappa = 0.42, F1 = 0.82), and Linear Bayes Normal Classifier (LBNC) (kappa = 0.34, F1 = 0.70). Additionally, single channel ECG, EMG, and EDA, as well as three-channel multimodal models were more diagnostic for emotion recognition. The agitation detection for dementia patients was addressed in [66]. The detection of agitation is a significant aid for caregivers of dementia patients. Physiological signals such as HR, EDA, and ST were monitored. Two SVM architectures based on a confidence measure are proposed such as confidence-based SVM and confidence-based multilevel SVM. The proposed method obtained an accuracy of 91.4% compared to 90.9% achieved with the traditional SVM. Negative emotions such as sadness, fear, surprise, and stress have been identified in [56]. EDA, ECG, ST, and PPG were recorded. The study used audio–visual clips for emotional stimuli and five machine learning algorithms for classification such as LDA (one of the linear models), CART of decision tree model, Self Organizing Map (SOM) of NN, Naïve Bayes of probability model, and SVM of nonlinear model. Experimental results showed an accuracy of 100% for SVM, 84% for CART, 76.2% for Naïve Bayes, 51.2% for SOM, and 50.7% for LDA.

A DL algorithm to extract relevant features from EDA and BVP has been proposed in [57]. It can handle discrete and continuous signals and consists of convolutional layers to extract significant features from the raw data, which bypasses the need for manual ad hoc feature extraction. Emotional states such as relaxation, anxiety, excitement, and fun were analyzed from players of a 3D game. The algorithm consists of a deep model that comprises a multilayered CNN to extract the relevant features to further feed a single-layer perceptron (SLP) to predict the affective states. Denoising auto-encoders were used to train the CNN. Then, the SLP is trained using backpropagation in order to map the CNN outputs to the affective values. It was found that the fusion between skin conductance and BVP with DL techniques outperforms standard and automatic feature extraction techniques (i.e., statistical features) across all the analyzed affective states. Another approach using these two signals as well as EMG was explored in [69]. A mental trainer experiment was conducted to select stable features for individual emotional states across several situations. Two rounds were run, finding useful physiological features classification in both rounds (70.1%) compared to other features that performed only in the first round (53%). Emotional states of the valence-arousal-dominance (VAD) model were induced such as negative valence/high arousal/low dominance (NHL) and positive valence/low arousal/high dominance (PLH). Feedforward ANN with two hidden layers was employed for classification. EDA along with EMG and PPG signals was employed to detect emotional states from video clips in [64]. A detector focus on affective events in real time was proposed. It captures affective events and associates them a binary valence (positive or negative). Multiple modalities to build complex rules using Gaussian Process Classifiers (GPCs) are used. Experimental results showed around 80% accuracy for event detection, and between 80% and 90% accuracy for binary valence prediction.

RESP signals have shown to reflect emotional states. However, they are affected by motion artifacts, thus limiting reliable affective state detection. Hence, a method to extract Emotion Elicited Segments (EESs) from RESP signals is proposed in [65]. Emotional changes such as love, sadness, joy, anger, and fear were extracted. The EESs segments contain reliable information to determine accurately the affective state of a subject. To extract the EESs segments, Mutual Information-Based Emotion Relevance Feature Ranking based on the Dynamic Time Warping Distance (MIDTW) is applied, as well as a Constraint-based Elicited Segment Density (CESD) analysis. The segment-based emotion analysis was evaluated using k-NN method, and the Probabilistic Neural Network (PNN) method. A leave-one emotion-one-person-out cross-validation method was implemented in the two methods. The advantage of using segment-based analysis lies in noise can be eliminated more effectively from the RESP signal. Experimental results showed an accuracy performance of 88%. RESP signal along with EMG, ECG, and EDA

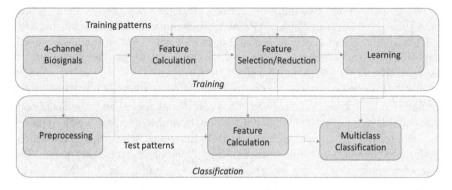

Fig. 6 Block diagram of the scheme of emotion-specific multilevel dichotomous classification (EMDC) proposed in [17]

were analyzed in [17] for emotional changes. Musical induction propitiated real emotional changes. Four emotional states were classified using extended linear discriminant analysis (pLDA), (1) positive/high arousal, (2) negative/high arousal, (3) negative/low arousal, and (4) positive/low arousal. The authors developed an emotion-specific multilevel dichotomous classification (EMDC) scheme and compared its performance with multiclass classification using the pLDA. The block diagram of the proposed scheme is depicted in Fig. 6. Experimental results showed correct classification ratio (CCR) of 95% for subject-dependent (i.e., three subjects) and 70% for subject-independent (features from all subjects were merged and normalized) classification.

Another approach is presented in [67]. An automatic multiclass arousal/valence classifier was implemented. Physiological signals such as ECG, EDA, and RESP were collected while affective states were induced using images gathered from IAPS. The sets of images have five levels of arousal dimension and five levels of valence dimension, including a reference level in both dimensions. Experimental results showed an accuracy greater than 90% for emotion recognition when nonlinear features are extracted. Such accuracy was achieved after 40-fold cross-validation steps for both dimensions and using a QDC classifier. The authors compared several classifiers such as LDC, Mixture of Gaussian (MOG), k-NN, Kohonen Self Organizing Map (KSOM), MPL, and QDC, where QDC showed better performance.

4 Available Databases for the Emotion Recognition Task

At present, few available databases use physiological signals for emotional state detection. They use emotional stimulus such as video, images, and situations to induce emotional changes. The emotional states have been categorized using the dimensional labeling as depicted in Figs. 2 and 3. Table 3 shows a list of

Table 3 List of available databases for emotional states detection using physiological signals

Database	Number of subjects	Physiological signals	Stimulus	Emotional states
DEAP [71]	32	EEG, EMG, RESP, ST, PPG, and EDA	Music videos	Arousal, valence and dominance
MAHNOB-HCI [72]	30	ECG, EEG, RESP, and ST	Fragments of movies and pictures	Arousal, and valence
MIT Media Lab Sentics Data [73]	1 (several segments)	BVP, EMG, respiration and EDA	Imagery	Neutral, anger, hate, grief, love, romantic love, joy, and reverence
MIT Media Lab Driver Stress Data [25]	17	ECG, EDA, EMG, and RESP	Rest, highway, and city drives	Low, medium, and high stress
HUMAINE [74]	Multiple datasets	ECG, EDA, ST, and RESP	Audiovisual	Several states across datasets
RECOLA [75]	46	EDA, ECG,	Video clips	Arousal, and valence
BioVid Emo DB [76]	86	EDA, ECG, and EMG	Film clips	Amusement, sadness, anger, disgust, and fear
ASCERTAIN [77]	58	ECG, EDA, and EEG	Videos	Arousal, valence, engagement, liking, and familiarity

available databases for emotional state recognition, which describes the number of subjects, the recorded physiological signals, the employed stimulus, and the detected emotional states. The interested reader can refer to the respective reference for complete information about the databases.

5 Challenges and Future Research Directions

The development of cheaper and less intrusive physiological methods has become the physiological signals important in real-world applications [58]. The use of these signals for the emotional detection task can solve issues suffered by other methods [38]. Video capture for facial expression recognition using computer vision techniques can be problematic in free environments; movement and gesture analysis are highly influenced by noise; speech analysis is not useful in situations where the user is silent and is affected by noise [27]; and facial expression and speech signals can be faked [78]. The physiological signals are collected through noninvasive sensors attached to the user's body and are relatively free from privacy concerns (compared to camera-based applications) [27]. They are less susceptible to social masking compared to face and voice since they are spontaneous and less controllable reactions [78], which is important for applications such as deception detection and autism treatment [58]. However, burgeoning applications using physiological signals and machine and/or DL techniques have raised a number of challenges that need to be addressed. Some of the most pressing are mentioned as follows:

- **Physiological data collection and physiological patterns:** Recordings from physiological signals are still invasive since the users have to be in contact with electrodes for some kind of signals. Those electrodes affect the measurement due to they are highly susceptible to motion artifacts. Even though several researches have been conducted using several measures to identify emotions, it has been highlighted in [58] that too many measurements could incur in interference to the users and not be favorable for practical applications. In addition, although physiological analysis is robust (not controllable by the user), one disadvantage is the signal variance across and within users. The development of independent emotional detection systems is a nontrivial problem [27]. Researches have tried to build user-independent models to generalize to new users. However, this is challenging since physiological patterns differ from user to user and depend on the situation [40]. Those models are built using physiological data from multiple users that is expected to generalize to novel subjects. The advantage is that user-specific calibration is not required, but the challenge relies on different subjects will have different physiological patterns for the same emotion. Physiological signals differ from user to user and from situation to situation [17]. Consequently, a trade-off between precision and generalization is essential [58].
- **Data availability:** In DL applications, a big amount of label data is required to train the network. This is not always achieved in healthcare applications. The training phase can be time consuming if the application does not count with

high computational resources. In addition, learning models can be affected by convergence issues and overfitting [23]. On the other hand, several emotional detection systems present their results based on experimental methods that induce emotions artificially. However, it is not clear if similar accuracies would be performed in naturalistic scenarios [79]. Existing datasets for emotional states stimulations such as IAPS and IADS are commonly used. However, those datasets provide standardized methods to classify the physiological information. The subjects have to think about what they feel, thus occurring in an inherent bias. Hence, real-life emotions can be more difficult to detect because they can be ambiguous and originated unconsciously in self-reported methods [10]. Obtaining the ground truth of physiological signals is a critical problem in emotional state research. The emotions cannot be felt or perceived directly from the raw data, which leads difficulties in data annotations. Hence, a universal dataset is difficult to collect [17]. The fact that different databases use a different experimental setup makes difficult to compare results across several approaches. The collection of several physiological signals from a large number of subjects is challenging [11]. Hence, there is a need of publicly available databases that allow to produce results that can be comparable for approaches using different databases.

- **Data preprocessing:** Additional signal processing is necessary to attenuate the noise in physiological signals. The signals may include random artifacts (stationary signals) being problematic for processing methods such as Fast Fourier Transform (FFT). To overcome this limitation, wavelet transform has been used to analyze transients, nonstationary, and time-varying phenomena [59]. In approaches based on DL, the raw input data cannot be used directly in many applications. A preprocessing, or normalization is required before training, which also requires more resources and human expertise. In addition, the configuration of hyper parameters, size, and number of filters in CNN is a blind process that requires a correct validation [23]. Therefore, for practical applications, it is necessary to build miniaturized noninvasive sensors with built-in denoising filters in order to improve the signal quality and reduce the preprocessing computational cost [17].

- **Feature extraction:** Unsupervised learning has been used for feature extraction, clustering, or dimensionality reduction [23]. Ad hoc feature extraction techniques require a parameter tuning phase in the training process to provide suitable set of features [57]. However, this parameter tuning phase can affect the performance of the application, thus imposing reliable techniques for feature extraction. It is a challenging task to identify which physiological signals are more diagnostic of emotional states [58], as well as it is difficult to map the physiological patterns onto specific emotions [17].

- **Feature selection:** A main issue in emotion recognition from physiological signals is to identify the reliable features to discriminate emotions. Feature selection methods allow extracting the most suitable feature subset from available features for a specific task, thus avoiding overfitting and redundancy. The three different selection methods for feature selection are wrapper, filter, and embedded. Wrapper consists in using predictive models to assign a score to each feature subset. A model is trained with each subset to be then tested on the rest of the dataset. According to the performance, a score is assigned to each subset, being chosen the subset with the best score. In filter methods, in turn, measurement metrics such as mutual information and inter-/intra-class distance from a dataset are used to score the subsets. Finally, the embedded methods select the feature subset at the same time that the model construction. Several feature subset selection algorithms have been proposed in the literature, including genetic algorithm (GA), sequential forward selection (SFS), sequential floating forward selection (SFFS), sequential backward selection (SBS), n-best individuals, perceptron, Fisher projection, principal component analysis (PCA), and genetic feature selection, to name a few [17, 57]. Analysis of variance (ANOVA) and linear regression are the most used common tools to identify the most relevant features for emotional state detection. However, these approaches assume that the physiological signals and the emotional states have a linear relationship [61]. The assumption is that DL can extract reliable feature sets compared to features extracted through automatic selection since they do not guarantee an optimal convergence for the model. The advantage is DL can be applied directly to the raw data in any signal type (not limited to discrete signals) since some techniques require discrete signals (data mining techniques [80]). Furthermore, DL can reduce signal resolution across their architectures more efficiently compared to Hidden Markov Models and Dynamic Bayesian Networks. However, ANN has been considered as black boxes, which makes difficult the interpretation of the learned model. Therefore, appropriate visualization method for these kinds of networks is required in order to interpret neural network-based features [57].

- **Classification methods:** Even though there is a large number of classifiers employed for emotion recognition based on physiological signals, there is not a consensus about which of these algorithms is more reliable for a particular emotional state recognition application [70]. The best classification method strongly depends on the characteristics of the dataset. This argument was reinforced in [17] with a comparative study performed over 20 different machine learning algorithms evaluated on real datasets. Linear classifiers have shown to perform successfully in emotion recognition classification [17]. The training data in classification algorithms constrains their performance. They use different models for the data. For example, k-NN algorithm is useful for nonlinear boundaries between classes and require large datasets to be accurate. In addition, decision trees require large datasets for a good performance. One limitation for SVMs is that they require a very careful parameter selection. Lastly, the Naïve Bayes classifier assumes independency between features, which is not achieved in physiological signals taken from the same user [70].
- **Emotional representation models:** The main issues in emotional state detection applications are representation, detection, and classification of users' emotions [1]. Emotion description models based on discrete categories (i.e., happiness, sadness, fear, anger, disgust, and surprise) have a precise mapping between the

sensed data and the emotional models. However, those discrete categories do not represent individuals' everyday activities [1]. It is not easy to model human emotions since all humans express their emotions in a different way. The discrete model can be problematic because of blended emotions cannot be represented effectively in those discrete categories. Hence, multiple dimensions or scales can be used to classify emotions such as continuous scales (e.g., pleasant–unpleasant, attention–rejection) [17, 78]. The use of a 2D space to represent emotions can carry loss of information. Some emotions cannot be distinguished (e.g., fear and anger) or lie outside the space (e.g., surprise). Hereafter, a special training is required to use that dimensional labeling [9].

- **Existing healthcare applications:** They record and analyze patients' physiological signals to monitor patients' mobility, and assist them in emergency situations. However, those solutions focus only on medical healthcare aspects and not in users' emotional states. More research is needed in this aspect since there are evidences that emotions could influence users' physical health [1]. A simple system to classify automatically users' emotional states is still missing [20]. Existing solutions in emotional state detection have been done in controlled environments. That detection in an uncontrolled environment is challenging. Hence, several different emotion-related sources need to be combined to improve accuracy [81]. It is required suitable technology that aids to reduce healthcare cost and improves the quality of healthcare services. Technology that helps in how to define, detect, model, and represent emotional states of people, and then use that information to improve the healthcare systems is needed [1]. In addition, emotional states detection approaches that interpret and analyze human emotions without users' intentions are required. It is essential to implement human-centered designs instead of computed-centered designs. Human-centered designs must detect users' affective behavior to interact with them based on that behavioral information [9]. Those approaches have to be accurate, robust to artifacts, and adapt to practical applications [17].
- **Integration within smart cities:** Emerging Internet of Things (IoT) and big data technologies have opened doors for the building of smart cities. IoT is an extension of the existing internet where many things (i.e., sensors and actuators) are connected to the Internet using machine to machine (M2M) architectures, artificial intelligence (AI), wireless sensor networks (WSN), and semantic technologies [82]. Smart cities make the traditional networks more flexible and sustainable through the use of technology in order to benefit the citizens. They consist of smart components in terms of infrastructure, transportation, health, technology, and energy [83]. Smart healthcare applications within the smart cities are necessary to meet the needs of the citizens. Connected physiological sensors will allow monitoring in real time the citizens' health condition anywhere. Hence, the incorporation of accurate emotional states detection systems within the smart cities will allow improving the quality of life and well-being, thus addressing mental health problems through event detection, and providing feedback for therapies, and treatments. However, to this end, it is required to address several IoT and smart cities challenges such as network heterogeneity, where it is

required to guarantee the coexistence among several networks (e.g., WLAN, Bluetooth, ZigBee), security and privacy issues, quality of service (QoS) requirements, trust, social acceptance, development of intelligent signal processing and sensing algorithms, standardization for interoperability, development of wireless technologies, and to guarantee energy efficiency, to name a few.

6   Conclusion

This chapter discusses the importance of emotional state detection from physiological signals in order to improve quality of life and well-being from citizens that can be implemented into the smart city concept. It shows relevant works on this area, as well as some used databases in this study. The importance of this topic lies in the fact that mental health is an important factor of health condition. It has been shown that negative emotions can carry undesirable health problems or even death. Consequently, the incorporation of accurate emotional state detection applications within the smart cities will aid to alleviate mental disorders, stress problems, or mental health. The things (i.e., sensors and actuators) connected to Internet will allow monitoring in real-time physiological signals from citizens and detect on time any anomaly and take actions in order to prevent or control health situations. It was found several works using machine and/or DL techniques that address this research topic. However, several issues are still under study to make these applications more trustworthy and efficient to detect events and prevent undesired consequences. In addition, several challenges have to be addressed in order to implement these emotional detection systems within the smart cities.

References

1. T. Taleb, D. Bottazzi, N. Nasser, A novel middleware solution to improve ubiquitous healthcare systems aided by affective information. IEEE Trans. Inf. Technol. Biomed. **14**(2), 335–349 (2010)
2. D. Tobón, T. Falk, M. Maier, Context awareness in WBANs: a survey on medical and non-medical applications. IEEE Wirel. Commun. **20**(4), 30–37 (2013)
3. P. Bellavista, D. Bottazzi, A. Corradi, R. Montanari, Challenges, opportunities and solutions for ubiquitous eldercare, in *Web Mobile-Based Applications for Healthcare Management* (IGI Global, 2007), pp. 142–165
4. B. Arnrich, C. Setz, R. La Marca, G. Tröster, U. Ehlert, What does your chair know about your stress level? IEEE Trans. Inf. Technol. Biomed. **14**(2), 207–214 (2010)
5. T.R. Bennett, J. Wu, N. Kehtarnavaz, R. Jafari, Inertial measurement unit-based wearable computers for assisted living applications: a signal processing perspective. IEEE Signal Process. Mag. **33**(2), 28–35 (2016)
6. S. Greene, H. Thapliyal, A. Caban-Holt, A survey of affective computing for stress detection: evaluating technologies in stress detection for better health. IEEE Consum. Electr. Mag. **5**(4), 44–56 (2016)

7. O.C. Santos, R. Uria-Rivas, M. Rodriguez-Sanchez, J.G. Boticario, An open sensing and acting platform for context-aware affective support in ambient intelligent educational settings. IEEE Sensors J. **16**(10), 3865–3874 (2016)
8. G. Rebolledo-Mendez, A. Reyes, S. Paszkowicz, M.C. Domingo, L. Skrypchuk, Developing a body sensor network to detect emotions during driving. IEEE Trans. Intell. Transp. Syst. **15**(4), 1850–1854 (2014)
9. Z. Zeng, M. Pantic, G.I. Roisman, T.S. Huang, A survey of affect recognition methods: audio, visual, and spontaneous expressions. IEEE Trans. Pattern Anal. Mach. Intell. **31**(1), 39–58 (2009)
10. A. Hariharan, M.T.P. Adam, Blended emotion detection for decision support. IEEE Trans. Hum. Mac. Syst. **45**(4), 510–517 (2015)
11. H. Al Osman, T.H. Falk, Multimodal affect recognition: current approaches and challenges, in *Emotion and Attention Recognition Based on Biological Signals and Images* (InTech, 2017), pp. 59–86
12. M.A. Hogg, D. Abrams, Social cognition and attitudes, in *Psychology*, 3rd edn. ed. by G.N. Martin, N.R. Carlson, W. Buskist (Pearson Education Limited, 2007), pp. 684–721
13. P. Ekman, About brows: emotional and conversational signals. Hum. Ethol. 163–202 (1979)
14. P. Ekman, W.V. Friesen, P. Ellsworth, *Emotion in the Human Face: Guidelines for Research and an Integration of Findings* (Elsevier, 2013)
15. H.-J. Go, K.-C. Kwak, D.-J. Lee, M.-G. Chun, Emotion recognition from the facial image and speech signal, in *SICE 2003 Annual Conference*, (2003)
16. D. Sander, D. Grandjean, K.R. Scherer, A systems approach to appraisal mechanisms in emotion. Neural Netw. **18**(4), 317–352 (2005)
17. J. Kim, E. André, Emotion recognition based on physiological changes in music listening. IEEE Trans. Pattern Anal. Mach. Intell. **30**(12), 2067–2083 (2008)
18. H. Schlosberg, Three dimensions of emotion. Psychol. Rev. **61**(2), 81–88 (1954)
19. B.L. Fredrickson, R.W. Levenson, Positive emotions speed recovery from the cardiovascular sequelae of negative emotions. Cognit. Emot. **12**(2), 191–220 (1998)
20. A. Greco, G. Valenza, L. Citi, E.P. Scilingo, Arousal and valence recognition of affective sounds based on electrodermal activity. IEEE Sensors J. **17**(3), 716–725 (2017)
21. G. Valenza, L. Citi, C. Gentili, A. Lanata, E.P. Scilingo, R. Barbieri, Characterization of depressive states in bipolar patients using wearable textile technology and instantaneous heart rate variability assessment. IEEE J. Biomed. Health Inform. **19**(1), 263–274 (2015)
22. J. Ressel, A circumplex model of affect. J. Pers. Soc. Psychol. **39**, 1161–1178 (1980)
23. D. Ravi, C. Wong, F. Deligianni, M. Berthelot, J. Andreu-Perez, B. Lo, G.-Z. Yang, Deep learning for health informatics. IEEE J. Biomed. Health Inform. **21**(1), 4–21 (2017)
24. J.T. Cacioppo, Introduction: emotion and health, in *Handbook of Affective Sciences*, (Oxford University Press, New York, 2003), pp. 1047–1052
25. J.A. Healey, R.W. Picard, Detecting stress during real-world driving tasks using physiological sensors. IEEE Trans. Intell. Transp. Syst. **6**(2), 156–166 (2005)
26. R.W. Picard, Affective medicine: technology with emotional intelligence, in *Future of Health Technology* (IOS Press, 2002), pp. 69–84
27. R. Gravina, G. Fortino, Automatic methods for the detection of accelerative cardiac defense response. IEEE Trans. Affect. Comput. **7**(3), 286–298 (2016)
28. M. Murugappan, M. Rizon, R. Nagarajan, S. Yaacob, I. Zunaidi, D. Hazry, EEG feature extraction for classifying emotions using FCM and FKM. Int. J. Comp. Commun. **1**(2), 21–25 (2007)
29. Y.-P. Lin, C.-H. Wang, T.-P. Jung, T.-L. Wu, S.-K. Jeng, J.-R. Duann, J.-H. Chen, EEG-based emotion recognition in music listening. IEEE Trans. Biomed. Eng. **57**(7), 1798–1806 (2010)
30. *Harvard Health Publications*, Harvard medical school, 18 March 2016. [Online] https://www.health.harvard.edu/staying-healthy/understanding-the-stress-response. Accessed 2 Aug 2017
31. D. Lincoln, Correlation of unit activity in the hypothalamus with EEG patterns associated with the sleep cycle. Exp. Neurol. **24**(1), 1–18 (1969)

32. R.J. Davidson, G.E. Schwartz, C. Saron, J. Bennett, D. Goleman, *Frontal Versus Parietal EEG Asymmetry During Positive and Negative Affect* (Cambridge University Press, New York, 1979)
33. R.H. Chowdhury, M.B. Reaz, M.A.B.M. Ali, A.A. Bakar, K. Chellappan, T.G. Chang, Surface electromyography signal processing and classification techniques. Sensors **13**(9), 12431–12466 (2013)
34. A. Nakasone, H. Prendinger, M. Ishizuka, Emotion recognition from electromyography and skin conductance, in *Proceedings of the 5th International Workshop on Biosignal Interpretation* (2005)
35. B.M. Appelhans, L.J. Luecken, Heart rate variability as an index of regulated emotional responding. Rev. Gen. Psychol. **10**(3), 229–240 (2006)
36. R.B. Singh, G. Cornélissen, A. Weydahl, O. Schwartzkopff, G. Katinas, K. Otsuka, Y. Watanabe, S. Yano, H. Mori, Y. Ichimaru, Circadian heart rate and blood pressure variability considered for research and patient care. Int. J. Cardiol. **87**(1), 9–28 (2003)
37. A.H. Kemp, A.R. Brunoni, I.S. Santos, M.A. Nunes, E.M. Dantas, R. Carvalho de Figueiredo, A.C. Pereira, A.L. Ribeiro, J.G. Mill, R.V. Andreao, Effects of depression, anxiety, comorbidity, and antidepressants on resting-state heart rate and its variability: an ELSA-Brasil cohort baseline study. Am. J. Psychiatr. **171**(12), 1328–1334 (2014)
38. R.W. Levenson, P. Ekman, W.V. Friesen, Voluntary facial action generates emotion-specific autonomic nervous system activity. Psychophysiology **27**(4), 363–384 (1990)
39. S.D. Kreibig, Autonomic nervous system activity in emotion: a review. Biol. Psychol. **84**(3), 394–421 (2010)
40. H. Al Osman, H. Dong, A. El Saddik, Ubiquitous biofeedback serious game for stress management. IEEE Access **4**, 1274–1286 (2016)
41. M.D. van der Zwaag, J.H. Janssen, J.H. Westerink, Directing physiology and mood through music: validation of an affective music player. IEEE Trans. Affect. Comput. **4**(1), 57–68 (2013)
42. S. Khalfa, P. Isabelle, B. Jean-Pierre, R. Manon, Event-related skin conductance responses to musical emotions in humans. Neurosci. Lett. **328**(2), 145–149 (2002)
43. R.W. Picard, S. Fedor, Y. Ayzenberg, Multiple arousal theory and daily-life electrodermal activity asymmetry. Emot. Rev. **8**(1), 62–75 (2016)
44. M.-Z. Poh, N.C. Swenson, R.W. Picard, A wearable sensor for unobtrusive, long-term assessment of electrodermal activity. IEEE Trans. Biomed. Eng. **57**(5), 1243–1252 (2010)
45. H. Fukushima, H. Kawanaka, M.S. Bhuiyan, K. Oguri, Estimating heart rate using wrist-type photoplethysmography and acceleration sensor while running, in *Annual International Conference of the IEEE Engineering in Medicine and Biology Society (EMBC)* (2012)
46. A.A. Alian, K.H. Shelley, Photoplethysmography. Best Pract. Res. Clin. Anaesthesiol. **28**, 395–406 (2014)
47. L. Peter, N. Noury, M. Cerny, A review of methods for non-invasive and continuous blood pressure monitoring: pulse transit time method is promising? Irbm **35**(5), 271–282 (2014)
48. B. Padasdao, E. Shahhaidar, C. Stickley, O. Boric-Lubecke, Electromagnetic biosensing of respiratory rate. IEEE Sensors J. **13**(11), 4204–4211 (2013)
49. E. Shahhaidar, B. Padasdao, R. Romine, O. Boric-Lubecke, Piezoelectric and electromagnetic respiratory effort energy harvesters, in *35th Annual International Conference of the IEEE EMBS*, Osaka, Japan (2013)
50. C.J. Wientjes, Respiration in psychophysiology: methods and applications. Biol. Psychol. **34**(2), 179–203 (1992)
51. J. Johnson, Bilateral finger temperature and the low of initial value. Psychophysiology **24**, 666–669 (1978)
52. P. Vos, P. De Cock, V. Munde, K. Petry, W. Van Den Noortgate, B. Maes, The tell-tale: what do heart rate; skin temperature and skin conductance reveal about emotions of people with severe and profound intellectual disabilities? Res. Dev. Disabil. **33**(4), 1117–1127 (2012)
53. A. Greco, G. Valenza, A. Lanata, G. Rota, E.P. Scilingo, Electrodermal activity in bipolar patients during affective elicitation. IEEE J. Biomed. Health Inform. **18**(6), 1865–1873 (2014)

54. M. Kumar, D. Arndt, S. Kreuzfeld, K. Thurow, N. Stoll, R. Stoll, Fuzzy techniques for subjective workload-score modeling under uncertainties. IEEE Trans. Syst. Man Cybern. B Cybern. **38**(6), 1449–1464 (2008)

55. M. Nardelli, G. Valenza, A. Greco, A. Lanata, E.P. Scilingo, Recognizing emotions induced by affective sounds through heart rate variability. IEEE Trans. Affect. Comput. **6**(4), 385–394 (2015)

56. E.-H. Jang, B.-J. Park, S.-H. Kim, J.-H. Sohn, Emotion classification based on physiological signals induced by negative emotions: discrimination of negative emotions by machine learning algorithm, in *9th IEEE International Conference on Networking, Sensing and Control (ICNSC)* (2012)

57. H.P. Martinez, Y. Bengio, G.N. Yannakakis, Learning deep physiological models of affect. IEEE Comput. Intell. Mag. **8**(2), 20–33 (2013)

58. O. AlZoubi, S.K. D'Mello, R.A. Calvo, Detecting naturalistic expressions of nonbasic affect using physiological signals. IEEE Trans. Affect. Comput. **3**(3), 298–310 (2012)

59. G. Chanel, C. Rebetez, M. Bétrancourt, T. Pun, Emotion assessment from physiological signals for adaptation of game difficulty. IEEE Trans. Syst. Man Cybern. A Syst. Humans **41**(6), 1052–1063 (2011)

60. W. Wen, G. Liu, N. Cheng, J. Wei, P. Shangguan, W. Huang, Emotion recognition based on multi-variant correlation of physiological signals. IEEE Trans. Affect. Comput. **5**(2), 126–140 (2014)

61. M. Swangnetr, D.B. Kaber, Emotional state classification in patient–robot interaction using wavelet analysis and statistics-based feature selection. IEEE Trans. Hum. Mac. Syst. **43**(1), 63–75 (2013)

62. R. Jenke, A. Peer, M. Buss, Feature extraction and selection for emotion recognition from EEG. IEEE Trans. Affect. Comput. **5**(3), 327–339 (2014)

63. C.A. Frantzidis, C. Bratsas, M.A. Klados, E. Konstantinidis, C.D. Lithari, A.B. Vivas, C.L. Papadelis, E. Kaldoudi, C. Pappas, P.D. Bamidis, On the classification of emotional biosignals evoked while viewing affective pictures: an integrated data-mining-based approach for healthcare applications. IEEE Trans. Inf. Technol. Biomed. **14**(2), 309–318 (2010)

64. J. Fleureau, P. Guillotel, Q. Huynh-Thu, Physiological-based affect event detector for entertainment video applications. IEEE Trans. Affect. Comput. **3**(3), 379–385 (2012)

65. C.-K. Wu, P.-C. Chung, C.-J. Wang, Representative segment-based emotion analysis and classification with automatic respiration signal segmentation. IEEE Trans. Affect. Comput. **3**(4), 482–495 (2012)

66. G.E. Sakr, I.H. Elhajj, H.A.-S. Huijer, Support vector machines to define and detect agitation transition. IEEE Trans. Affect. Comput. **1**(2), 98–108 (2010)

67. G. Valenza, A. Lanata, E.P. Scilingo, The role of nonlinear dynamics in affective valence and arousal recognition. IEEE Trans. Affect. Comput. **3**(2), 237–249 (2012)

68. S.K. Hadjidimitriou, L.J. Hadjileontiadis, Toward an EEG-based recognition of music liking using time-frequency analysis. IEEE Trans. Biomed. Eng. **59**(12), 3498–3510 (2012)

69. S. Walter, J. Kim, D. Hrabal, S.C. Crawcour, H. Kessler, H.C. Traue, Transsituational individual-specific biopsychological classification of emotions. IEEE Trans. Syst. Man Cybern. Syst. **43**(4), 988–995 (2013)

70. Imotions, *What is GSR (Galvanic Skin Response) and How Does It Work?*, 12 May 2015. [Online] https://imotions.com/blog/gsr/. Accessed 2 Aug 2017

71. S. Koelstra, C. Muhl, M. Soleymani, J.-S. Lee, A. Yazdani, T. Ebrahimi, T. Pun, A. Nijholt, I. Patras, Deap: a database for emotion analysis; using physiological signals. IEEE Trans. Affect. Comput. **3**(1), 18–31 (2012)

72. M. Soleymani, J. Lichtenauer, T. Pun, M. Pantic, A multimodal database for affect recognition and implicit tagging. IEEE Trans. Affect. Comput. **3**(1), 42–55 (2012)

73. R.W. Picard, E. Vyzas, J. Healey, Toward machine emotional intelligence: analysis of affective physiological state. IEEE Trans. Pattern Anal. Mach. Intell. **23**(10), 1175–1191 (2001)

74. E. Douglas-Cowie, R. Cowie, I. Sneddon, C. Cox, O. Lowry, M. Mcrorie, J.-C. Martin, L. Devillers, S. Abrilian, A. Batliner, et al., The HUMAINE database: addressing the collection

and annotation of naturalistic and induced emotional data, in *Affective Computing and Intelligent Interaction*, (Springer, Berlin, 2007), pp. 488–500

75. F. Ringeval, A. Sonderegger, J. Sauer, D. Lalanne, Introducing the RECOLA multimodal corpus of remote collaborative and affective interactions, in *10th IEEE International Conference and Workshops on Automatic Face and Gesture Recognition (FG)*, Shanghai, China (2013)

76. L. Zhang, S. Walter, X. Ma, "BioVid Emo DB": a multimodal database for emotion analyses validated by subjective ratings, in *IEEE Symposium Series on Computational Intelligence (SSCI)*, Athens, Greece (2016)

77. University of Trento, Italy, in *Multimedia and Human Understanding Group (MHUG)* [Online] http://mhug.disi.unitn.it/wp-content/ASCERTAIN/ascertain.html. Accessed 10 Aug 2017

78. G. Chanel, J. Kronegg, D. Grandjean, T. Pun, Emotion assessment: arousal evaluation using EEG's and peripheral physiological signals, in *Multimedia Content Representation, Classification and Security* (2006), pp. 530–537

79. S. Afzal, P. Robinson, Natural affect data: collection and annotation, in *New Perspectives on Affect and Learning Technologies* (Springer, 2011), pp. 55–70

80. H. P. Martínez and G. N. Yannakakis, "Mining multimodal sequential patterns: a case study on affect detection," in *Proceedings of the 13th international conference on multimodal interfaces*, 2011.

81. M.I.o. Technology, *Affective Computing*, MIT [Online] http://affect.media.mit.edu/. Accessed 5 June 2017

82. T. Hui, S.R. Simon, D.S. Daniel, Major requirements for building Smart Homes in Smart Cities based on Internet of Things technologies. *Futur. Gener. Comput. Syst.* **76**, 358–369 (2017)

83. U.R. Acharya, K.P. Joseph, N. Kannathal, C.M. Lim, J.S. Suri, Heart rate variability: a review. *Med. Biol. Eng. Comput.* **44**(12), 1031–1051 (2006)

Toward Uniform Smart Healthcare Ecosystems: A Survey on Prospects, Security, and Privacy Considerations

Hadi Habibzadeh and Tolga Soyata

Abstract A plethora of interwoven social enablers and technical advancements have elevated smart healthcare from once a supplemental feature to now an indispensable necessity crucial to addressing intractable problems our modern cities face, which range from gradual population aging to ever surging healthcare expenses. State-of-the-art smart healthcare implementations now span a wide array of smart city applications including smart homes, smart environments, and smart transportation to take full advantage of the existing synergies among these services. This engagement of exogenous sources in smart healthcare systems introduces a variety of challenges; chief among them, it expands and complicates the attack surface, hence raising security and privacy concerns. In this chapter, we study the emerging trends in smart healthcare applications as well as the key technological developments that give rise to these transitions. Particularly, we emphasize threats, vulnerabilities, and consequences of cyberattacks in modern smart healthcare systems and investigate their corresponding proposed countermeasures.

Keywords Privacy · Security · Wearable sensors · Access control · Authentication

1 Introduction

With the world slowly recovering from the last economic recession in 2007 [1, 2], which occurred in parallel with the gradual population aging and the prevalence of chronic diseases such as osteoarthritis and diabetes in epidemic proportions [3, 4], smart healthcare—often portrayed as a panacea for improving healthcare quality and reducing its ever-increasing expenses—has been recently gaining unprecedented momentum. Further driven by impressive breakthroughs in the Internet of Things

H. Habibzadeh (✉) · T. Soyata
University at Albany, SUNY, Albany, NY, USA
e-mail: hhabibzadeh@albany.edu; tsoyata@albany.edu

© Springer Nature Switzerland AG 2020   75
A. El Saddik et al. (eds.), *Connected Health in Smart Cities*,
https://doi.org/10.1007/978-3-030-27844-1_5

(IoT) and smart city technologies, smart healthcare (or alternatively electronic health or e-health) has shown massive potential to bring *continuous*, *real-time*, and *personalized* health services to masses, thereby substantially decreasing the burden of already under-staffed healthcare centers [5]. Indeed, the proliferation of a wide array of e-health services ranging from clinical-grade [6, 7] to fitness [8, 9] to logistical and infrastructure [10, 11] applications is a testament to the growth of this field.

The interplay of these social impetuses and technological advancements has now paved the way for the emergence of next-generation implementations, where healthcare services are not merely restricted to continuous monitoring of physiological parameters. Instead, they operate in tandem with non-healthcare aspects of a smart city—such as smart homes and smart environments [12]—to provide comprehensive care. This transition is transpiring in a broader context and outside the locus of smart healthcare. For example, in a future smart city, a wearable remote ECG monitoring system [13] can automatically contact emergency units at the onset of a heart attack. Then, an autonomous defibrillator ambulance [14] can be dispatched to help the patient. Traffic status can be manipulated to minimize ambulance travel time [15], thereby increasing the survival chance of the patient. Although this simple scenario falls under the smart healthcare umbrella (judging by its purpose), it involves other smart city services such as smart transportation. Additionally, considering the proliferation of smart electric vehicles, this scenario indirectly engages the smart grid [16]. Such a *unified single IoT infrastructure* is yet to be realized, however, recent developments in the IoT signal its beginnings.

This transition introduces numerous challenges and opportunities. It renders smart healthcare an even more interdisciplinary field, where the effectiveness of implementations hinges on a close cooperation among engineers, physicians, patients, city authorities, businesses, etc. Establishing such a communication among healthcare constituents, however, has become a major obstacle against its progression [17]. Furthermore, inflating the sphere of e-health substantially increases the breadth and complexity of the attack surface, which poses serious security and privacy concerns, particularly, considering the gravity of the task, which involves citizens' safety and well-being. The latter case has recently become more alarming in the aftermath of increasing attacks that target critical healthcare infrastructure such as hospitals [18]. The extent and intensity of these breaches, often conducted for extortion purposes, have created an aura of distrust and skepticism between smart healthcare and its users. Neglecting these apprehensions can indeed delay the widespread acceptance of smart healthcare.

We dedicate this study to security and privacy considerations of these emerging smart healthcare applications. To this end, we first investigate the latest trends in smart healthcare applications in Sect. 2 to see how the most recent research works in the literature take advantage of existing symbiotic relationship among e-health and various aspects of modern smart cities. We then analyze the overall structure of such services and discuss the underlying technical developments that have fueled this transition in Sect. 3. We study these enablers from the standpoint of sensing, communication, and data processing and elaborate on how emerging technologies such as crowd-sensing, non-dedicated sensing, low-power short-range communication, machine learning, and deep learning solutions are driving smart healthcare toward its bright future. These nascent technologies, however, introduce security concerns. We review these vulnerabilities in Sect. 4 by discussing the latest attacks and threats against real-world implementations. Protecting smart healthcare applications from these ever-increasing threats and vulnerabilities requires a holistic approach. To this end, Sect. 5 provides a summary of some of the most prevalent attacks that target in-field individual components of smart healthcare along with their common countermeasures. Section 6 focuses on approaches that aim to protect the entirety of the system, particularly by providing services such as access control, authentication, and authorization. Sections 7 and 8 provide a discussion of existing unresolved challenges and concluding remarks, respectively.

2 Smart Healthcare Applications

Increasing public awareness about the importance of personalized, continuous, and efficient healthcare, coupled with recent breakthroughs in the IoT arena has made the scene ready for the emergence of a diverse range of smart healthcare applications. A substantial number of proposed services aim to provide a decision-support framework for physicians and specialists, thereby helping them with disease prevention, diagnosis, and therapy [19]. Such *clinical-grade* applications involve accurate data acquisition and processing that must comply with stringent procedures and standards enforced by specialized organizations such as American Diabetes Association (ADA) [20, 21] and American Heart Association (AHA) [22, 23]. Considering that these strict requirements can become prohibitive for many investors and researchers, a parallel branch of smart healthcare oriented toward *non-clinical* applications is gaining momentum. These services often include noninvasive monitoring devices such as smartwatches and wristbands to help users keep track of their activities, to promote healthier lifestyles. Alternatively, a wide variety of non-clinical applications are designed to provide continuous care for elderly and people with disabilities. Finally, instead of providing real-time and personalized healthcare, the third category of e-health aims to facilitate communication among healthcare's multiple constituents, including patients, physicians, specialists, hospitals' staff, and emergency units. In this section, we study smart healthcare applications under these three categories: (i) Clinical, (ii) Non-clinical, and (iii) Logistical applications.

As discussed in Sect. 1, the boundaries among these applications are narrowing. Investors and researchers must become cognizant of numerous challenges and complications this integration of a wide variety of smart city services poses. We discuss the significance of this in Sect. 3. This transition also introduces various security and privacy concerns. For example, a hardware-level attack to a smart healthcare device by an insider not only compromises health related private data but can also endanger the entire network, leaving the home network and other smart city services (such as smart home devices) vulnerable to cyberattacks [24]. We elaborate on major security and privacy concerns in Sections 5 and 6.

2.1 Clinical-Grade Healthcare Applications

Measuring major physiological parameters in clinical settings is traditionally conducted by trained staff and personnel via typically expensive and invasive monitoring systems. Although accurate—which is a fundamental requirement in these applications—traditional methods fail to provide continuous monitoring, which is becoming increasingly more relevant to the prevalence of chronic diseases [25]. Furthermore, measurements conducted in controlled environments of hospitals and laboratories do not sufficiently reflect patients' actual physical status in their day-to-day life. Numerous smart healthcare systems are proposed to address these requirements. The outputs of these services are directly used by physicians and specialists for prevention, diagnosis, and therapy purposes, which highlights the strict accuracy and reliability requirements of clinical smart healthcare. Unfortunately, however, noninvasive, inexpensive, and real-time monitoring does not yield high sensing accuracy. A part of these shortcomings can be offset by the utilization of advanced preprocessing and data processing techniques, which are now an integral component of every smart healthcare system. Nonetheless, as even occasional failures (false negatives) can lead to catastrophic outcomes, clinical-grade monitoring systems notoriously suffer from high false positive rates [26]. We provide more details on smart healthcare data processing in Sect. 3.3.

A large portion of clinical-grade smart healthcare applications uses continuous monitoring to detect specific events. Specifically, given the increasing share of heart failures, a wide range of applications targeting cardiovascular diseases (CVD) are proposed in the literature. For example, the authors in [27] propose a cloud-based ECG monitoring system that assists with diagnosing cardiovascular diseases by classifying heart activity into *normal, premature, ventricular contractions,* and *other.* The classification is carried out by a 30-neuron artificial neural networks (ANN) based on QRS complex features. In a telemonitoring scenario, processed information can be transmitted to a physician to assist them with decision making. This is, however, a non-trivial task as the sheer size of information collected in real-time continuous systems can readily inundate physicians and specialists. Effectively representing processing results has been subject to extensive research [28–30]. For example, a novel "QT-Clock" is presented in [31] that can summarize ECG data collected in a 24-h interval, facilitating prolonged QTc diagnoses considerably.

Although valuable, continuous sensing alone is insufficient in many cases, as a wide array of chronic diseases (such as diabetes) can only be contained through exhaustive adaptations in daily lifestyle. For such scenarios, comprehensive smart healthcare services have been developed to facilitate patient-physician collaboration, control their diet and medicine intake, and potentially recommend physical activities [32]. Aside from normal monitoring, such systems must analyze the environment and detect patients' activities, while meeting the requirements and recommendation of specialized groups. Data pertaining to patient progress and alerts indicating a critical event can be shared in real-time with a physician to provide telemonitoring [32]. Some IoT-based healthcare systems even involve automatic medicine administration, thereby ensuring perfect scheduling and exact dosage without requiring patient's diligence. An implantable example of such devices is implemented in [33]. In spite of its invasive implantation, such methods can increase patients' comfort in long-run (particularly, as opposed to traditional glucose monitoring that involves taking blood samples by *finger sticking*). We further discuss advantages and disadvantages of such methods in Sect. 3.1.

2.2 Non-clinical Healthcare Applications

Clinical-grade applications inherently entail extreme accuracy and reliability, as even occasional errors can bring about grave consequences. Many researchers and investors prefer to explore new horizons of smart healthcare free of these stringent requirements and standards. Furthermore, developing applications for the entire population (healthy and non-healthy) provides further investment motivation by promising a larger market. These major enablers have stimulated the emergence of non-clinical applications, which mostly focus on improving users' lifestyles. Relatively looser regulations in non-clinical applications directly translate to cost reduction and improved noninvasiveness—both of which are integral requirements for these applications. This field has received substantial momentum with the advancement of smart portable devices such as smartphones, smartwatches, and smart glasses. Despite their rather casual implementations, the contribution of this branch of healthcare to prevention, diagnoses, and rehabilitation of diseases must not be underestimated. In this section, we review notable example developments in this field.

A typical non-clinical smart healthcare application involves wearable sensors that collect data on a variety of physiological and environmental parameters. Sensors can take different forms depending on target applications and their requirements. For instance, textile wearable sensors worn around feet and ankles transmit inertia measurements over Bluetooth Low Energy (BLE) to a smartphone; where Support Vector Machine (SVM) algorithm classifies user's gait as either normal or *foot drop* [34]. Achieving accuracies between 71% and 98%, such an application can expedite rehabilitation process [35]. Indeed, as discussed earlier, the new generation of the smart healthcare applications employ various aspects of smart city to improve their usability. An example of such an application is provided in [8], where a combination of participatory sensing and existing sensing infrastructure in environmental monitoring, air quality monitoring, and smart transportation is used to suggest a suitable exercise route. By considering pollution, traffic, the difficulty of the terrain, ultraviolet (UV) radiation index, and temperature, the proposed application uses collaborative filtering (CF) to classify routes into three categories (danger, caution, idle) based on the physical status and health condition of the user. An ambient assisted living (AAL) targeting outdoor activities of the elderly and people with disability is developed in [36]. The proposed system is based on crowed-sensing and assists users with navigation, finding urgent health attention, providing help while afflicted with confusion, and routine tasks such as making calls and passing across streets. It can also classify user's status into various categories including *OK*, *Fallen*, *Wandering*, *Risk of Getting Lost*, etc. This example clearly shows how the implementation of an effective modern smart healthcare application can extend to not only multiple smart city infrastructures but also various social considerations.

Not all the non-clinical application focus on continuous personalized monitoring. Particularly, the prevalence of new technologies such as virtual reality (VR) and augmented reality (AR) has resulted in a variety of rehabilitation services. Particularly, VR-based video games proposed in [37] and [38] provide affordable home-based setups to accelerate rehabilitation of stroke patients with impaired arms. This directly translates to significant cost reduction by minimizing the involvement of trained personnel and special equipment.

2.3 Logistical and Infrastructure Healthcare Applications

Ubiquitous smart healthcare has created the "big data" problem, where transmission, storage, and processing of a large amount of data pose multiple challenges. Parallel to data acquisition research, many have redirected their focus to address these big data-related challenges, thereby completing the puzzle of the *uniform smart healthcare ecosystem*. For example, multi-agent systems (MAS) based on semantic comprehension can facilitate data sharing among various hospitals [39], even when the size of stored information and its distribution increases. However, in addition to its sheer size, the large number of stakeholders in smart city ecosystems also poses various challenges. An effective infrastructure is required to share data among patients, hospitals, insurance companies, pharmacies, and emergency units. Although cloud-based implementations are typically considered the natural choice in these scenarios, they raise genuine security and privacy concerns. Encryption and watermarking are proposed to protect data transfers to and from cloud servers [40]. We detail smart healthcare security considerations in Sections 5 and 6.

In addition to data sharing, some smart health applications aim to increase the efficiency of hospitals by introducing the *smart hospital* concept. An example of such system is developed in [41]. The system embodies a diverse range sensing nodes such as RFID tags, smartphones, and wireless sensor networks (WSNs) to collect information regarding the location and progress of each patient as well as their major biomarkers. The developed system allows patients with both registration and follow-up and helps them navigate within the building. Implementing such a smart environment in hospitals can reduce waiting time and costs while increasing the quality of provided services. Additionally, some applications can merely focus on facilitating face-to-face interaction between patients and physicians [17], which can be particularly of assistance to the elderly and people with disability, as they cannot make frequent visits to hospitals.

Some government agencies monitor social networks for early detection of outbreaks. This solution can effectively reduce the costs of expensive existing methods (which mostly rely on a network of physicians and pharmacies) and help with detecting outbreaks in their early stages, thereby substantially increasing the chances of its containment. Particularly, detecting seasonal influenza outbreaks via social networks seems to be quite effective [42]. Multiple examples of similar works are provided in [43], which discusses the application of the artificial intelligence to the data collected from social networks for *computing* the health status of the society (e.g., via prediction of outbreaks, measuring the efficacy of countermeasures, etc.).

2.4 Summary

Smart healthcare applications can be categorized into (i) clinical, (ii) non-clinical, and (iii) logistical and infrastructure applications. Clinical-grade services aim to assist healthcare stakeholders with prevention, diagnoses, therapy, and rehabilitation of various diseases. Non-clinical applications target personal healthcare to promote a healthier lifestyle. Logistical applications mostly focus on hospital automation and facilitate patient-physician collaboration. The dissimilarities in scopes of these applications diversify their requirements and priorities. Table 1 summarizes the

Table 1 A comparison of smart healthcare major branches: (i) clinical, (ii) non-clinical, and (iii) logistical and infrastructure applications

Application	Priorities (high to low)	Example services
Clinical (Sect. 2.1)	High-accuracy	Glucose monitoring [44]
	Robust security	Respiration monitoring [45]
	Privacy protection	Hypertension monitoring [46]
	Non-invasive	
	Low-cost	
Non-clinical (Sect. 2.2)	Non-invasive	Diet control [47]
	Low-cost	In-home rehabilitation [37]
	Privacy protection	Stress monitoring [48]
	Robust security	
	High-accuracy	
Logistical (Sect. 2.3)	Robust security	Smart hospital [49]
	Privacy protection	Medical data sharing [50]
	High-accuracy	Telemedicine [51]
	Non-invasive	
	Low-cost	

This table contrasts the priorities and characteristics of each category. Priorities are listed based on decreasing importance for each category. For example, clinical-grade devices aim to provide high accuracy, even if that increases their costs and invasiveness. In contrast, non-clinical fitness services can decrease accuracy in favor of lower cost and lower invasiveness. *Example Services* lists some of the example implementations of each application idiosyncrasies of each category. Particularly, the importance of five underlying characteristics of such systems is investigated: accuracy, security, privacy, non-invasiveness, and expense. For example, many clinical applications can trade off expense to increase accuracy. In contrary, the expense is the main criterion for many commercialized and non-clinical services (hence its priority is set to *high* in the table).

3 System Architecture

Despite its relatively short record, smart healthcare (as a subcategory of smart city and IoT) has been subject to profound changes. The early implementation of smart health was mostly centered around three components: Data acquisition and sensing, data concentration and aggregation, and data processing, storage, and visualization. Closest to the user, data acquisition involves a diverse range of sensing devices that collect raw data on user's multiple biomarkers. Due to stringent requirements on noninvasiveness, battery life, and ease-of-use (including weight and size), these sensing devices are incapable of providing intense computing. More importantly, these sensors oftentimes operate as stand-alone devices, implying that they do not have access to the entire acquired data. The most expedient solution is to outsource calculations to computationally-capable servers, where demanding data processing algorithms and long-term data storage can be provided free of the constraints sensing devices face. Direct cloud access, however, is typically far beyond the capabilities of sensing devices. This problem is typically circumvented through a hierarchal implementation, where an intermediary component bridges the gap between data acquisition and the cloud. This conduit provides transparent cloud connectivity via local wireless personal area networks (WPANs) and wireless body area networks (WBANs), thereby substantially removing communication burden from sensors. An abstract depiction of this architecture is shown in Fig. 1.

This classic architecture of smart healthcare sufficiently addresses application requirements. Particularly, hierarchal implementation is proven to be effective against system's large scale, rapid, and constant data generation, and extreme (and growing) heterogeneity. The cloud-based implementation also ensures *deep value*, where invaluable information can be revealed by combining data from multiple sources (data fusion). The backbone of this architecture, therefore, remains applicable to new-generation smart health applications as well; however, recent developments in the IoT field have resulted in significant modifications in implementation details. For example, the emergence of smart portable devices has introduced the mobile-health (m-health, as opposed to electronic-health or e-health) concept, where new sensing platforms such as the participating and non-dedicated sensing [52] have revolutionized the data acquisition component. Furthermore, as discussed in Sect. 2, smart healthcare is growing beyond its traditional definition. Similar evolution is transpiring in other smart city applications. These developments portend a uniform IoT ecosystem. Considering the functionality, this ecosystem

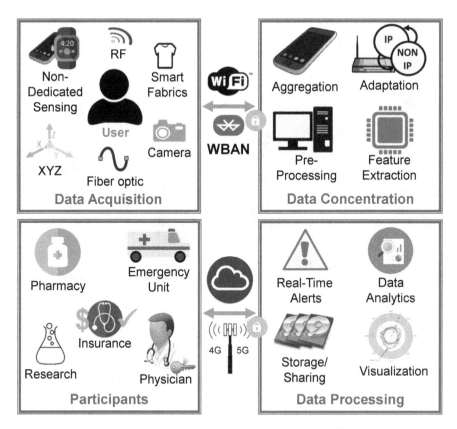

Fig. 1 Functionality of the smart healthcare infrastructure can be thought of as having three categories: (i) Data Acquisition involves dedicated and non-dedicated sensing to collect information about users and their surrendering environment, (ii) Data Concentration performs rudimentary data processing and bridges the local network with the cloud, and (iii) Data Processing stores, analyzes, and visualizes the data over an either distributed or non-distributed platform. The results are shared with various participants including physicians, insurance companies, pharmacies, etc

can be structured based on a four-component model. An *infrastructure* component gathers raw data and transfers them to the cloud for processing. *Utility* component provides application-specific services for parochial services such as smart health, smart transportation, AQ monitoring, etc. *Social development* component conflates individual applications to provide social services such as comprehensive healthcare, education, and entertainment [12]. Finally, *security and privacy* components must be spread over all building blocks of the system to ensure its robustness against cyber threats and security flaws. An abstract representation of this paradigm is depicted in Fig. 2. In the rest of this section, we study each component of smart healthcare in details and investigate how recent developments in smart city arena have affected its implementation. A thorough and complete review of the most recent advances in the smart city system architecture can be found in [53].

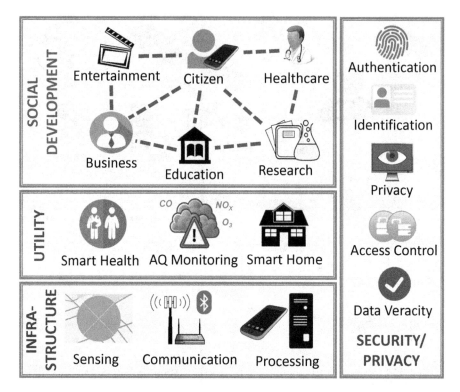

Fig. 2 A demonstration of state-of-the-art smart healthcare applications. Such systems encompass four components: (i) Infrastructure involves sensing, communication, and processing platforms, (ii) Utility employs the infrastructure toward parochial smart city applications, (iii) Social Development ensures interoperability among stand-alone applications, hence taking advantage of existing synergies, (iv) Security and Privacy protects the entire system from privacy leaks and cyber threats

3.1 Data Acquisition and Sensing

This component of the smart healthcare architecture embodies a variety of sensing devices, which aim to provide continuous, noninvasive, accurate, and inexpensive raw data acquisition of physiological and environmental parameters. These strict requirements coupled with a harsh deployment environment pose various restrictions on sensor weight, cost, size, and computational and communication capabilities. Hence, limited resource availability is the major consideration in data acquisition design and implementation. Similar to other aspects of smart healthcare, data acquisition component has been subject to gradual evolution. As explained in [3], the first generation of smart health sensing typically revolved around data acquisition from a limited number of sensors such as electrocardiogram (ECG) patches and pulse oximeters. It was soon discovered that *data fusion* in a multi-sensory setting can effectively reveal hidden information at the expense of increased computational complexity (a trade-off worth making especially in the cloud-based architecture with abundant resources) [54, 55]. The recent generation of data acquisition implementations are centered around the same premise, however, they incorporate non-traditional sources of data such as patients' historical records, research results, and laboratories experiments [56]. Although this approach further complicates the challenges regarding the big data management, it adds substantial value to applications' performance, as systems tend to evince emergent characteristics.

Multiple enablers have fueled these developments in data acquisition. Advances in solid-state physics and VLSI design have increased the computational capability of smart sensors while reducing their power dissipation. In the meantime, recent breakthroughs in material sciences have resulted in the emergence of bio-compatible and flexible printed circuit boards (PCBs) [57]. Complementary to these, novel energy harvesting solutions have remarkably mitigated the limited power availability, thereby improving sensors' noninvasiveness and accelerating the emergence of perpetual data acquisition [58–60]. Finally, smart healthcare sensing has received significant momentum with the proliferation of smart portable devices and novel solutions such as crowd-sensing and non-dedicated data acquisition [52].

Being the backbone of data acquisition component, sensors are typically implemented in three forms: *ambient sensors*, *wearable sensors*, and *implantable sensors*. Ambient sensors can collect users' information from a distance, which minimizes their invasiveness. Cameras are the most common type of ambient sensors. When used with powerful image processing techniques, camera-based solutions can be applied to a wide spectrum of applications. For example, the system proposed in [61] uses smartphones' embedded cameras to capture changes in ambient light intensity caused by breathing-induced body movements. These changes can be processed to reveal information about tidal volume and respiration rate. Indeed, this approach is substantially less invasive and more cost-efficient than standard clinical methods such as trained personal observation, Doppler radars, and spirometry. However, cameras are susceptible to the noise induced by other light sources, suffer from a limited line of sight, and raise privacy concerns [62]. This has motivated some researchers to investigate RF-based sensors as a strong candidate for ambient sensing. Various studies show that users' movements caused by falling [63], respiration [64], and heartbeats [65] interfere with RF signals (particularly, Received Signal Strength (RSS) indicator). RF sensors address many limitations of cameras, however, the filed is still in its fledgling state and many proposed solutions are tested in highly controlled environments.

Wearable sensors must remain in close proximity of users' bodies. Some may require direct contact with the skin, while others may not. For example, the authors in [66] propose a cuffless wearable sensor for blood pressure monitoring based on photoplethysmograph (PPG) signals captured by pulse oximeters. Clearly, the proposed system excels clinical approaches, which involve trained physicians and sphygmomanometer—and require patients to wear a cuff around their arm—in terms of ease-of-use and continuous data acquisition. Pulse oximeters are typically worn at the fingertips, which can become cumbersome in the long-term use. A study conducted in [67] shows that when coupled with advanced image processing techniques, built-in cameras of smartphones can also be employed to capture PPG signals. Furthermore, conducted studies in [68] and [69] prove the applicability of pulse oximeters to blood oxygen saturation monitoring applications. Other commonly used wearable sensors include dry and non-contact ECG patches [70] and Inertial Measurement Units (IMUs), which include multi-axis accelerometers, gyroscopes, and force sensors [71].

Once implanted within the body, in-vivo sensors can collect data and administer medicines accurately, without requiring any intervention from users. In spite of their invasive installation process, in-vivo sensors outperform their wearable alternatives in terms of ease-of-use in long-term operation. For example, an implantable device capable of glucose monitoring and injecting insulin is proposed in [33] for diabetic patients. The device can operate for 180 days after insertion when performing data measurements every 2 min. Limited power availability is the bane of in-vivo sensors. A study conducted in [72] proposes an implantable blood pressure monitoring system that is powered by RF backscattering; hence it can operate for an extended period. However, the sensor includes a wearable pair that continuously transmits wireless power to the device. Table 2 summarizes our discussion about most commonly used sensors in smart healthcare data acquisition.

Table 2 Sensors used in smart healthcare data acquisition component can be categorized into *ambient*, *wearable*, and *implantable* devices

Type	Advantages and disadvantages	Example applications
Ambient sensors	⇑ Minimal invasiveness ⇑ Cost-efficient ⇓ Limited accuracy ⇓ Privacy concerns ⇓ Interference susceptibility	Respiration monitoring (camera) [61] Blood oxygen monitoring (camera) [73] Fall detection (RF) [63] Heart beat monitoring (RF) [65] Respiration monitoring (WiFi) [64]
Wearable sensors	⇑ High flexibility ⇑ Cost-efficient ⇑ Non-invasive ⇓ Security concerns ⇓ Limited accuracy ⇓ Uncomfortable	BP monitoring (pulse oximeter) [74] Muscle activity monitoring (textile) [75] Seismocardiography (accelerometer) [76] Electrocardiography (ECG) [77] Fall detection (IMU) [71]
In-vivo sensors	⇑ High accuracy ⇑ Comfortable ⇓ Invasive ⇓ Limited battery life ⇓ Uncomfortable	Glucose monitoring (abdominal tissue) [33] BP monitoring (femoral artery) [72]

Ambient sensors are typically used for casual fitness-related applications. Wearable sensors can be used for both clinical and non-clinical purposes, while implantable (in-vivo) sensors are most suitable for clinical applications due to their unmatched accuracy

3.2 Data Concentration and Aggregation

Data concentration and aggregation component facilitates cloud access by creating a virtual conduit between in-field sensors and the cloud. Breaking the distance between these two components and placing the data concentrator close to sensing devices transfer the communication burden from sensors to the concentrator. Therefore, concentrators are typically provisioned to be relatively resourceful—sometimes grid-connected—computers that are not constrained with limitations of field devices. This approach is readily implementable, as a single concentrator can cater to many sensors. A concentrator establishes a short-range wireless with sensors, over which filed devices can upload their data and receive command and control messages from the cloud. Once a communication link is established, a concentrator provides three fundamental services to its associated sensor nodes: *preprocessing and aggregation, protocol adaptation*, and *cloudlet services*.

Radio Access Technologies (RATs) Establishing a connection between sensors and the concentrator faces the typical challenges of IoT and smart city communication. The power availability limitation is the main setback. Data is also highly heterogeneous; an application might involve multi-media, text-based, scalar, and real-time data, with each type demanding a specific quality of service management. Furthermore, as many smart healthcare applications are event-based (such as fall detection, heart attack prediction, etc.), the network traffic is highly bursty and unpredictable. Finally, security and privacy considerations are also of utmost importance. When combined with 3Vs (veracity, volume, and velocity) of the smart city communication [78], satisfying these requirements entails many challenges. A variety of WBAN and WPAN protocols are proposed in the literature. However, ZigBee, Bluetooth Low Energy, and WiFi have received the widest adoption. ZigBee (developed by ZigBee Alliance [79]) has for long been considered the de facto standard for WPAN implementations, due to its low complexity, acceptable reliability, low energy consumption, and decent data rate and range ($\leq$250 kbps and $\leq$100 m). This standard, however, suffers from multiple shortcomings. First, the performance of ZigBee deteriorates with the number of nodes [80]. More importantly, as ZigBee operates in the same frequency band as WiFi and due to its relatively lower transmission power, the standard is known to evince poor WiFi compatibility [81]. This can become a prohibitive limitation considering the ever-increasing popularity of WiFi. These limitations have inclined some researchers toward IEEE 802.11 (WiFi) standard, which provides remarkable throughput and unmatched ubiquity. Nonetheless, WiFi is not originally designed for smart city dense networks. Its performance decreases with the network density. Additionally, WiFi consumes orders of magnitude more energy than its low-power alternatives. BLE [82] is indeed the shining star of smart healthcare applications. It can provide relatively high data rates ($\leq$2 Mbps) and decent coverage ($\approx$ 70 m) [83]. In addition to its high energy efficiency (study conducted in [84] shows that a small coin battery can power a BLE-powered sensor for about a year in an activity recognition application), the popularity of BLE can be mostly attributed to its unparalleled ubiquity, as many portable devices such as smartphones, laptops, and smartwatches shipped with embedded BLE compatibility. BLE, however, cannot be configured in the mesh topology, which limits its scalability and arises security and privacy concerns [85].

Expected to be available in 2020, the fifth generation of mobile communication (5G) promises a low-delay (less than 1 ms), long-range, low-energy (90% reduction in comparison to 4G), high-rate (up to 10 Gbps), and resilient connectivity for smart city applications [86]. The 5G's ability to provide diverse QoS and Quality of Experience (QoE) management coupled with its compatibility with both massive Machine Type Communication (mMTC) and Ultra-Reliable Low Latency Communication (URLLC) [87] promises great opportunities to dovetail smart healthcare and other smart city applications. To these, we should also add features such as impressive mobility support (500 kmph) [88], Device to Device communication [89, 90], and Licensed-Assisted Access (LAA) [91], all of which are critical to cross-application comprehensive healthcare services. Overall, taking into the account the close ties of cellular networks with smart cities [92], the share and importance of such RATs in the smart healthcare is expected to grow.

Data Preprocessing and Aggregation Two inherent characteristics of smart healthcare communication motivate data preprocessing and aggregation. First, the dense deployment of sensors often results in duplicates or values that are in the close vicinity of each other. For example, built-in accelerometers of a user's smartwatch and smartphone typically measure and report the same value, which implies some degrees of redundancy. The other contributing factor can be associated with event-based nature of many healthcare applications, where all the sensors deployed in an application generate a tide of data upon occurrence of an event. In these scenarios, having multiple sensors that report the same event represents redundancy. The data preprocessing and aggregation component aims to reduce long-range communication burden by detecting and reducing these redundancies. This, however, requires this component to perform basic calculations on raw data (such as max, min, mean, and average), which inexorably increases the energy consumption of the node. However, as communication is notably more demanding than computation—in terms of energy consumption—data aggregation can lead to a notable reduction in the overall power dissipation. Similarly, rudimentary data preprocessing can be applied to raw data to eliminate outliers and erroneous samples. Particularly, if the resource availability of the concentrator allows it, early event detection techniques and feature extraction methods can result in major reductions in network traffic. The data aggregation and preprocessing introduce multiple challenges. For example, whether the energy consumption reductions caused by aggregating are enough to offset computation power demand remains dependent on the application. Multiple models, however, are proposed in the literature to evaluate these trade-offs [93]. Furthermore, aggregating faulty samples with normal ones can vitiate veracity of measurements, as one corrupt recording can contaminate the entire sample [94].

Cloudlet A new approach to hierarchal smart healthcare involves deployment of relatively powerful machines in the close vicinity of field devices [95]. Often termed as *cloudlet*, these machines can execute complicated data processing algorithms, offer extensive long-term data storage, and manage network operation [96], thereby minimizing the dependence of the application on the cloud [97]. This architecture improves various aspects of the application. For example, reducing the physical distance among sensors, users, and servers increases various aspects of QoS. Additionally, cloudlet-based applications can resume their operation in the absence of Internet connectivity, thereby providing offline services.

3.3 Data Processing: Structure and Algorithms

Sophisticated data analysis algorithms form the engine that drives smart healthcare toward once-unimaginable boundaries. These algorithms, nonetheless, are demanding and require access to a vast pool of data gathered from various sources—some of it is even not part of smart healthcare sphere, e.g., AQ data, traffic status, social networks, etc. This naturally calls for cloud-based implementations. We dedicate this section to major characteristics of this cloud-based architecture, studying not only the implementation but also various services it offers.

Structure and Framework Centralized cloud-based servers are the mainstream approach for data processing; they can well satisfy the ever-increasing demand of reliable computation by providing resourceful, always-on, flexible, scalable, and affordable (by benefiting from economy of scale) data processing and storage platforms. It is important to acknowledge that the term *centralized* is used loosely in this context, as almost all cloud-based servers are structured by an interconnection of a multitude resourceful machines (sometimes, physically distant from each other). However, as such services are typically offered by the same entity (Cloud Service Provider (CSP)) under the same policy, we consider them as centralized units (as opposed to massively distributed m-health services). CSP and the administration that controls a smart healthcare application can be the same entities, which yields to a *private* cloud implementation. In contrary, it is often more affordable to lease a *public* server form third-party CSPs, which share their resources with a multitude of subscribers. This, however, poses various security and privacy concerns [98]. The list of public CSPs, which customers can choose from is ever growing, as now the major tech companies provide their own processing services, including the Google Cloud IoT platform [99], Microsoft Azure IoT [100], Amazon AWS [101], and IBM Watson IoT [102] to name a few. These services not only provide a hardware platform for hosting data storage and processing but also offer off-the-shelf data analytics algorithms, visualization tools, and a spectrum of APIs for controlling end-devices; hence paving the way for the softwarization of the data plane [103]. Finally, for applications that require a middle-ground, hybrid implementations can be suggested, where sensitive data are stored and processed in private servers while demanding algorithms and long-term storage of the bulk of data are outsourced to public servers [104].

Alternatively, the diffusion of computationally capable smart portable devices, such as smartphones and smartwatches, gives rise to nascent m-health architecture, where computations are offloaded to a large number of distributed, heterogeneous devices. By putting volunteering individuals in charge of the communication and processing, the m-health substantially depresses operating costs while giving rise to flexibility and scalability of the system (epically when paralleled with non-dedicated sensing [52]). Multiple drawbacks, however, can be associated with this implementation. Aside from complications of incentivizing individuals, security and privacy considerations must also be addressed. Furthermore, the high entropy in device properties and stochastic nature of the network make it substantially difficult to guarantee the availability of the system [105]. Further curbing the applicability of distributed approaches, not all data processing algorithms are executable in a massively parallel fashion.

Machine Intelligence Software Core Whether distributed or centralized, public or private, the cloud must provide two fundamental services (aside from data storage): (i) data analytics and (ii) data visualization.

Data analytics refers to machine learning [106] and deep learning algorithms that extract valuable information from the pile of apparently unrelated raw data, thereby facilitating decision making by performing the descriptive, diagnostic, predictive, and prescriptive analysis. The data processing component must deliver these services while meeting the 5Vs (Veracity, Volume, Velocity, Variety, and Value) [78] requirements of IoT applications. Additionally, considering the gravity of the task—which directly affects the well-being of users—the machine intelligence must deliver exceptional accuracy (particularly in terms of low false-negatives) as well as immunity to noise [107]. Once such a platform is established, invaluable services can be provided to users. For example, the study conducted in [108] uses Support Vector Machine (SVM) to categorize voices recorded by numerous sensors such as smartphones and voice recorders with the objective of detecting Parkinson's Diseases (PD) in early stages (as PD causes speech impairments). Multiple features such as lowest and highest frequencies, jitter, perturbation, and amplitude are used for the classification. The SVM is executed by a centralized server, which shares the processing results with a physician. Being incorporated with other smart city services, the server can also collect traffic information to facilitate access and expedite emergency response when required. The system proposed in [109] uses cameras to capture head images, from which various features such as head movements, blinking rate, and facial expressions are extracted. These features are then combined with data obtained from user's usage of social networks to classify their mood into three separate states [109]. Using logistic regression, the authors achieve an accuracy of almost 90%. Aiming to improve the efficiency of emergency rooms, the authors of [110] propose an RFID-based patient localization technique based on k-means and Random Forest. Using this hybrid approach, they report an accuracy of 98%, showing the efficacy and robustness of hybrid and hierarchal implementations. These example data analytics applications clearly accentuate the integral role of machine intelligence in the consolidation of smart healthcare with other smart city applications.

In response to the growth of the m-health, many research works in the literature have investigated the distributed implementation of data analytics [111–113]. Particularly, clustering solutions evince great potential for distributed implementations. Nonetheless, such approaches negatively affect various aspects of the system, with the communication plane typically receiving the brunt of the performance degradation, as distributed algorithms heavily rely on data exchange among nodes. Finally, once processed, the information must be output to participants in forms of recommendations, action control, and particularly, visualization. An effective approach to the latter is rife with myriad complications. First, the massive size of the extracted information calls for data abstraction and summarization. For example, the study conducted in [31] proposes a novel visualization solution for condensing 24-h heart rate data into a simple graph, helping physicians detect Long QT (LQT) syndrome. Second, various participants of the e-health system seek different information; therefore, data visualized for (say) patients differ substantially from those prepared for physicians. These two requirements necessitate a *hierarchal* and *personalized* presentation.

4 Smart Healthcare Vulnerabilities

Aside from its myriad advantages, the diffusion of smart healthcare (and IoT in general) in various dimensions of our healthcare system brings about multiple detrimental side effects. Particularly, by increasing the *attack surface*, this transition leaves security, safety, and privacy of the users vulnerable to cyberattacks. The extent of these vulnerabilities ranges from security flaws in individual smart devices to weaknesses in underlying infrastructures such as hospitals. For example, in 2017, Food and Drug Administration (FDA) issued a warning regarding the susceptibility of pacemakers and cardiac devices to intrusion and privacy breaches [114]. Fortunately, no specific attack exploiting these flaws was reported; nonetheless, considering the gravity of these devices to patients, such security threats cause genuine concerns and retard proliferation of smart healthcare devices.

Further adding to the security and privacy concerns, an increasing number of attacks are now targeting underlying health infrastructures. For example, in 2017, attackers used a ransomware to cut access to computers in a hospital in Los Angeles [115]. The hospital regained access only after paying $17,000 to the attackers. Although this incident did not directly threat hospitalized patients, it interfered with the admittance of new patients to the emergency center. Even more unsettling, in the same year, the so-called *WannaCry* ransomware affected UK's National Health Services (NHS), which led to "massive shutdowns and inconveniences to the country's health care infrastructure" [116]. Similar extortion-oriented attacks have been reported across the globe [117], including a $55,000 ransom attack to a hospital in Greenfield, Indiana in 2018 [114]. Indeed, the interwoven structure of smart healthcare further exacerbates the situation, as the dispersion of even seemingly insignificant data can create security considerations. For example, it is known that fitness-related data can reveal sensitive information pertaining to military zones [118].

Considering the smart healthcare's inflating sphere of influence, it can be expected that the frequency and extent of such attacks continue to increase for the foreseeable future. This can depress the social acceptance of such applications and impede the prevalence of smart healthcare and its many advantages. Consequently, a massive amount of effort has been undertaken to strengthen the security and privacy aspects of this domain. These efforts can be subsumed under technical and non-technical (social) categories. The former involves applying security preserving techniques to different components of the architecture shown in Fig. 2, while the latter includes regulations passed by policymakers to legally oblige system developers to protect the privacy and security of their users. Health Insurance Portability and Accountability Act (HIPAA) and the European Data Protection Directive 95/46/EC [119] are the most eminent examples of such regulations. In this chapter, we focus on the former category.

The underlying contributing factor to security and privacy vulnerabilities of smart health can be ascribed to the service-oriented design approach of developers, who oftentimes neglect the security aspects of their systems to expedite the development and employment process. Still being its infancy, many smart healthcare products and services—whether commercial or not—are developed somehow as proof-of-concept prototypes to assess the feasibility of new ideas and evaluate their social acceptance. Furthermore, unlike performance metrics such as battery life, memory size, and physical dimensions, the security and privacy metrics are difficult to quantify and advertise [120]. This leaves some producers reluctant to heavily invest in these areas. It is, therefore, not surprising to see that many of these products regard security and privacy as *features* rather than an integral part of the system [121].

Although the maturity of IoT coupled with the rising awareness about security (fueled by recent attacks) has mitigated this problem to some extent, older vulnerable devices entail long-lasting repercussions by adding to the security *heterogeneity* of the system. The security heterogeneity is a multi-faceted problem that substantially complicates the fulfillment of a protective initiative. Following the preceding discussion, one aspect of this non-uniformity can be associated with the amalgamation of the older generation and insecure devices with newer (typically) secure ones. By creating weak links, this provides adversaries with the opportunity to exploit vulnerabilities of the former group to compromise the entire network. From another perspective, this heterogeneity evinces itself in data and user access requirements [122]; some data are inherently more sensitive than others. For example, video and audio-based information are more prone to attacks than air quality parameters. Nonetheless, when fused together, even unimportant data can disclose critical information about users [118]. User non-uniformity implies that a complex smart healthcare system involves numerous stakeholders from patients to their physicians to insurance companies to emergency units. These users require various levels of data access, which often change dynamically based on the context [123]. Indeed, managing these heterogeneities is an onerous task.

Addressing these intricate security and privacy considerations in the smart city must be carried out in accordance with the limited resource availability of smart sensors, implying that many existing sophisticated techniques are not applicable to smart healthcare applications. This adds another dimension to the security and privacy problem, where these requirements must be met without adversely affecting the experience of the user. This dimension is sometimes referred to as *Quality of Protection (QoP)* [124]. Additionally, aside from intentional cyberattacks, smart health applications must also offer higher reliability, resilience, and self-healing features. Finally, even devices with robust security mechanisms may fail to protect users' data, unless both users and system administrators meticulously enforce security recommendations [120]. Increasing the awareness among various stakeholders is, therefore, critical to any holistic security framework.

The standardization of security and privacy protection mechanisms poses yet another challenge in securing smart healthcare services. Currently, the available solutions are highly fragmented, as a universal standard is yet to be adopted. This fragmentation occurs in each service of the smart city (including smart healthcare) but the problem will be more pronounced in entangled future ecosystems that involve a wide variety of smart city services. Indeed, the emergence of higher-level security services provided by CoAP, DTLS, IPSec, etc. can partially abate these concerns. Nonetheless, interoperable access control, identification, authentication, and trustworthiness assessment are yet to emerge. The major policymakers and standardization groups are aware of these shortcomings and have undertaken various efforts to standardize IoT security (e.g., ITU-T Y.2060, Y.2066, Y.2067, Y. 2075, etc. [125]). Particularly, ITU-T Y.2075 and ITU-T H860 target smart healthcare applications, the former defines the requirements for e-health monitoring, while the latter regulates multimedia data exchange [126].

Any effective protective solution must overcome the aforesaid challenges to satisfy various requirements that are subsumed under the general term, *security*, including [127, 128]:

- *Confidentiality* protects data against privacy leaks, eavesdropping, and unauthorized access.
- *Availability* implies that data must be made available to authorized users at their behest with least amount of delay possible.
- *Data integrity* detects and amends data manipulations, either intentional (caused by adversaries) or unintentional (caused by networking errors) ones.
- *Interoperability* facilitates authorized information sharing among various participants of the healthcare system.
- *Identification* limits the data access to the authorized users.
- *Authorization* verifies the legitimacy of data and users.
- *Data loss immunity* enables the system to recover to its original state after a partial loss of data.
- *Privacy* cuts access to the data for the irrelevant users.

Smart healthcare applications are particularly vulnerable to identity-based attacks. Unfortunately, traditional PIN-based authentication techniques are proven to be inadequate in many applications considering that (i) smart healthcare ecosystems involve a large number of stakeholders and (ii) many users are elderly, who might not easily remember their credentials. Various solutions are proposed to relax this requirement (e.g., using RFID tags [129]). In addition to identity-based threats, many smart healthcare systems are vulnerable to service attacks (Denial of Service), which can result in catastrophic consequences [130]. The following sections provide a more detailed study of some of the major threat models in smart healthcare applications.

5 Security and Privacy of Field Devices

As discussed in Sect. 4, regarding security and privacy protection mechanisms as supplementary *features* is the underlying cause of many existing vulnerabilities. Instead, security must be incorporated in the early phases of the design process as an integral component of the system. Furthermore, because it is the weakest link that determines the overall robustness of the system, any attempt to ensure security and protect privacy must include all components of the system. This latter consideration, however, is typically neglected, as developers often focus on the security of the communication and omit other components.

Cryptography is the backbone of the security and privacy protection in the sensing and communication planes. Particularly, taking advantage of its simplicity, many smart sensors are equipped with built-in Advanced Encryption Standard (AES) accelerators [131]. In case a more robust encryption is required, algorithms that use Elliptic Curve Cryptography (ECC), such as Elliptic Curve Digital Signature (ECDSA), can be employed. ECC security matches RSA, however, utilizing smaller keys renders it less resource demanding. ECDSA, however, involves complicated verification procedures, which shifts the computation burden to the cloud side [132]. These cryptography-based approaches can well improve device security against a wide variety of software-based attacks. However, they are oftentimes ineffective against hardware and side channel attacks. Additionally, many of these solutions are susceptible to attacks carried out by insiders [133].

5.1 Common Threats and Proposed Solutions

This section analyzes some of the major threats and the proposed solutions for ensuring security and privacy of field devices, by focusing on sensing and communication components. Instead of targeting the entirety of the system, most of the vulnerabilities studied in this section correspond with the system's individual components or at most aim at the underlying data collection network (as opposed to enforcing access control, identification, and authentication that involve higher-level component of the system (e.g., cloud), which are discussed in Sect. 6). The relative parochial scope of these threats, however, does not translate to ineffectiveness. Although we have separated the solutions and threats into two sections, a comprehensive security package must be uniformly spread over all levels.

Node capture involves insider adversaries tampering a node in the network, oftentimes through hardware changes (including uploading code through debugging pins or soldering hardware pieces to the device). Therefore, it requires physical access to the device. Once compromised, the adversary can read the memory content of the captured node, make it generate false data, or gain full control over its operation, which allows them to perform insider attacks targeting the entire network. Firmware verification—particularly hardware-based solutions that rely on Trusted Platform Modules [134]—and limiting access to debugging pins can provide some degree of immunity to such attacks [135].

Node replication is based on secret key information gained from captured nodes, which allows the adversary to insert multiple compromised nodes into the network mimicking the identity and credentials of the captured device. Replicated nodes (imposters) can generate wrong data, perform selective packet forwarding, and conduct sinkhole attacks [128]. Typically, location-based solutions, where neighbors of a node attest its legitimacy are used for detecting imposters. Network mobility and colluding replicas, however, can render these solutions rather impotent. More robust approaches, such as token exchange based on Artificial Immune System (AIS) can mitigate these problems [136].

Injection attacks involve adversaries uploading malicious firmware to the device (code injection) or tampering with nodes to generate incorrect data (data injection). The former can be mitigated by checking the validity of the firmware, whereas the latter is typically detected by "estimators" [133]. An estimator contrasts the values generated by a senor with the expected values. A substantial and persistent deviation from expected values indicates an attack. The efficacy of such solutions, however, is limited when adversaries have some familiarity with the network and the expected values. More sophisticated estimators based on Kalman filter and machine learning solutions are proposed in the literature to address these limitations [137, 138]. Injection attacks are particularly common in smart healthcare applications. For example, the study conducted in [139] shows the susceptibility of BLE (arguably, the most prevalent communication in smart healthcare applications) to these attacks.

Side channel attacks are carried out by inspecting parameters such as execution time, power consumption, and cache access patterns to gain information about sensitive information (e.g., secret keys). Side channel attacks can then render software-based encryption techniques rather ineffective. Decreasing the correlation between the key size and computations (such as Montgomery's multiplication [140]) as well as randomizing calculations [141] can substantially improve the immunity of the system against side-channel attacks [131].

Jamming is a well-known type of Denial of Service (DoS) attacks, which targets system's availability. To achieve this, adversaries use jammer devices to generate random RF signals that intentionally cause interference with data transmission, thereby decreasing the Signal-to-Noise Ratio (SNR). The complexity of jamming attacks increases with the knowledge of the adversaries about the network, which allows them to adjust their attack to the network's reaction. Countervailing jamming in such scenarios often involves game theory-based solutions that aim to detect an equilibrium between adversary's actions and network reactions [142]. Such solutions, however, typically take a toll on sensors' computational load and their energy consumption demands.

Denial of sleep (DoSL) is a link layer variant of DoS attacks. In DoSL, the adversary exploits security flaws to create packet collision, message overhearing, and idle listening to increase the energy consumption of smart sensors. Additionally, these attacks can be carried out simply by sending consecutive Request to Send (RTS) messages. DoSL accelerates battery drain. Knowing that battery replacement in many WSNs is cost prohibitive, this can lead to imminent shut down of such networks [143]. Securing the network against DoSL typically revolves around authentication and anti-replay mechanisms [144].

Vampire attacks reduce networks' expected lifetime by gradually draining sensors' batteries. Two aspects differentiate this attack from DoSL and resource exhaustion attacks; first, it typically targets long-term availability of the network and second, it exploits vulnerabilities of the network layer. Particularly, the malicious nodes generate and transmit packets that require higher-than-average routing and processing (e.g., by creating loops or establishing longer routes), hence increasing the power dissipation of the network. Vampire attacks can be mitigated by loop detection routing algorithms and optimal route re-computation as well as clean slate sensor routing protocols [145].

Black hole is a network layer DoS attack, where a malicious node exploits vulnerabilities in routing protocols such as Ad-hoc On-demand Distance Vector (AODV) and Dynamic Source Routing (DSR) to broadcast a fake shortest path to a destination. Eventually, this results in all the packets generated by the network to be redirected to the compromised node. The malicious device can then drop these packets (black hole attack) or forward a select number of them (selective black hole attack). Various solutions are proposed in the literature to countermeasure black hole attacks including sending data through multiple paths and establishing trusted routes based on the packet delivery ratio. Such solutions, however, increase power demand of the system and add to its complexity [146].

Man-in-the-middle, or equivalently *manipulation* [147], describes (typically) network layer data manipulation attacks, where an adversary alters data traveling from its source to destination. Particularly, joining procedure of new devices to the network is known to be susceptible to such attacks [148]. This is indeed a major challenge for smart healthcare systems as their dynamism implies frequent inclusion and exclusion of devices, providing adversaries ample opportunities to compromise the data. Network robustness against man-in-the-middle attacks can be increased by employing data encryption techniques (either symmetric or asymmetric), network layer authentication, and digest algorithms [149].

5.2 Specificities of Smart Healthcare Applications

A majority of the vulnerabilities discussed in Sect. 5.1 are inherited from IoT-based nature of modern smart healthcare applications. In addition to these vulnerabilities, there still exists a wide range of security concerns that directly stem from immanent characteristics of smart healthcare. Particularly, extent and diversity of smart health-care systems are proven to be the root cause of many such threats. A practical health-care system likely relies on users conventional smart devices such as smartphones and smartwatches to collect and relay data. These devices forward information to the cloud using a heterogeneous communication network that involves home and public WiFi as well as cellular communication. This creates ample opportunity for adversaries to compromise the system. For example, many smart existing services revolve around Android-powered devices. The conducted studies in [150] show how adversaries can steal critical information from these devices using screen-shot attacks. Additionally, it is known that WiFi and ZigBee (two most commonly-used communication technologies in WBAN) can be compromised using man-in-the-middle, DDos, and replay attacks [151]. Therefore, due to this heterogeneity, providing end-to-end security is oftentimes augmented by employing higher-level encryption (e.g., Constraint Application Protocol (CoAP) [152] in the application layer and IPSec and Datagram Transport Layer Security (DTLS) [153] in the transport layer). Lower level security solutions are also available. For example, IPv6 over Low power Wireless Personal Area Network (6LoPAN) uses AES to provide authentication and confidentiality (by adjusting the Auxiliary Security Header). Although effective, many of these solutions substantially increase power demand of existing healthcare devices. There are some existing works in the literature that aim to address this limitation by outsourcing demanding computations of these algorithms to more resourceful devices such as gateways [154].

5.3 Summary

This discussion of a select number of cyberattacks clearly shows their diversity, which evinces itself in terms of exploited vulnerabilities (hardware and software), adversaries intentions (e.g., crippling the network or stealing data), targeted layers (e.g., physical, link, and network), scale and possible repercussions. Emerging sensing and processing paradigms such as crowd-sensing and edge-processing fur-ther complicate smart healthcare security equation by adding additional unknowns such as participant trustworthiness [155]. Table 3 summarizes our discussion about crypto-level security concerns in smart healthcare applications.

Table 3 Summary of some threats against sensing and communication components of smart healthcare, their repercussions, and common solutions

Attacks	Target		Repercussions	Proposed solutions
	HW	SW		
Node capture	✓	✗	False data generation Secret key leakage Basis for other attacks	Limiting access to debugging pins/firmware verification (SW or HW)
Node replication	✓	✗	False data generation Basis for sink hole attack Packet drop	Neighbor attestation/toke exchange
Injection	✓	✗	False data generation Basis for node capture attack	Data verification by estimators
Jamming	✓	✗	Degraded QoS Increased energy demand Packet drop	Game theoretic traffic analysis
Side channel	✓	✓	Secret key leakage	Montgomery's multiplication/randomizing computations
DoSL	✗	✓	Battery drain	Authentication/replay attack protection
Vampire	✗	✓	Gradual battery drain	Routing loop detection/clean slate sensor routing
Black hole	✗	✓	Gradual battery drain Packet loss Privacy leakage	Multi-path routing/establishing trusted routes
Man in the middle	✗	✓	False data injection Packet loss Privacy leakage	Data encryption/authentication/digest algorithms

6 Access Control, Identification, and Authentication

The diffusion of cloud-based computing in smart healthcare systems explicitly implies a separation between data's host (where data is processed and stored) and their generators (users). Considering that cloud-based servers are typically owned and controlled by third-party entities, such separation causes genuine security and privacy concerns. Furthermore, taking advantage of economies of scale, cloud resources are shared among various applications and services, which increases incidents of privacy leakage and provides more opportunities for adversaries to compromise the system's security. In addition to protecting data against the threats discussed in Sect. 5, an impervious security system cannot be established without overcoming cloud security challenges.

A comprehensive protecting solution must be spread over all functionality of the cloud [156]: data processing, data retrieval, and data storage. The first requirement can be satisfied by Fully Homomorphic Cryptography (FHC) techniques, which allow computation on encrypted data [157, 158]. FHC, however, is computationally complex even for powerful cloud-based servers. Ensuring security of data during retrieval and storage is typically addressed by identification, authorization, and access control mechanisms. Scale, dynamism, and complexity of healthcare systems render many traditional solutions impractical. Hence, this field calls for innovative solutions, which we investigate in detail in this section.

6.1 Access Control

Traditional access control mechanisms (based on RSA, AES, and IDEA) are developed to provide secure one-to-one data sharing, which makes them suitable for classic applications such as file transfer and email exchange. The requirements of modern smart healthcare platforms, however, differ significantly from these traditional services, which involve a large number of participants with highly dynamic access privileges, which change with roles, time, location, etc. [159]. Indeed, multiple copies of data can be created to implement more resilient data sharing paradigms based on the traditional techniques; nonetheless, the sheer scale of the smart healthcare renders such approaches impractical. Attribute-Based Access Control (ABAC) can satisfy this requirement. Based on Attribute-Based Encryption (ABE, also called Fuzzy Identity-Based Encryption) [160], ABAC utilizes users' attributes (e.g., location, profession, affiliation, etc.) to create private keys. Therefore, the combination of various attributes allows fine-grained access control management. For example, the authors in [161] develop a cloud-based framework for ABE-based personal health record sharing that manages access control among various owners and users (including patients, physicians, family members, pharmacies, etc.). The proposed solution also provides attribute revocation (a user's access to a record must be terminated as soon as their attributes change) and relies on honest but curious servers.

6.2 Identification and Authentication

A robust authentication mechanism must ensure protection against a multitude of attacks including eavesdropping, online and offline password guessing, spoofing, man-in-the-middle, replay, and dictionary attacks. Even a single vulnerability against one of these threats suffices to undermine the overall efficacy of the authentication mechanism. This comprehensiveness inexorably entails hybrid solutions, as developing a non-hybrid solution capable of satisfying all these requirements is proven to be cumbersome. Additionally, authentication techniques must comply with immanent characteristics of eHealth cloud, particularly its distributed and multi-server implementation [162], while offering simple and secure account recovery as well as system restoration after disasters and breaches [163].

Traditionally, the authentication is carried out using passwords, which can always be stolen and guessed (especially low-entropy ones). Alternatively, two-factor authentication can address some of these concerns, where in addition to passwords, users must insert a smart card to verify their identity. This prevents passwords guessing, stealing, and sharing, as there is only a single card per user. This remote-access identity-based verification mechanism, however, is still susceptible to eavesdropping, password guessing, and smart key stealing [164]. Addressing these limitations, emerging biometrics-based solutions use physiological parameters (e.g., fingerprints, facial features, etc.) to identify and authenticate users. Additionally, in response to nascent trends in the digital health domain, such as socialization of smart objects [165] and their interplay with social media [166], biometrics-based solutions can now authenticate users based on their behavioral patterns including their use of social networks [167] and handwriting [168]. These two approaches are also referred to as *hard* and *soft* biometrics-based authentication [169]. Strong protection can be maintained by a hybrid utilization of both the behavioral and biometrics-based authentication, as opposed to replacing one with the other.

Maximizing the security robustness of smart healthcare systems, various three-factor authentication mechanisms, based on passwords, smart cards, and biometrics have been proposed in the literature. Utilizing strong encryption mechanism such as RSA, ECC, and Hash function (ECC is typically preferred due to its strong protection and small key size) under the hood, the three-factor authentication can provide immunity against a variety of attacks including guessing, eavesdropping, intercept, replay to name a few [170]. Aside from its many advantages, three-factor authentication is rather a complicated system, which impedes its widespread proliferation among the elderly and disabled. Both groups are major participants in healthcare systems. This calls for alternative approaches that are user-friendly and independent from peripheral devices such as smartphones and card readers. To this end, various ambient sensors (e.g., cameras and RFID) can extract users' biometrics to authenticate them, thereby creating a naked environment, where interactions between users and the environment take place directly and continuously [171].

6.3 Data Trustworthiness

The system's heterogeneity coupled with a large number of stakeholders in a typical smart healthcare application introduces an extra dimension in data security and privacy: *data trustworthiness*. Intentional (by adversaries) and unintentional (e.g., by faulty devices) incidents can inject fallible data in smart healthcare applications. Due to the gravity of the task, it is necessary to evaluate and assess the *trustworthiness* of the collected data. This problem is particularly emphasized in crowd-sensing applications. Two key factors determine data trustworthiness. The first one is ascribed to the accuracy of the sensors (typically embedded into participants' smart devices), while the second is typically associated with their *reputation* [172]. Social Network-Aided Trustworthiness Assurance (SONATA) is a notable solution to evaluate data trustworthiness in a crowd-sensing application [173]. In this solution, a community of participants that perform the same sensing task is used to evaluate trustworthiness through a voting-based approach, dynamically. The study conducted in [174] uses a similar approach, however, the authors further increase the reliability of the voting process by increasing the *voting clout* of a group of selected trustworthy participants.

Aside from the preceding discussion, the recent incidents regarding the privacy violation of users by some of the major services providers have also added a new aspect to trustworthiness in IoT and smart healthcare systems. In fact, many users and system administrators now prefer to sever their reliance on third-party service providers. This has inexorably motivated the emergence of decentralized solutions. Particularly, block-chain services are expected to play a significant role for securely storing medical records on a distributed platform. Existing research has proven the efficacy of block-chain technology in protecting users' privacy and security [175].

7 Future Directions and Open Issues

Although the current smart healthcare services are fragmented and disjoint, the newest trends and developments in IoT and the smart city hint at an imminent fusion of services and applications into a unified ecosystem. Multiple trends fuel this unification including (but not limited to) the prevalence of smart wearables and crowd-sensing platforms, the emergence of electric vehicles and smart home services, the growth of machine learning and deep learning algorithms, the advancements of cloud and fog computing, etc. To these, one should also add societal developments such as the global aging population, increasing technology-awareness in eastern and southern Asia, as well ever increasing market dominance of some technology giants. Establishing such an ecosystem, however, is contingent upon guaranteeing interoperability among myriad components of smart cities, which for years has been the bane of IoT-based services.

There are multiple emerging technologies that can facilitate interoperability in the context of smart healthcare and the smart city. For example, 5G has the potential to overcome the fragmentation in communication technologies, particularly, considering its intrinsic compatibility with existing common Radio Access Technologies (such as WiFi) using the Licensed Assisted Technology (LAA) [176]. When coupled with the profusion of smart wearable devices, it is not unreasonable to imagine that BLE/5G will be the de facto approach for short and long range communication, respectively.

Equivalently impressive is the evolution of the blockchain technology, which simultaneously addresses the security concerns and the challenges regarding the data storage and sharing in smart healthcare services. Additionally, this technology can pave the way to further the adoption of fog computing, which is yet another major pillar for future smart healthcare ecosystem. Despite its increasing popularity, however, the adoption of blockchain technology faces various challenges including ensuring the interoperability among different blockchains, protecting the security of the data when at least 50% of the network is compromised, and evaluating the trustworthiness of information [177].

In addition to the aforementioned challenges, standardization and security remain the main deterrence against the growth of smart healthcare ecosystem. Although multiple efforts have been undertaken to standardize data communication, sensing, storage, and processing are often get neglected, which negatively impacts the integration of services in these levels. The unification of smart healthcare services with each other, as well as sundry smart city applications, also exacerbates security and privacy concerns as it complicates the existing attack surface. Unfortunately, many major stakeholders fail to properly incorporate a comprehensive security protection system in their designs (perhaps because in some cases companies short-term financial interests are in contrast with their customers or maybe privacy and security features are not as *advertisable* as performance metrics). Despite the remarkable advancements in communication component, preserving security and privacy for effectively sharing and processing information still remains the major hindrance against the proliferation of ubiquitous smart healthcare.

8   Summary and Concluding Remarks

Despite their relatively short life, fledgling smart healthcare systems have evolved from simple monitoring services with a limited number of sensors to now complicated multi-faceted and multi-dimensional systems, that are interwoven seamlessly with various aspects of our lives in the post-ICT era. This article is dedicated to unraveling major enablers that have contributed to this transition, spanning from technical breakthroughs to their security and privacy repercussions. Emphasizing the convergence of various smart city applications into a unified ecosystem and focusing on the security and privacy ramifications of such trends, we study modern smart healthcare systems from the standpoint of the following aspects:

(i) Application, where we investigate existing works to show how clinical grade, fitness-related, and infrastructure applications are evolving and merging to form a unified healthcare ecosystem.

(ii) Architecture, where we discuss underlying technical advances that have fueled the evolution of the smart healthcare. We explain how the maturity of sensing devices has made available to our disposal a wide spectrum of inexpensive, resourceful, noninvasive, and bio-compatible sensors. To this, we should add viable alternatives such as crowd-sensing, which substantially reduce the expenses of large-scale sensing platforms. Additionally, we detail the contribution of emerging low-power and high-rate communication such as BLE to a reduction in communication expenses. Furthermore, we provide an analysis of the critical role of machine learning and deep learning algorithms in the realization of the smart healthcare ecosystem.

(iii) Vulnerabilities, where we examine the most recent cyberattacks targeting actual implementations to identify major vulnerabilities and weaknesses of smart healthcare applications.

(iv) Crypto-level security, where we detail security flaws of the sensing and communication components of the smart healthcare, with an emphasis on less conventional hardware and software attacks carried out by insiders.

(v) System-level security, where we address the vulnerabilities of the cloud, myriad challenges it faces in quest of protecting users' security and privacy, as well as the proposed solutions and their associated advantages and disadvantages.

Our study concludes by arguing that nothing more than security and privacy considerations blocks the path toward the realization of the future healthcare ecosystem. This concern can only be mitigated by implementing security protection mechanisms as an integral part of the system, added to the design in early stages, and spread uniformly over every single component of the system.

References

1. C.J. Truffer, S. Keehan, S. Smith, J. Cylus, A. Sisko, J.A. Poisal, J. Lizonitz, M.K. Clemens, Health spending projections through 2019: the recession's impact continues. Health Aff. **29**(3), 522–529 (2010)

2. D. Stuckler, S. Basu, M. Suhrcke, A. Coutts, M. McKee, The public health effect of economic crises and alternative policy responses in Europe: an empirical analysis. Lancet **374**(9686), 315–323 (2009)

3. J. Andreu-Perez, D.R. Leff, H.M.D. Ip, G.Z. Yang, From wearable sensors to smart implants- toward pervasive and personalized healthcare. IEEE Trans. Biomed. Eng. **62**(12), 2750–2762 (2015)

4. L.E. Hebert, P.A. Scherr, J.L. Bienias, D.A. Bennett, D.A. Evans, Alzheimer disease in the us population: prevalence estimates using the 2000 census. Arch. Neurol. **60**(8), 1119–1122 (2003)

5. M. Estai, Y. Kanagasingam, M. Tennant, S. Bunt, A systematic review of the research evidence for the benefits of teledentistry. J. Telemed. Telecare **24**(3), 147–156 (2017). 1357633X16689433

6. K.A. Al Mamun, M. Alhussein, K. Sailunaz, M.S. Islam, Cloud based framework for Parkinson's disease diagnosis and monitoring system for remote healthcare applications. Futur. Gener. Comput. Syst. **66**, 36–47 (2017)

7. A. Page, M. Hassanalieragh, T. Soyata, M.K. Aktas, B. Kantarci, S. Andreescu, Conceptualizing a real-time remote cardiac health monitoring system, in *Enabling Real-Time Mobile Cloud Computing Through Emerging Technologies*, ed. by T. Soyata (IGI Global, Hershey, 2015), pp. 1–34

8. F. Casino, C. Patsakis, E. Batista, F. Borràs, A. Martínez-Ballesté, Healthy routes in the smart city: a context-aware mobile recommender. IEEE Softw. **34**(6), 42–47 (2017)

9. B. Reeder, A. David, Health at hand: a systematic review of smart watch uses for health and wellness. J. Biomed. Inform. **63**, 269–276 (2016)

10. J. Tavares, T. Oliveira, Electronic health record patient portal adoption by health care consumers: an acceptance model and survey. J. Med. Internet Res. **18**(3), e49 (2016)

11. G. Manogaran, R. Varatharajan, D. Lopez, P.M. Kumar, R. Sundarasekar, C. Thota, A new architecture of internet of things and big data ecosystem for secured smart healthcare monitoring and alerting system. Futur. Gener. Comput. Syst. **82**, 375–387 (2018)

12. G. Muhammad, M. Alsulaiman, S.U. Amin, A. Ghoneim, M.F. Alhamid, A facial-expression monitoring system for improved healthcare in smart cities. IEEE Access **5**, 10871–10881 (2017)

13. E. Spanò, S.D. Pascoli, G. Iannaccone, Low-power wearable ECG monitoring system for multiple-patient remote monitoring. IEEE Sens. J. **16**(13), 5452–5462 (2016)

14. H. Samani, R. Zhu, Robotic automated external defibrillator ambulance for emergency medical service in smart cities. IEEE Access **4**, 268–283 (2016)

15. R. Sundar, S. Hebbar, V. Golla, Implementing intelligent traffic control system for congestion control, ambulance clearance, and stolen vehicle detection. IEEE Sens. J. **15**(2), 1109–1113 (2015)

16. F. Mwasilu, J.J. Justo, E.K. Kim, T.D. Do, J.W. Jung, Electric vehicles and smart grid interaction: a review on vehicle to grid and renewable energy sources integration. Renew. Sustain. Energy Rev. **34**, 501–516 (2014)

17. A. Alaiad, L. Zhou, Patients' Adoption of WSN-Based Smart Home Healthcare Systems: An Integrated Model of Facilitators and Barriers. IEEE Transactions on Professional Communication **60**(1), 4–23 (2017)

18. A.L. Young, M. Yung, Cryptovirology: the birth, neglect, and explosion of ransomware. Commun. ACM **60**(7), 24–26 (2017)

19. A. Page, S. Hijazi, D. Askan, B. Kantarci, T. Soyata, Research directions in cloud-based decision support systems for health monitoring using Internet-of-Things driven data acquisition. Int. J. Serv. Comput. **4**(4), 18–34 (2016)

20. American Diabetes Association, About Us: American Diabetes Association. http://www.diabetes.org/ Accessed 02 August 2018

21. P. Kakria, N.K. Tripathi, P. Kitipawang, A real-time health monitoring system for remote cardiac patients using smartphone and wearable sensors. Int. J. Telemed. Appl. **2015**, 8:8–8:8 (2015)

22. American Heart Association, Building healthier lives free of cardiovascular diseases and strokes. http://www.heart.org/HEARTORG/ Accessed 02 August 2018

23. R. Pandey, N.C. Dingari, N. Spegazzini, R.R. Dasari, G.L. Horowitz, I. Barman, Emerging trends in optical sensing of glycemic markers for diabetes monitoring. Trends Anal. Chem. **64**, 100–108 (2015)

24. O. Arias, K. Ly, Y. Jin, *Security and Privacy in IoT Era* (Springer, Cham, 2018), pp. 351–378

25. U.E. Bauer, P.A. Briss, R.A. Goodman, B.A. Bowman, Prevention of chronic disease in the 21st century: elimination of the leading preventable causes of premature death and disability in the USA. Lancet **384**(9937), 45–52 (2014)

26. B. Veeravalli, C.J. Deepu, D. Ngo, *Real-Time, Personalized Anomaly Detection in Streaming Data for Wearable Healthcare Devices* (Springer, Cham, 2017), pp. 403–426

27. X. Wang, Q. Gui, B. Liu, Z. Jin, Y. Chen, Enabling smart personalized healthcare: a hybrid mobile-cloud approach for ECG telemonitoring. IEEE J. Biomed. Health Inform. **18**(3), 739–745 (2014)
28. M. Chen, Y. Ma, J. Song, C.F. Lai, B. Hu, Smart clothing: connecting human with clouds and big data for sustainable health monitoring. Mobile Netw. Appl. **21**(5), 825–845 (2016)
29. V.L. West, D. Borland, W.E. Hammond, Innovative information visualization of electronic health record data: a systematic review. J. Am. Med. Inform. Assoc. **22**(2), 330–339 (2014)
30. A. Page, T. Soyata, J. Couderc, M. Aktas, B. Kantarci, S. Andreescu, Visualization of health monitoring data acquired from distributed sensors for multiple patients, in *IEEE Global Telecommunications Conference*, San Diego (2015), pp. 1–7
31. A. Page, M.K. Aktas, T. Soyata, W. Zareba, J. Couderc, QT clock to improve detection of QT prolongation in long QT syndrome patients. Heart Rhythm **13**(1), 190–198 (2016)
32. G. Fico, A. Fioravanti, M.T. Arredondo, J. Gorman, C. Diazzi, G. Arcuri, C. Conti, G. Pirini, Integration of personalized healthcare pathways in an ICT platform for diabetes managements: a small-scale exploratory study. IEEE J. Biomed. Health Inform. **20**(1) (2016), pp. 29–38
33. J.Y. Lucisano, T.L. Routh, J.T. Lin, D.A. Gough, Glucose monitoring in individuals with diabetes using a long-term implanted sensor/telemetry system and model. IEEE Trans. Biomed. Eng. **64**(9), 1982–1993 (2017)
34. J.D. Stewart, Foot drop: where, why and what to do? Pract. Neurol. **8**(3), 158–169 (2008)
35. M. Abtahi, S. Barlow, M. Constant, N. Gomes, O. Tully, S. D'Andrea, K. Mankodiya, MagicSox: an E-textile IoT system to quantify gait abnormalities. Smart Health **5–6**, 4–14 (2017)
36. A.C.B. Garcia, A.S. Vivacqua, N. Sánchez-Pi, L. Martí, J.M. Molina, Crowd-based ambient assisted living to monitor the elderly's health outdoors. IEEE Softw. **34**(6), 53–57 (2017)
37. M. da Silva Cameirão, S. Bermúdez i Badia, E. Duarte, P.F. Verschure, Virtual reality based rehabilitation speeds up functional recovery of the upper extremities after stroke: a randomized controlled pilot study in the acute phase of stroke using the rehabilitation gaming system. Restor. Neurol. Neurosci. **29**(5), 287–298 (2011)
38. P. Standen, K. Threapleton, A. Richardson, L. Connell, D. Brown, S. Battersby, F. Platts, A. Burton, A low cost virtual reality system for home based rehabilitation of the arm following stroke: a randomised controlled feasibility trial. Clin. Rehabil. **31**(3), 340–350 (2017). PMID: 27029939
39. N.H. Alkahtani, S. Almohsen, N.M. Alkahtani, G. Abdullah Almalki, S.S.Meshref, H. Kurdi, A semantic multi-agent system to exchange information between hospitals. Procedia Comput. Sci. **109**, 704–709 (2017). 8th International Conference on Ambient Systems, Networks and Technologies, ANT-2017 and the 7th International Conference on Sustainable Energy Information Technology, SEIT 2017, 16–19 May 2017, Madeira, Portugal
40. M.S. Hossain, G. Muhammad, Cloud-assisted industrial Internet of Things (IIoT) – enabled framework for health monitoring. Comput. Netw. **101**, 192–202 (2016). Industrial Technologies and Applications for the Internet of Things
41. X. Chen, L. Wang, J. Ding, N. Thomas, Patient flow scheduling and capacity planning in a smart hospital environment. IEEE Access **4**, 135–148 (2016)
42. A. Alessa, M. Faezipour, A review of influenza detection and prediction through social networking sites. Theor. Biol. Med. Model. **15**(1), 2 (2018)
43. L. Fernandez-Luque, M. Imran, Humanitarian health computing using artificial intelligence and social media: a narrative literature review. Int. J. Med. Inform. **114**, 136–142 (2018)
44. M.A. Al-Taee, W. Al-Nuaimy, Z.J. Muhsin, A. Al-Ataby, Robot assistant in management of diabetes in children based on the internet of things. IEEE Internet Things J. **4**(2), 437–445 (2017)
45. A.G. Ferreira, D. Fernandes, S. Branco, J.L. Monteiro, J. Cabral, A.P. Catarino, A.M. Rocha, A smart wearable system for sudden infant death syndrome monitoring, in *2016 IEEE International Conference on Industrial Technology (ICIT)* (2016), pp. 1920–1925

46. G. Janjua, D. Guldenring, D. Finlay, J. McLaughlin, Wireless chest wearable vital sign monitoring platform for hypertension, in *2017 39th Annual International Conference of the IEEE Engineering in Medicine and Biology Society (EMBC)* (2017), pp. 821–824
47. K. Kaiya, A. Koyama, Design and implementation of meal information collection system using IoT wireless tags, in *2016 10th International Conference on Complex, Intelligent, and Software Intensive Systems (CISIS)* (2016), pp. 503–508
48. S. Clarke, L.G. Jaimes, M.A. Labrador, mStress: a mobile recommender system for just-in-time interventions for stress, in *2017 14th IEEE Annual Consumer Communications Networking Conference (CCNC)* (2017), pp. 1–5
49. A. Gomez-Sacristan, M.A. Rodriguez-Hernandez, V. Sempere, Evaluation of quality of service in smart-hospital communications. J. Med. Imaging Health Inform. **5**(8), 1864–1869 (2015)
50. B. Fabian, T. Ermakova, P. Junghanns, Collaborative and secure sharing of healthcare data in multi-clouds. Inf. Syst. **48**, 132–150 (2015)
51. P. Dayal, N.M. Hojman, J.L. Kissee, J. Evans, J.E. Natale, Y. Huang et al., Impact of telemedicine on severity of illness and outcomes among children transferred from referring emergency departments to a children's hospital PICU. Pediatr. Crit. Care Med. **17**(6), 516–521 (2016). https://doi.org/10.1097/PCC.0000000000000761
52. M. Habibzadeh, Z. Qin, T. Soyata, B. Kantarci, Large scale distributed dedicated- and non-dedicated smart city sensing systems. IEEE Sens. J. **17**(23), 7649–7658 (2017)
53. M. Habibzadeh, T. Soyata, B. Kantarci, A. Boukerche, C. Kaptan, Sensing, communication and security planes: a new challenge for a smart city system design. Comput. Netw. **144**, 163–200 (2018)
54. M. Liggins II, D. Hall, J. Llinas, *Handbook of Multisensor Data Fusion: Theory and Practice* (CRC Press, Boca Raton, 2017)
55. G. Fortino, S. Galzarano, R. Gravina, W. Li, A framework for collaborative computing and multi-sensor data fusion in body sensor networks. Inf. Fusion **22**, 50–70 (2015)
56. Y. Zhang, M. Qiu, C.W. Tsai, M.M. Hassan, A. Alamri, Health-CPS: healthcare cyber-physical system assisted by cloud and big data. IEEE Syst. J. **11**(1), 88–95 (2017)
57. H.L. Peng, J.Q. Liu, H.C. Tian, B. Xu, Y.Z. Dong, B. Yang, X. Chen, C.S. Yang, Flexible dry electrode based on carbon nanotube/polymer hybrid micropillars for biopotential recording. Sens. Actuators A Phys. **235**, 48–56 (2015)
58. M. Habibzadeh, M. Hassanalieragh, A. Ishikawa, T. Soyata, G. Sharma, Hybrid solar-wind energy harvesting for embedded applications: supercapacitor-based system architectures and design tradeoffs. IEEE Circuits Syst. Mag. **17**(4), 29–63 (2017)
59. M. Habibzadeh, M. Hassanalieragh, T. Soyata, G. Sharma, Solar/wind hybrid energy harvesting for supercapacitor-based embedded systems, in *IEEE Midwest Symposium on Circuits and Systems*, Boston (2017), pp. 329–332
60. M. Habibzadeh, M. Hassanalieragh, T. Soyata, G. Sharma, Supercapacitor-based embedded hybrid solar/wind harvesting system architectures, in *Proceedings of the 30th IEEE International System-on-Chip Conference*, Munich (2017)
61. B.A. Reyes, N. Reljin, Y. Kong, Y. Nam, K.H. Chon, Tidal volume and instantaneous respiration rate estimation using a volumetric surrogate signal acquired via a smartphone camera. IEEE J. Biomed. Health Inf. **21**(3), 764–777 (2017)
62. K. Arning, M. Ziefle, "get that camera out of my house!" conjoint measurement of preferences for video-based healthcare monitoring systems in private and public places, in *Inclusive Smart Cities and e-Health*, ed. by A. Geissbühler, J. Demongeot, M. Mokhtari, B. Abdulrazak, H. Aloulou (Springer, Cham, 2015), pp. 152–164
63. S. Kianoush, S. Savazzi, F. Vicentini, V. Rampa, M. Giussani, Device-free RF human body fall detection and localization in industrial workplaces. IEEE Internet Things J. **4**(2), 351–362 (2017)
64. X. Liu, J. Cao, S. Tang, J. Wen, P. Guo, Contactless respiration monitoring via off-the-shelf WiFi devices. IEEE Trans. Mob. Comput. **15**(10), 2466–2479 (2016)

65. F. Adib, H. Mao, Z. Kabelac, D. Katabi, R.C. Miller, Smart homes that monitor breathing and heart rate, in *Proceedings of the 33rd Annual ACM Conference on Human Factors in Computing Systems. CHI '15* (ACM, New York, 2015), pp. 837–846

66. M. Kachuee, M.M. Kiani, H. Mohammadzade, M. Shabany, Cuffless blood pressure estimation algorithms for continuous health-care monitoring. IEEE Trans. Biomed. Eng. **64**(4), 859–869 (2017)

67. D.L. Carnì, D. Grimaldi, A. Nastro, V. Spagnuolo, F. Lamonaca, Blood oxygenation measurement by smartphone. IEEE Instrum. Meas. Mag. **20**(3), 43–49 (2017)

68. C.Y. Huang, M.C. Chan, C.Y. Chen, B.S. Lin, Novel wearable and wireless ring-type pulse oximeter with multi-detectors. Sensors **14**(9), 17586–17599 (2014)

69. S. Acharya, A. Rajasekar, B.S. Shender, L. Hrebien, M. Kam, Real-time hypoxia prediction using decision fusion. IEEE J. Biomed. Health Inform. **21**(3), 696–707 (2017)

70. V.P. Rachim, W.Y. Chung, Wearable noncontact armband for mobile ECG monitoring system. IEEE Trans. Biomed. Circuits Syst. **10**(6), 1112–1118 (2016)

71. P. Müller, M.A. Bégin, T. Schauer, T. Seel, Alignment-free, self-calibrating elbow angles measurement using inertial sensors. IEEE J. Biomed. Health Inform. **21**(2), 312–319 (2017)

72. N.J. Cleven, J.A. Müntjes, H. Fassbender, U. Urban, M. Görtz, H. Vogt, M. Gräfe, T. Göttsche, T. Penzkofer, T. Schmitz-Rode, W. Mokwa, A novel fully implantable wireless sensor system for monitoring hypertension patients. IEEE Trans. Biomed. Eng. **59**(11), 3124–3130 (2012)

73. D. Shao, C. Liu, F. Tsow, Y. Yang, Z. Du, R. Iriya, H. Yu, N. Tao, Noncontact monitoring of blood oxygen saturation using camera and dual-wavelength imaging system. IEEE Trans. Biomed. Eng. **63**(6), 1091–1098 (2016)

74. T.M. Seeberg, J.G. Orr, H. Opsahl, H.O. Austad, M.H. Røed, S.H. Dalgard, D. Houghton, D.E.J. Jones, F. Strisland, A novel method for continuous, noninvasive, cuff-less measurement of blood pressure: evaluation in patients with nonalcoholic fatty liver disease. IEEE Trans. Biomed. Eng. **64**(7), 1469–1478 (2017)

75. B. Zhou, M. Sundholm, J. Cheng, H. Cruz, P. Lukowicz, Measuring muscle activities during gym exercises with textile pressure mapping sensors. Pervasive Mob. Comput. **38**, 331–345 (2017). Special Issue IEEE International Conference on Pervasive Computing and Communications (PerCom) 2016

76. A.Q. Javaid, H. Ashouri, A. Dorier, M. Etemadi, J.A. Heller, S. Roy, O.T. Inan, Quantifying and reducing motion artifacts in wearable seismocardiogram measurements during walking to assess left ventricular health. IEEE Trans. Biomed. Eng. **64**(6), 1277–1286 (2017)

77. A. Page, O. Kocabas, T. Soyata, M.K. Aktas, J. Couderc, Cloud-based privacy-preserving remote ECG monitoring and surveillance. Ann. Noninvasive Electrocardiol. **20**(4), 328–337 (2014)

78. M. Habibzadeh, A. Boggio-Dandry, Z. Qin, T. Soyata, B. Kantarci, H. Mouftah, Soft sensing in smart cities: handling 3Vs using recommender systems, machine intelligence, and data analytics. IEEE Commun. Mag. **56**(2), 78–86 (2018)

79. ZigBee Alliance, ZigBee Alliance Web page (2017). http://www.zigbee.org/. Accessed 10 November 2017

80. T. de Almeida Oliveira, E.P. Godoy, Zigbee wireless dynamic sensor networks: feasibility analysis and implementation guide. IEEE Sens. J. **16**(11), 4614–4621 (2016)

81. Y. Kim, S. Lee, S. Lee, Coexistence of ZigBee-based WBAN and WiFi for health telemonitoring systems. IEEE J. Biomed. Health Inform. **20**(1), 222–230 (2016)

82. Bluetooth Special Interest Group (SIG), Core Specifications - Bluetooth Technology Website (2017). https://www.bluetooth.com/specifications/bluetooth-core-specification. Accessed 17 October 2017

83. M. Collotta, G. Pau, A novel energy management approach for smart homes using bluetooth low energy. IEEE J. Sel. Areas Commun. **33**(12), 2988–2996 (2015)

84. A. Basalamah, Sensing the crowds using bluetooth low energy tags. IEEE Access **4**, 4225–4233 (2016)

85. O. Bello, S. Zeadally, M. Badra, Network layer inter-operation of device-to-device communication technologies in Internet of Things (IoT). Ad Hoc Netw. **57**(C), 52–62 (2017)

86. M. Agiwal, A. Roy, N. Saxena, Next generation 5G wireless networks: a comprehensive survey. IEEE Commun. Surv. Tutorials **18**(3), 1617–1655 (2016)
87. N.A. Johansson, Y.P.E. Wang, E. Eriksson, M. Hessler, Radio access for ultra-reliable and low-latency 5G communications, in *2015 IEEE International Conference on Communication Workshop (ICCW)* (June 2015), pp. 1184–1189
88. O. Galinina, S. Andreev, M. Komarov, S. Maltseva, Leveraging heterogeneous device connectivity in a converged 5G-IoT ecosystem. Comput. Netw. **128**(Supplement C), 123–132 (2017). Survivability Strategies for Emerging Wireless Networks
89. M.N. Tehrani, M. Uysal, H. Yanikomeroglu, Device-to-device communication in 5G cellular networks: challenges, solutions, and future directions. IEEE Commun. Mag. **52**(5), 86–92 (2014)
90. J. Qiao, X.S. Shen, J.W. Mark, Q. Shen, Y. He, L. Lei, Enabling device-to-device communications in millimeter-wave 5G cellular networks. IEEE Commun. Mag. **53**(1), 209–215 (2015)
91. A. Mukherjee, J.F. Cheng, S. Falahati, H. Koorapaty, D.H. Kang, R. Karaki, L. Falconetti, D. Larsson, Licensed-assisted access LTE: coexistence with IEEE 802.11 and the evolution toward 5G. IEEE Commun. Mag. **54**(6), 50–57 (2016)
92. M. Habibzadeh, W. Xiong, M. Zheleva, E.K. Stern, B.H. Nussbaum, T. Soyata, Smart city sensing and communication sub-infrastructure, in *IEEE Midwest Symposium on Circuits and Systems*, Boston (Aug 2017), pp. 1159–1162
93. Y. Lu, P. Kuonen, B. Hirsbrunner, M. Lin, Benefits of data aggregation on energy consumption in wireless sensor networks. IET Commun. **11**(8), 1216–1223 (2017)
94. P. Sridhar, A.M. Madni, M. Jamshidi, Hierarchical aggregation and intelligent monitoring and control in fault-tolerant wireless sensor networks. IEEE Syst. J. **1**(1), 38–54 (2007)
95. U. Shaukat, E. Ahmed, Z. Anwar, F. Xia, Cloudlet deployment in local wireless networks: motivation, architectures, applications, and open challenges. J. Netw. Comput. Appl. **62**(Supplement C), 18–40 (2016)
96. Y. Chen, Y. Chen, Q. Cao, X. Yang, Packetcloud: a cloudlet-based open platform for in-network services. IEEE Trans. Parallel Distrib. Syst. **27**(4), 1146–1159 (2016)
97. T. Soyata, H. Ba, W. Heinzelman, M. Kwon, J. Shi, Accelerating mobile cloud computing: a survey, in *Communication Infrastructures for Cloud Computing*, ed. by H.T. Mouftah, B. Kantarci (IGI Global, Hershey, 2013), pp. 175–197
98. M. Almorsy, J. Grundy, I. Müller, An analysis of the cloud computing security problem (2016). Preprint arXiv:1609.01107
99. Google LLC, Cloud IoT Core, Google Cloud Platform. https://cloud.google.com/iot-core/
100. Microsoft Corp., Microsoft Azure Cloud Computing Platform and Services. https://azure.microsoft.com/en-us/
101. Amazon Inc., Amazon Web Services (AES) - Cloud Computing Services. https://aws.amazon.com/
102. IBM Corp., IBM Watson Internet of Things (IoT). https://www.ibm.com/internet-of-things
103. L. Hu, M. Qiu, J. Song, M.S. Hossain, A. Ghoneim, Software defined healthcare networks. IEEE Wirel. Commun. **22**(6), 67–75 (2015)
104. J. Li, Y.K. Li, X. Chen, P.P. Lee, W. Lou, A hybrid cloud approach for secure authorized deduplication. IEEE Trans. Parallel Distrib. Syst. **26**(5), 1206–1216 (2015)
105. P.T. Endo, A.V. de Almeida Palhares, N.N. Pereira, G.E. Goncalves, D. Sadok, J. Kelner, B. Melander, J.E. Mangs, Resource allocation for distributed cloud: concepts and research challenges. IEEE Netw. **25**(4), 42–46 (2011)
106. S. Hijazi, A. Page, B. Kantarci, T. Soyata, Machine learning in cardiac health monitoring and decision support. IEEE Comput. Mag. **49**(11), 38–48 (2016)
107. S. Li, L. Da Xu, X. Wang, Compressed sensing signal and data acquisition in wireless sensor networks and internet of things. IEEE Trans. Ind. Inform. **9**(4), 2177–2186 (2013)
108. M. Alhussein, Monitoring Parkinson's disease in smart cities. IEEE Access **5**, 19835–19841 (2017)
109. D. Zhou, J. Luo, V.M. Silenzio, Y. Zhou, J. Hu, G. Currier, H.A. Kautz, Tackling mental health by integrating unobtrusive multimodal sensing, in *AAAI* (2015), pp. 1401–1409

110. L. Calderoni, M. Ferrara, A. Franco, D. Maio, Indoor localization in a hospital environment using random forest classifiers. Expert Syst. Appl. **42**(1), 125–134 (2015)
111. J. Qin, W. Fu, H. Gao, W.X. Zheng, Distributed k-means algorithm and fuzzy c-means algorithm for sensor networks based on multiagent consensus theory. IEEE Trans. Cybern. **47**(3), 772–783 (2017)
112. W. Kim, M.S. Stanković, K.H. Johansson, H.J. Kim, A distributed support vector machine learning over wireless sensor networks. IEEE Trans. Cybern. **45**(11), 2599–2611 (2015)
113. M.M.A. Patwary, D. Palsetia, A. Agrawal, W.k. Liao, F. Manne, A. Choudhary, A new scalable parallel DBSCAN algorithm using the disjoint-set data structure, in *2012 International Conference for High Performance Computing, Networking, Storage and Analysis (SC)* (Nov 2012), pp. 1–11
114. FDA Safety Communication, Cybersecurity Vulnerabilities Identified in St. Jude Medical's Implantable Cardiac Devices and Merlin@home Transmitter: FDA Safety Communication. https://www.fda.gov/MedicalDevices/Safety/AlertsandNotices/ucm535843.htm. Accessed 03 December 2018
115. B. Barrett, Hack Brief: Hackers are Holding an LA Hospital's Computers Hostage. https://www.wired.com/2016/02/hack-brief-hackers-are-holding-an-la-hospitals-computers-hostage/. Accessed 12 March 2018
116. S. Balasubramanlan, The Global Cyberattack and the Need to Revisit Health Care Cybersecurity. https://www.huffingtonpost.com/entry/lessons-learned-the-global-cyberattack-the-need_us_591a1ac5e4b086d2d0d8d1ed. Accessed 12 March 2018
117. S. Larson, Why Hospitals are so Vulnerable to Ransomware Attacks. http://money.cnn.com/2017/05/16/technology/hospitals-vulnerable-wannacry-ransomware/index.html. Accessed 19 March 2018
118. J. Rogers, Fitness Tracking Data on Strava App Reveal US Military Bases Details, Sparking Security Concerns. http://www.foxnews.com/tech/2018/01/29/fitness-tracking-data-on-strava-app-reveal-us-military-bases-details-sparking-security-concerns.html. Accessed 19 March 2018
119. J.L. Fernández-Alemán, I.C. Señor, P. Ángel Oliver Lozoya, A. Toval, Security and privacy in electronic health records: a systematic literature review. J. Biomed. Inform. **46**(3), 541–562 (2013)
120. C. Cerrudo, An emerging us (and world) threat: cities wide open to cyber attacks. Securing Smart Cities (2015)
121. O. Arias, J. Wurm, K. Hoang, Y. Jin, Privacy and security in internet of things and wearable devices. IEEE Trans. Multi-Scale Comput. Syst. **1**(2), 99–109 (2015)
122. H. Takabi, J.B.D. Joshi, G.J. Ahn, Security and privacy challenges in cloud computing environments. IEEE Secur. Priv. **8**(6), 24–31 (2010)
123. A.B. Budurusubmi, S.S. Yau, An effective approach to continuous user authentication for touch screen smart devices, in *IEEE International Conference on Software Quality, Reliability and Security (QRS)* (Aug 2015), pp. 219–226
124. K. Zhang, K. Yang, X. Liang, Z. Su, X. Shen, H.H. Luo, Security and privacy for mobile healthcare networks: from a quality of protection perspective. IEEE Wirel. Commun. **22**(4), 104–112 (2015)
125. I. Hwang, Y. Kim, Analysis of security standardization for the internet of things, in *2017 International Conference on Platform Technology and Service (PlatCon)* (Feb 2017), pp. 1–6
126. P. Kumari, M. López-Benítez, G.M. Lee, T. Kim, A.S. Minhas, Wearable internet of things - from human activity tracking to clinical integration, in *2017 39th Annual International Conference of the IEEE Engineering in Medicine and Biology Society (EMBC)* (July 2017), pp. 2361–2364
127. J. Rajamäki, R. Pirinen, Towards the cyber security paradigm of ehealth: resilience and design aspects. AIP Conf. Proc. **1836**(1), 020029 (2017)
128. J. Lin, W. Yu, N. Zhang, X. Yang, H. Zhang, W. Zhao, A survey on internet of things: architecture, enabling technologies, security and privacy, and applications. IEEE Internet Things J. **4**(5), 1125–1142 (2017)

129. B. Ondiege, M. Clarke, G. Mapp, Exploring a new security framework for remote patient monitoring devices. Computers **6**(1), 11 (2017)
130. M.A. Ferrag, L. Maglaras, A. Derhab, A.V. Vasilakos, S. Rallis, H. Janicke, Authentication schemes for smart mobile devices: threat models, countermeasures, and open research issues (2018). Preprint arXiv:1803.10281
131. O. Kocabas, T. Soyata, M.K. Aktas, Emerging security mechanisms for medical cyber physical systems. IEEE/ACM Trans. Comput. Biol. Bioinform. **13**(3), 401–416 (2016)
132. Z. Liu, J. Großschädl, Z. Hu, K. Järvinen, H. Wang, I. Verbauwhede, Elliptic curve cryptography with efficiently computable endomorphisms and its hardware implementations for the Internet of Things. IEEE Trans. Comput. **66**(5), 773–785 (2017)
133. K. Zhang, J. Ni, K. Yang, X. Liang, J. Ren, X.S. Shen, Security and privacy in smart city applications: challenges and solutions. IEEE Commun. Mag. **55**(1), 122–129 (2017)
134. X. Wang, C. Konstantinou, M. Maniatakos, R. Karri, Confirm: detecting firmware modifications in embedded systems using hardware performance counters, in *Proceedings of the IEEE/ACM International Conference on Computer-Aided Design. ICCAD '15* (IEEE, Piscataway, 2015), pp. 544–551
135. S. Agrawal, M.L. Das, A. Mathuria, S. Srivastava, Program integrity verification for detecting node capture attack in wireless sensor network, in *Information Systems Security*, ed. by S. Jajoda, C. Mazumdar (Springer, Cham, 2015), pp. 419–440
136. L.S. Sindhuja, G. Padmavathi, Replica node detection using enhanced single hop detection with clonal selection algorithm in mobile wireless sensor networks. J. Comput. Netw. Commun. **2016**, 1:1–1:1 (2016)
137. L. Hu, Z. Wang, Q.L. Han, X. Liu, State estimation under false data injection attacks: security analysis and system protection. Automatica **87**, 176–183 (2018)
138. A. Abbaspour, K.K. Yen, S. Noei, A. Sargolzaei, Detection of fault data injection attack on UAV using adaptive neural network. Procedia Comput. Sci. **95**, 193–200 (2016)
139. M. Ryan, et al., Bluetooth: with low energy comes low security. WOOT **13**, 4–4 (2013)
140. C. Mclvor, M. McLoone, J.V. McCanny, Fast Montgomery modular multiplication and RSA cryptographic processor architectures, in *Conference Record of the Thirty-Seventh Asilomar Conference on Signals, Systems and Computers, 2004*, vol. 1 (IEEE, Piscataway, 2003), pp. 379–384
141. A. Boscher, E.V. Trichina, H. Handschuh, Randomized RSA-based cryptographic exponentiation resistant to side channel and fault attacks (20 March 2012) US Patent 8139763
142. Y. Li, L. Shi, P. Cheng, J. Chen, D.E. Quevedo, Jamming attacks on remote state estimation in cyber-physical systems: a game-theoretic approach. IEEE Trans. Autom. Control **60**(10), 2831–2836 (2015)
143. M. Brownfield, Y. Gupta, N. Davis, Wireless sensor network denial of sleep attack, in *Proceedings from the Sixth Annual IEEE SMC Information Assurance Workshop* (June 2005), pp. 356–364
144. D.R. Raymond, R.C. Marchany, S.F. Midkiff, Scalable, cluster-based anti-replay protection for wireless sensor networks, in *Information Assurance and Security Workshop, 2007. IAW'07. IEEE SMC* (IEEE, Piscataway, 2007), pp. 127–134
145. E.Y. Vasserman, N. Hopper, Vampire attacks: draining life from wireless ad hoc sensor networks. IEEE Trans. Mob. Comput. **12**(2), 318–332 (2013)
146. Y. Liu, M. Dong, K. Ota, A. Liu, Activetrust: secure and trustable routing in wireless sensor networks. IEEE Trans. Inf. Forensics Secur. **11**(9), 2013–2027 (2016)
147. H. Suo, J. Wan, C. Zou, J. Liu, Security in the Internet of Things: a review, in *2012 International Conference on Computer Science and Electronics Engineering (ICCSEE)*, vol. 3 (IEEE, Piscataway, 2012), pp. 648–651
148. M.J. Covington, R. Carskadden, Threat implications of the Internet of Things, in *2013 5th International Conference on Cyber Conflict (CyCon)* (IEEE, Piscataway, 2013), pp. 1–12
149. D. Puthal, S. Nepal, R. Ranjan, J. Chen, Threats to networking cloud and edge datacenters in the Internet of Things. IEEE Cloud Comput. **3**(3), 64–71 (2016)

150. S.M. Muzammal, M.A. Shah, H.A. Khattak, S. Jabbar, G. Ahmed, S. Khalid, S. Hussain, K. Han, Counter measuring conceivable security threats on smart healthcare devices. IEEE Access **6**, 20722–20733 (2018)
151. C. Kolias, A. Stavrou, J. Voas, I. Bojanova, R. Kuhn, Learning Internet-of-Things Security "Hands-On". IEEE Secur. Priv. **14**(1), 37–46 (2016)
152. C. Bormann, Z. Shelby, K. Hartke, Constrained application protocol (coap), draft-ietf-core-coap-18 (2013)
153. E. Rescorla, N. Modadugu, Datagram transport layer security version 1.2. Technical report (2012)
154. S.R. Moosavi, T.N. Gia, E. Nigussie, A.M. Rahmani, S. Virtanen, H. Tenhunen, J. Isoaho, End-to-end security scheme for mobility enabled healthcare internet of things. Futur. Gener. Comput. Syst. **64**, 108–124 (2016)
155. A. Zhang, L. Wang, X. Ye, X. Lin, Light-weight and robust security-aware D2D-assist data transmission protocol for mobile-health systems. IEEE Trans. Inf. Forensics Secur. **12**(3), 662–675 (2017)
156. J. Shen, D. Liu, J. Shen, Q. Liu, X. Sun, A secure cloud-assisted urban data sharing framework for ubiquitous-cities. Pervasive Mob. Comput. **41**, 219–230 (2017)
157. S. Tonyali, K, A., N. Saputro, A.S. Uluagac, M. Nojoumian, Privacy-preserving protocols for secure and reliable data aggregation in IoT-enabled smart metering systems. Futur. Gener. Comput. Syst. **78**(Part 2), 547–557 (2018)
158. O. Kocabas, T. Soyata, Towards privacy-preserving medical cloud computing using homomorphic encryption, in *Enabling Real-Time Mobile Cloud Computing through Emerging Technologies*, ed. by T. Soyata (IGI Global, Hershey, 2015), pp. 213–246
159. K. Yang, Z. Liu, X. Jia, X.S. Shen, Time-domain attribute-based access control for cloud-based video content sharing: a cryptographic approach. IEEE Trans. Multimedia **18**(5), 940–950 (2016)
160. T. Jung, X.Y. Li, Z. Wan, M. Wan, Control cloud data access privilege and anonymity with fully anonymous attribute-based encryption. IEEE Trans. Inform. Forensics Secur. **10**(1), 190–199 (2015)
161. M. Li, S. Yu, Y. Zheng, K. Ren, W. Lou, Scalable and secure sharing of personal health records in cloud computing using attribute-based encryption. IEEE Trans. Parallel Distrib. Syst. **24**(1), 131–143 (2013)
162. S.R. Moosavi, T.N. Gia, A.M. Rahmani, E. Nigussie, S. Virtanen, J. Isoaho, H. Tenhunen, SEA: a secure and efficient authentication and authorization architecture for IoT-based healthcare using smart gateways. Procedia Comput. Sci. **52**, 452–459 (2015). The 6th International Conference on Ambient Systems, Networks and Technologies (ANT-2015), the 5th International Conference on Sustainable Energy Information Technology (SEIT-2015)
163. A. Sahi, D. Lai, Y. Li, Security and privacy preserving approaches in the ehealth clouds with disaster recovery plan. Comput. Biol. Med. **78**, 1–8 (2016)
164. D. Mishra, A. Chaturvedi, S. Mukhopadhyay, Design of a lightweight two-factor authentication scheme with smart card revocation. J. Inform. Secur. Appl. **23**, 44–53 (2015)
165. L.E. Holmquist, F. Mattern, B. Schiele, P. Alahuhta, M. Beigl, H.W. Gellersen, Smart-its friends: a technique for users to easily establish connections between smart artefacts, in *International Conference on Ubiquitous Computing* (Springer, Berlin, 2001), pp. 116–122
166. L. Ding, P. Shi, B. Liu, The clustering of internet, internet of things and social network, in *2010 3rd International Symposium on Knowledge Acquisition and Modeling (KAM)* (IEEE, Piscataway, 2010), pp. 417–420
167. M.L. Gavrilova, F. Ahmed, S. Azam, P.P. Paul, W. Rahman, M. Sultana, F.T. Zohra, *Emerging Trends in Security System Design Using the Concept of Social Behavioural Biometrics* (Springer, Cham, 2017), pp. 229–251
168. J. Tian, Y. Cao, W. Xu, S. Wang, Challenge-response authentication using in-air handwriting style verification. IEEE Trans. Dependable Secure Comput. **PP**(99), 1–1 (2018)

169. M. Sultana, P.P. Paul, M. Gavrilova, A concept of social behavioral biometrics: motivation, current developments, and future trends, in *International Conference on Cyberworlds* (IEEE, Piscataway, 2014), pp. 271–278

170. L. Zhang, S. Zhu, S. Tang, Privacy protection for telecare medicine information systems using a chaotic map-based three-factor authenticated key agreement scheme. IEEE J. Biomed. Health Inform. **21**(2), 465–475 (2017)

171. T. Kumar, A. Braeken, M. Liyanage, M. Ylianttila, Identity privacy preserving biometric based authentication scheme for naked healthcare environment, in *2017 IEEE International Conference on Communications (ICC)* (May 2017), pp. 1–7

172. C. Prandi, S. Ferretti, S. Mirri, P. Salomoni, Trustworthiness in crowd-sensed and sourced georeferenced data, in *2015 IEEE International Conference on Pervasive Computing and Communication Workshops (PerCom Workshops)* (IEEE, Piscataway, 2015), pp. 402–407

173. B. Kantarci, K.G. Carr, C.D. Pearsall, SONATA: social network assisted trustworthiness assurance in smart city crowdsensing. Int. J. Distrib. Syst. Technol. **7**(1), 59–78 (2016)

174. M. Pouryazdan, B. Kantarci, T. Soyata, H. Song, Anchor-assisted and vote-based trustworthiness assurance in smart city crowdsensing. IEEE Access **4**, 529–541 (2016)

175. T.M. Fernández-Caramés, P. Fraga-Lamas, A review on the use of blockchain for the internet of things. IEEE Access **6**, 32979–33001 (2018)

176. Y. Huo, X. Dong, W. Xu, M. Yuen, Cellular and WiFi co-design for 5G user equipment (2018). Preprint arXiv:1803.06943

177. M.N. Kamel Boulos, J.T. Wilson, K.A. Clauson, Geospatial blockchain: promises, challenges, and scenarios in health and healthcare. Int. J. Health Geogr. **17**(1), 25 (2018)

Biofeedback in Healthcare: State of the Art and Meta Review

Hawazin Faiz Badawi and Abdulmotaleb El Saddik

Abstract This chapter consists of five main sections. It begins by discussing the scope of utilizing biofeedback technology in healthcare systems. Then, it presents a brief history of biofeedback technology and previous reviews. The second section highlights the sensory technology in biofeedback systems by presenting the different types of sensors and their features. The third section explores recent research of biofeedback-based healthcare systems by presenting a range of applications in different fields combined with the utilized sensors. The fourth section discusses the challenges and issues that affect the deployment of biofeedback in healthcare systems. The last section concludes this review.

Keywords Biofeedback · Healthcare · Systems · Applications · Sensors · State of the art · Classification · Challenges

1 Introduction

Promoting health and well-being is one of the major goals of preventive healthcare research. Biofeedback considers a promising and accepted method in this field [1]. It aims to promote well-being and help to prevent and treat physiological and psychological diseases. It has been recognized by many medical institutions and Mayo Clinic [2] is one of them. It defines biofeedback as "a technique you can use to learn to control your body's functions, such as your heart rate. With biofeedback, you're connected to electrical sensors that help you receive information (feedback) about your body (bio)." Also, Mayo Clinic [2] lists a set of physical and mental diseases that can be managed by biofeedback, which highlights its importance, and discusses how biofeedback is a safe technique. Therefore, this technique can be utilized outside clinics and hospitals to benefit patients and healthy individuals.

H. F. Badawi · A. El Saddik (✉)
Multimedia Communications Research Laboratory (MCRLab), University of Ottawa, Ottawa, ON, Canada
e-mail: hbada049@uottawa.ca; elsaddik@uottawa.ca

© Springer Nature Switzerland AG 2020   113
A. El Saddik et al. (eds.), *Connected Health in Smart Cities*,
https://doi.org/10.1007/978-3-030-27844-1_6

The incredible evolution in the wearable technologies opens doors for developing biofeedback systems that enhance individuals' awareness about their health.

The following subsections provide a historical background of the biofeedback technique and discuss the previous reviews.

1.1 Biofeedback Techniques: Background

Historically, this technique has been used extensively for thousands of years in various forms such as yoga and other meditation practices [1]. In 1969, the term "biofeedback" was introduced at the first annual meeting of the Biofeedback Research Society as the acquiring of biological feedback using electrical instruments [3].

The biofeedback techniques evolved and currently classify as "Clinical Biofeedback" and "Ubiquitous Biofeedback." Clinical biofeedback was coined in 1975 [4] and defined as "a type of operant conditioning wherein, with the help of a trained therapist, an individual can learn to control specific physiological functions by changing the thoughts and perceptions that produce them" [1]. Thus, the clinical biofeedback requires a clinical setup and a coach to help the patients in understanding their physiological functions. Some of the early clinical biofeedback experiments found in [5, 6]. According to the Mayo Clinic, biofeedback technique is recognized as a complementary medicine for many physical and mental health illnesses such as anxiety or stress, asthma, and headache [2].

In contrast to the clinical biofeedback, Ubiquitous Biofeedback (U-Biofeedback) was coined in 2014 [1] and defined as "a system that utilizes software tools to provide continuous and long term management of physiological processes. Such systems are typically part of the user environment or worn on the subject's body. They do not require the user to attend clinical sessions in order to benefit from biofeedback techniques." Thus, the U-Biofeedback provides a huge advantage for people to track their health status conveniently. Some examples of the developed U-Biofeedback systems are systems for stress management in [1, 7], physical activity advisory system in [8], the respiratory biofeedback system in [9], sleep management system in [10], and the diet advisor system in [11].

Continuous evolution of sensors encouraged healthcare researchers to develop novel biofeedback systems. They vary in their purposes from sensing respiratory systems [12], and body motion [13], to provide biofeedback training [14]. Further discussion of biofeedback systems and the utilized sensors is provided in Sects. 2 and 3.

1.2   Biofeedback Technology: Previous Reviews

Researchers have been keen to review the related literature since the emergence of biofeedback concept. Research in [15] is one of the initial reviews on biofeedback training. It discusses the clinical applications in which biofeedback training proves its efficiency. It started by presenting the cases where the biofeedback training is well-accepted, which are muscle retraining, elimination of subvocal speech while reading and elimination of tension headaches. Then, it discussed the cases where the biofeedback training shows promising results but have not been proved yet. They are elimination of cardiac arrhythmias, lowering blood pressure, and reducing seizure frequency. It concluded by listing the cases where the results are not sufficient to draw conclusions from the available evidence.

The book in [16] is the first comprehensive review on biofeedback-related literature. According to [17], this book includes 2292 citations referred to different biofeedback training research such as those on human and animal work, cybernetics and control systems, and EEG and consciousness.

In addition to generic reviews, many research focus on reviewing specific areas of biofeedback applications in healthcare. For example, the review in [18] discusses the prediction of biofeedback performance in EMG biofeedback studies. It starts by investigating the efficiency of using the locus of control in predicting performance in different biofeedback cases. Then, it shows the results and issues of this usage in EMG biofeedback. Another review in [19] discusses the case of utilizing temperature biofeedback in migraine treatment. It identifies the three required skills in the biofeedback training to optimize self-control in clinical sessions. It concludes by stating that the findings of using this type of biofeedback for migraine treatment are not encouraging and further improvements are needed. The review in [20] discusses the efficacy of biofeedback in minimizing chronic pain. It reviews a collection of research that recommends biofeedback training as one of the psychological techniques in pain management.

With the beginning of the millennium, many reviews present the promising results of utilizing biofeedback as an alternative treatment for various diseases such as addictive disorders [21], anxiety disorders [22], temporomandibular disorder [23], eating disorders [24], and headache disorders [25]. Recent reviews emphasize positive findings for more diseases such as Bladder Bowel Dysfunction [26], Tinnitus [27], Parkinson's Disease [28], chronic constipation [29], and anxiety and depression [30].

A collection of recent reviews is shown in Table 1. We collected them by running the following query in Scopus [31], which resulted in 66 reviews:

TITLE-ABS-KEY ("Biofeedback" AND "Healthcare" AND "Literature" OR "Review").

Table 1 shows the review title, publishing year, the review type in terms of having the "biofeedback" as major topic of the review, where it is mentioned in the title, abstract and author keywords, or minor, where it is mentioned in one of them,

Table 1 Summary of biofeedback-related literature reviews

Review title—reference	Year	Title	Abstract	Author keywords	Biofeedback Major	Biofeedback Minor	Health condition
Digital technology and mobile health in behavioral migraine therapy: A narrative review—[32]	2018		✓			✓	Behavioral migraine therapy
A cross-sectional review of the prevalence of integrative medicine in pediatric pain clinics across the United States—[33]	2018			✓		✓	Pediatric pain
Immersion of virtual reality for rehabilitation—Review—[34]	2018			✓		✓	Rehabilitation
The effectiveness of biofeedback therapy in managing bladder bowel dysfunction in children: A systematic review—[26]	2018	✓	✓	✓	✓		Bladder bowel dysfunction in children
Feedback-based treatments for eating disorders and related symptoms: A systematic review of the literature—[24]	2018		✓	✓	✓		Eating disorders (EDs) and EDs-related symptoms
Systematic review of biofeedback interventions for addressing anxiety and depression in children and adolescents with long-term physical conditions—[30]	2018	✓	✓	✓	✓		Anxiety and depression
EULAR revised recommendations for the management of fibromyalgia—[35]	2017			✓		✓	Fibromyalgia
Psychological therapy for people with tinnitus: A scoping review of treatment components—[27]	2017		✓			✓	Tinnitus
Biofeedback treatment of chronic constipation: Myths and misconceptions—[29]	2016	✓	✓	✓	✓		Chronic constipation
Post-stroke hip fracture in older people: A narrative review—[36]	2016		✓			✓	Post-stroke hip fracture
Fecal incontinence: A review of current treatment options—[37]	2016			✓		✓	Fecal incontinence

(continued)

Table 1 (continued)

Review title—reference	Year	Title	Abstract	Author keywords	Biofeedback Major	Biofeedback Minor	Health condition
The integrative management of PTSD: A review of conventional and CAM approaches used to prevent and treat PTSD with emphasis on military personnel—[38]	2015	✓				✓	Post-traumatic stress disorder (PTSD)
Conservative management for postprostatectomy urinary incontinence—[39]	2015	✓	✓			✓	Urinary incontinence
Inducible laryngeal obstruction during exercise: Moving beyond vocal cords with new insights—[40]	2015	✓				✓	Inducible laryngeal obstruction during exercise
Non-surgical treatment of urinary incontinence—[41]	2015	✓				✓	Urinary incontinence
Dystonia—[42]	2014	✓				✓	Dystonia
A review of the clinical evidence for complementary and alternative therapies in Parkinson's disease—[28]	2014			✓		✓	Parkinson's disease
A systematic review of neurofeedback as a treatment for fibromyalgia syndrome symptoms—[43]	2014	✓	✓	✓	✓		Fibromyalgia syndrome
Outcomes in non-surgical management for bowel dysfunction—[44]	2014			✓		✓	Bowel dysfunction
The role of anorectal investigations in predicting the outcome of biofeedback in the treatment of faecal incontinence—[45]	2013	✓	✓	✓	✓		Faecal incontinence
Stress management techniques in the prison setting—[46]	2013			✓		✓	Stress in prison
Nonpharmacologic, complementary, and alternative interventions for managing chronic pain in older adults—[47]	2013			✓		✓	Chronic pain in older adults
Biomedical risk assessment as an aid for smoking cessation—[48]	2012			✓		✓	Smoking cessation
Interventions for improving coordination of reach to grasp following stroke: A systematic review—[49]	2012	✓				✓	Stroke

thus it discussed as an intervention or alternative method, and the health condition discussed in the review.

This amount of reviews reflects the high interest of utilizing clinical biofeedback in the healthcare field, which is one of the motivations to conduct this state-of-the-art meta review.

2 Biofeedback and Sensory Technologies

Sensors are the backbone of the biofeedback-based healthcare systems that aim to manage physical and mental health issues. This section provides an overview of them followed by the state-of-the-art sensory technologies utilized in biofeedback-based healthcare systems.

2.1 Sensors Overview

The developed sensory technologies and wireless communications play a critical role in healthcare systems. They can facilitate the patient's treatment and promote individuals well-being toward a healthy lifestyle. By continuous monitoring of vital signals, biofeedback-based personal healthcare systems represent a convenient solution for coexisting with many chronic diseases such as cardiac disorders, hypertension, and diabetes.

Nowadays, sensors represent the borders between the physical objects in real world and their digital twins in the virtual world. In fact, they characterize the digital twin according to the characteristics list of digital twin in [50]. They can be defined as "a device that converts a physical phenomenon into an electrical signal" [51]. Different types of sensors have been utilized extensively in healthcare systems, where they are often called biosensors. Their capabilities are improving continuously due to their critical role in biofeedback training. This improvement includes physical and technical aspects of the sensor such as size and accuracy of the collected data. Thus, leading companies compete to develop high-quality sensors and related products in terms of accuracy, reliability, and user-friendly design. Philips [52] and General Electric [53] are examples of companies develop sensory products for clinical biofeedback. Regarding the U-Biofeedback, many products exist, which utilize single or multiple sensors, to be used in U-Biofeedback systems as a source of data. Wearable technologies produced by different companies such as Garmin watches [54], Fitbit trackers [55], and Oura rings [56] are equipped with various sensors such as ECG, accelerometer, and body temperature sensors. Such products provide a huge amount of personalized data which is a key factor in biofeedback-based healthcare systems. Historically, EMG and EEG sensors are examples of initially utilized sensors in the clinical biofeedback systems [57].

Different quality parameters are used to evaluate sensors in healthcare systems because they vary in accordance with their function whether it is a simple function or a complex one. Size, weight, shape, fabricating materials, battery life, and portability are examples of physical parameters. One of the most important parameters is sampling rate, which can be defined as the number of electrical signals samples that are taken per time unit and measured by Hertz (Hz) [58]. Other parameters that are used to evaluate biosensors are [59] invasiveness, obtrusiveness, and mobility. Invasiveness is a parameter that is used to determine sensor's ability to perform its function with or without the need of intrusion in patient's skin. Obtrusiveness is the parameter that is used to determine whether the design of a sensor is obtrusive or not and therefore will affect the patient's appearance or not. Mobility is the parameter that is used to determine sensor's ability to function in different locations and under different circumstances.

Thus, sensors could be classified based on the quality parameters, the operating method either as wire or wireless sensors, and their function in accordance to the application field such as biosensors in the medical field, and mechanical sensors in industrial field [51]. The following subsection discusses biosensors that track involuntary organs and blood systems in a human body.

2.2 Involuntary and Blood Sensors

We proposed these names to provide common classes that can adopt the biosensors used for tracking physical features of a human body such as involuntary organs and blood circulation. This will also facilitate the classification of existing and newly developed sensors in the healthcare field. Figure 1 shows the biosensors that belong to each class. They are explained by stating the function, the types (if exists), and the state of the art.

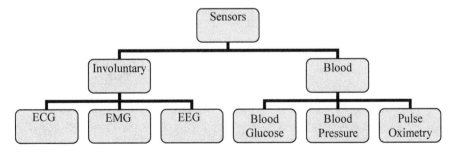

Fig. 1 The proposed classification and the sensors under each class

2.2.1 Involuntary Sensors

This class includes sensors that are used to monitor and measure the electrical pulses resulted from the contraction and relaxation of involuntary organs in the human body, which are heart, muscles, and brain.

ECG Sensors

ECG (Electrocardiograph) is a graphical record of the heart electrical activity that is used by healthcare providers to assess the heart status and diagnose diseases if exist [60, 61]. ECG sensors, which called electrodes, are attached to specific parts of patient's skin (e.g., chest, arms, and legs) to monitor and record the electrical impulses that are resulted from continuous cycle of contraction and relaxation of cardiac muscle [60, 61]. A typical ECG signal is illustrated in Fig. 2 [62].

The ECG function can be explained through three main stages (Fig. 3), which are collecting, converting, and transmitting ECG signals. In short, analog ECG converts to its digital equivalent using Analog to Digital Converter (ADC) to be processed and transmitted to a peripheral device for diagnostic purposes. Figure 3 depicts the working method of ECG sensors abstractly.

Nowadays, there are many types of ECG devices and can be classified in several ways. One way is to classify ECG devices as a Standard ECG and Continuous ECG [63]. This classification is based on the number of electrodes and the ECG signal sampling duration. Another way is classifying ECG devices based on the transmitting way of ECG signals from sensors to monitoring device, which is often located in healthcare provision area (e.g., hospitals and clinics). Based on this concept, there are wired ECG sensors and wireless ECG sensors. Wireless ECG monitoring systems use various communication technologies to transmit ECG signals such as those systems mentioned in [63–66]. Also, the materials used in ECG electrodes manufacturing lead to the presence of new classification of ECG sensors. It is "wet" and "dry" ECG sensors [64]. Many leading companies worldwide

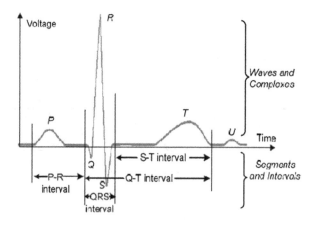

Fig. 2 A typical ECG signal, source [62]

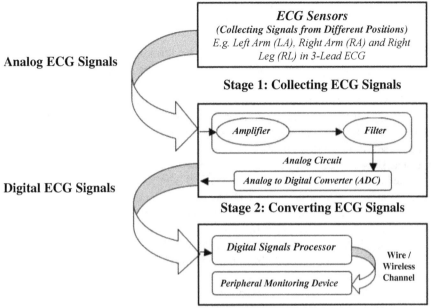

Fig. 3 The three main stages of ECG function

dedicated their efforts to manufacture reliable ECGs such as Philips [67], Ericsson [68], Schiller [69], General Electric [70], and Nokia [71].

There are many quality parameters that characterize each device. The most important parameters for this type of sensors are number of leads in each device, type of electrodes in term of "wet" or "dry" in addition to the general parameters mentioned in Sect. 2.1.

The increased number of victims due to the cardiovascular diseases motivated many research groups worldwide to improve ECG technology. Some research focus on designing smart ECG sensors such as [72–74] while others focus on enhancing the ECG operating environment such as improving the networks used for connecting wireless ECG sensors [63]. The research in [72] focused on developing a wireless ECG smart sensor to detect life-threatening events. It proposed a smart sensor that provides, at a very low cost, sufficient functionality to give indication of life-threatening events to the first responders. The research in [73] also developed a wireless ECG system for continuous event recording and communicating to a clinical alarm station. This system is designed for arrhythmia diagnostic purposes and worked by transmitting ECG signals to a Hand Held Device (HHD) and then to a remote Clinical Alarm Station (CAS) in emergency cases. The research in [74] focused on a wireless Tele-Home-Care system and developed a wearable ECG recording system for continuous arrhythmia monitoring. It aims to provide freedom of movement for patients while they are under continuous monitoring.

Other researches that aim to support the freedom of movement for the patients are found in [62, 64]. The system in [64] is an ultra-wearable, wireless, low power while the system in [62] is a novel wearable ECG monitoring system based on Active-Cable and intelligent electrodes for ubiquities healthcare.

Regarding the improvement of ECG surrounding environments, there are many research groups that focus on medical sensor networks including the transmission of ECG signals between sensors and diagnosing stations, ECG signals processing, and ECG electrodes. One of the pioneer groups [63] focused on enhancing medical sensor networks. They developed a combined hardware and software platform for medical sensor networks, called CodeBlue. They used it to develop several wireless medical sensors including ECG [63]. Their motivation was the urgent need for reliable medical sensor networks, which offer a high degree of security, a wide range of data rates, node mobility, and support multicast routing topologies. Regarding the ECG signals transmission, researchers in [75] designed and developed an ECG sensor that transmits medical data to a cell phone where they are displayed and stored. The Bluetooth is used to achieve this task and provide continuous monitoring of a patient heart anywhere cellular coverage is available. Considering the ECG signals processing, there is a research group that developed an open-source ECG analysis software to reduce the duplication of efforts for developing basic beat detection and classification software. The developed open-source QRS software has sensitivities and positive productivities close to 99% [76].

Some research groups focused on defining a unified format for the processing and storage of digital ECG recordings. The system in [77] is an example of such research. They developed a multi-manufacturer ECG viewer based on SCP-ECG standard. Regarding the ECG electrodes, researchers in [78] compared between wet, dry, and insulating bioelectric recording electrodes. Three main points motivated them: the inconvenient use of an electrolyte, the toxicological concerns with electrolyte gels, and the performance limitations of wet electrodes. They concluded that the performance of dry and insulating electrodes is better than wet one.

Many leading companies focused on manufacturing improved ECG sensors such as Philips [67], SHILLER [69], and General Electric [70] provide many types of ECG sensors that are classified based on patient situation and location.

EMG Sensors

EMG sensor is used to capture and measure electrical signals generated by contraction and relaxation of muscles such as skeletal muscles [60]. It is one of the sensors that are commonly involved in the Body Area Network. Also, EMG sensors have a critical role in nerve conduction studies due to the strong relationship between muscles and neuron systems [60]. In fact, nerve cells control body muscles by sending electrical impulses, which cause specific reaction from each muscle [60]. Consequently, abnormal reactions of the body muscles considered as a direct indicator of nerves and muscles disorders [60] such as balance abnormalities. In addition, EMG signals used to analyze the biomechanics of human or animal movement, in addition, to control or mimic a human gait for artificial equipment manufacturing [79].

EMG electrodes have three different types, which are surface electrodes, intramuscular electrodes, and needle electrodes that are utilized in surface EMG (SEMG), wire EMG, and needle EMG techniques, respectively [58, 80]. Each technique provides specific information that plays an important role in particular applications. For example, information provided by SEMG can be used in many applications such as ergonomics, rehabilitation, sport, and geriatric medicine [80].

Usually, EMG electrodes made from traditional disposable metallic and needed a specific glue to be placed upon the targeted muscle [81]. EMG sensors continuously improved to be in a compact size, wireless, noninvasive [82], and wearable such as EMG garments [81].

Regarding the functionality, EMG sensors adopt a similar method to those in ECG and EEG sensors [81]. The sampling rate is the main quality parameter that is used to evaluate EMG performance, which differs if the rectification performed prior to sampling and storing data or not [58]. Rates of 50–100 Hz are sufficient if rectification is performed while 800 Hz is the minimal rate required in the opposite case [58]. Other quality parameters differ based on electrode type [58]. For example, the quality parameters of surface electrodes are electrode material, size, shape, use of gel or paste, inter-electrode distance, electrode location, and orientation upon the muscle.

Many research groups dedicated their efforts to improve EMG sensors due to their critical role in electromyography and kinesiology. One of the well-known contributions is the "Standards for Reporting EMG Data," which was developed by Dr. Roberto Merletti, endorsed by the International Society of Electrophysiology and Kinesiology (ISEK) in 1999 and published in the Journal of Electromyography and Kinesiology (JEK) [58]. Also, the European Community has three different projects on SEMG [80].

In general, research efforts classify into two trends: one trend focuses on dealing with the issues and limitations related to EMG sensors such as large size and necessity of wires, while another trend focuses on improving EMG sensors capabilities to develop useful applications. Projects in [82, 83] are examples of the first trend while projects in [84–87] are examples of the second trend.

EEG Sensors
EEG sensor is used to detect and monitor signals within the human brain [60]. It is one of the sensors that is commonly involved in the Body Area Network. It performs its function by attaching small electrodes at multiple locations on the human's scalp [60]. The potential difference between the signal electrode placed on the scalp and a reference electrode is calculated and a conductive paste is used to minimize noises [88]. Then, the brain's electrical signals sensed by these sensors are processed in a similar way to ECG.

EEG sensors have three main types: routine EEG, continuous EEG, and ambulatory EEG (AEEG). Routine EEG typically monitors the patient's brain waves for 20 min, which is often not sufficient for reflecting the actual state of diagnostic disorder such as epilepsy [89]. To overcome this disadvantage, the continuous EEG is proposed as a standard. However, it requires clinical admission, which is expensive and takes the patient away from the home convenience [89]. To overcome these disadvantages, the ambulatory EEG is invented as a tool that monitors the patient status at home [89]. It has several advantages such as continuous recording up to 72 hours in addition to reasonable cost and ease of use [89].

Regarding the quality parameters of EEG, the sampling rate is the main one in addition to the size, weight, and the portability. The International Federation in Electroencephalography and Clinical Neurophysiology defined a standard called the 10–20 electrode placement system. It states that the range of sampling rate is 100–200 Hz and 128 Hz is the typical value [88]. This standard also determines the electrode names with correspondence to their locations on the scalp [88].

Many research dedicated the efforts to improve EEG sensors, especially the AEEG. Researchers in [90] focused on limited battery issue in AEEG. They started by stating the main drawbacks that still exist even after AEEG usage. The huge amount of data resulted from continuous recording, and a large number of required wires are examples of these drawbacks. They affect battery life, neurologist time, increases AEEG weight, and reduces its portability [90]. Therefore, the researchers suggested the wireless AEEG as a solution for the last drawbacks [90]. Also, they compared three different techniques of data reduction in order to overcome limited battery constraint. The techniques are: reduce the quality of the recording, use compression algorithms on the row data, and discontinuous recording [90]. They aim to determine the suitable technique by checking if the technique reduces the analysis time, sensitivity percentage, and data reduction percentage. They concluded that the third technique is the most suitable one to produce proper data for transmission and analysis purposes in addition to save battery life. Also, they recommended to use the online selection technique to save transmission and analysis time in case of long-term recording [90]. After this study, this research group introduced a real-time data reduction algorithm in [91] based on discontinuous recording technique. The basic idea of this algorithm is discarding the non-interesting part of EEG recording through the online transmission and only the potential part is saved for diagnosing purposes [91]. They applied this algorithm on an EEG dataset that contains 982 expert marked events in 4 days of data. The results show that 90% of events can be recorded correctly even with 50% of data reduction [91]. The goal behind this algorithm is to have direct, low power, and hardware implementation with reduced data, which in turn can be used in different BAN applications [91]. Also, they aimed to enhance EEG sensors to be wearable [92]. Another research focused on developing a Data-Driven Decision Support System (DSS) for EEG signals acquisition and parallel elaboration by proposing AmI-GRID environment [93]. The proposed environment can be utilized in many medical applications and will increase efficiency, accuracy, knowledge, and speed of explanation processes of EEG signals [93]. Also, it represents the main characteristics of Data-Driven DSS, which are improved patient safety, improved quality of care, and improved efficiency in healthcare delivery [93]. Figure 4 shows the different types under each involuntary sensor.

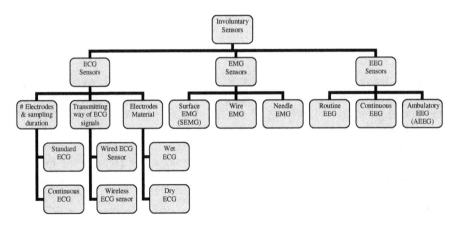

Fig. 4 Involuntary sensors and their types

2.2.2 Blood Sensors

This class includes sensors that are used to monitor and measure blood medical properties, which are blood glucose, blood pressure, and oxygen concentration in the bloodstream.

Blood Glucose Sensors

Blood glucose (BG) sensor is one of the most important sensors in healthcare area. It is used to monitor the glucose concentration, which is also called blood sugar [60], in the bloodstream. In fact, BG sensor plays a critical role in monitoring diabetics who are vulnerable to dangerous diseases such as eye and skin diseases.

BG sensors are classified mainly into invasive and noninvasive sensors. Invasive sensors measure glucose level by placing a blood drop from a patient's finger on a strip that contains chemicals sensitive to the glucose in the blood sample [94]. Then, an optical meter (glucometer) is used to analyze the blood sample and display a numerical result [60]. For healthy people, this result ranges between 3.5 and 6.1 mM [95].

A noninvasive BG sensor is invented to meet the need for monitoring the glucose level in diabetics continuously without the pain associated with the traditional method. Researchers and developers utilized the available technologies such as infrared technology and optical sensing to develop this type of sensors [60]. A comprehensive study of noninvasive blood glucose measurement (NIGM) sensors with assessments of the technologies used to develop them are shown in [96]. The technologies used for continuous and noninvasive monitoring of glucose concentration include Radio Frequency (RF) [97, 98] and spiral designs inspired from ring resonators [99]. They rely on the fact that detected change in the electrical properties of the blood is a result of a change in the glucose level in the blood, which can be used as an indicator of this level [100]. Another study [101] of NIGM sensor is developed based on analyzing the spectroscopic measurements. It proved that BG concentration is one of the parameters that can be predicted from the spectroscopic data resulted from mathematical modeling. In this study, the NIGM sensor uses three different models: two internal models to improve accuracy of measuring BG and one to improve robustness [101].

The study in [95] uses Near Infrared (NIR) absorption spectroscopy technique to measure BG by implanting a miniaturized optical BG sensor. It works by sensing the change of photon absorption in the blood after metabolism, which reflects the glucose concentration variations. One of the important challenges that face implantable sensors is the availability of sufficient power source in a reasonable size. One of the promising solutions is the technology that converts the thermal energy in human body into electrical power that can be used to operate such sensors [95].

Some studies suggested analyzing the breath of patient to determine BG level such as the study in [102]. It proposed a method to prove this fact with an error margin of 20.13% due to the small number of people participated in the experiment. The noninvasive measurement is performed by analyzing the acetone existing in the exhaled breath with the support of electronic nose system that is based on quartz crystal microbalance (QCM) sensors [102]. Their role in this system is to sense the low-level concentration of acetone and then compare the obtained data with the BG value [102]. The researchers believed that this method is a promising relief for diabetics who need to take the blood samples frequently per day [102].

Also, researchers in [99] proposed a novel sensor configuration to measure BG concentration using microwave measurement techniques. They choose a single-spiral microstrip sensor, which operates in the microwave frequency range. They provided results that support the feasibility of this method as a significant, robust, and economical solution for the challenges of noninvasive measurements [99].

From the previous overview, we can notice that there are several quality parameters for BG sensors. Sensor's shape, fabricating materials, technology in use, energy source are some of these quality parameters in addition to sampling rate like other types of sensors.

Blood Pressure Sensors

Blood pressure (BP) sensor is one of the noninvasive sensors that play a significant role in a body area network and in the healthcare field in general. It is used to monitor and measure the systolic and diastolic human blood pressure, which is the main cause behind several dangerous diseases [60].

BP sensors can be classified into two main categories: invasive and noninvasive sensors. Invasive sensors are implanted inside the patient's body while noninvasive sensors are not. The noninvasive sensors can be classified into two types: cuff-based and cuff-less sensors. Cuff-less sensor provides a high degree of free movement for patients. Unlike the Cuff-less sensor, the cuff-based sensor requires specific positions to provide accurate blood pressure readings and it is based on oscillometric technology.

Many technologies have been utilized to manufacture BP sensors. For example, researchers in [103] used piezoelectric technology with a specific transistor to model a BP sensor due to its ability to detect the sounds and pressure, which are the required parameters to measure BP. Another example is the usage of Fabry–Perot Interferometers (FPI) technology to develop a BP sensor due to its sensitivity to changes in the length of optical path [104]. Researchers in [104] developed a fiber optic pressure sensor that is also a noninvasive, cuff-based BP sensor and the initial results were promising.

Researchers in [105] developed an actual wearable, cuff-less noninvasive blood pressure (NIBP) sensor. It is a lightweight, compact, unobtrusive, and miniaturized sensor. They used the photoplethysmographic (PPG) technology to develop this sensor that provides the blood pressure readings regardless of the patient posture [105]. They achieved this feature by using MEMS accelerometers to perform the task in a stable and reliable way [105].

Another work [106] developed a new approach to measure the four components of blood pressure, which are systolic blood pressure (SBP), diastolic blood pressure (DBP), mean arterial pressure (MAP), and Pulse Pressure (PP) by using a radial artery tonometry pressure sensor combined with a Korean traditional medical concept [106]. They estimated the BP by evaluating many parameters such as Applied Pressure (AP) and elasticity of wrist tissue.

Researchers in [107] developed a new approach that offers continuous monitoring based on the Pulse Arrival Time (PAT) in addition to analyze the impact of posture on the PAT measure [107]. They declared the importance of context information about body posture and physical activities to interpret PAT measurements in unconstrained scenarios [107]. In contrast, researchers in [108] developed a method for continuous sensing of the blood pressure regardless of patients posture. They stated that the accuracy and calibration of this sensor depend on two points: a true anatomical model of the patient and an ability to eliminate noise resulted from movements that are not related to heartbeat [108].

Research in [109, 110] are good examples of efforts toward developing invasive BP sensors. In [109], researchers developed an invasive system that consists of an implant, which consists of a sensor chip and a telemetric unit; and an external reader station. The system provides energy to the implant wirelessly [109]. The initial results were promising in term of sensor calibration for those who need continuous and long-term monitoring [109]. Researchers in [110] also developed a system for invasive BP using the PTT concept for measuring the BP completely inside the body. The developed system avoids the risk of thrombosis because the sensor system installed around the artery [110]. The initial results were satisfactory and they open new horizons for advancement in invasive BP measurements.

Many research efforts dedicated to develop noninvasive continuous BP monitoring systems, such as [111] and [112]. In [111], researchers used CMOS-based tactile sensor for continuous noninvasive cuff-less BP measuring by developing a novel monolithic sensor. In a similar way, researchers in [112] developed a method for continuous non-disturbing monitoring of BP by deployment of two different sensors: a novel magnetoelastic skin curvature sensor and standard ECG electrodes. They declared the ability of developed method to determine the qualitative assessment of the BP.

Pulse Oximetry

Pulse oximetry is one of the most used sensors in the healthcare area known as SpO_2. It is used to measure the arterial oxygen saturation in the individual's blood in addition to three more parameters, which are heart rate, respiration rate, and arterial carbon monoxide "saturation" [113].

In general, pulse oximetry sensors can be classified as invasive and noninvasive sensors. The invasive sensors are used for long-term and continuous monitoring. The researchers in [113] developed a new ear sensor for mobile, continuous, and long-term pulse oximetry called Circumcision Pulse Oximetry. They chose the ear canal to implant the sensor because it considered a stable environment against intensive movements and acceleration. They compared this new principle for invasive pulse oximetry with the principles of noninvasive pulse oximetry, which are reflectance and transmission principles [113]. By this design, they overcame the mobility constraints and satisfied the three requirements to develop optimal sensors, which are invisibility, unobtrusiveness, and mobility [113]. Also, they listed some examples of medical applications where the mobile pulse oximetry can be utilized. They are sleep apnea, obstructive disease, and asthma monitoring in addition to other useful applications such as mobile SaO_2 monitoring for firefighters and extreme mountain climbers. Another research in [114] proposed a novel long-term implantable pulse oximetry system. It works by wrapping an optical transparent elastic cuff directly around an arterial blood vessel.

The noninvasive pulse oximetry is known as a small clip, which contains the sensor, attached to the individual's finger, earlobe, or toe [60]. It can be worn in many other forms such as a ring [56], a wrist bracelet [55], or an adhesive patch [115]. This sensor works by emitting a light signal that passes through the skin. Based on the light absorption of oxygenated hemoglobin and the total hemoglobin in atrial blood, the result is expressed as a percentage of oxygenated hemoglobin to the total amount of hemoglobin [60]. Researchers in [115] developed a portable real-time wireless pulse oximetry system. They reduced the size and cost by using ZigBee wireless technology. The sensor node of this system worn on the wrist and fingertip. The results of using this system for in-home patients were satisfactory in terms of comfortable in daily life [115]. Researchers in [116] also developed a similar wearable reflectance system that is worn on the wrist and fingertip with extra feature, which is low-power consumption. Fingertip pulse oximetry has the main disadvantage, which is the possibility of fatal infections due to reusing it with many patients where it contacts the skin directly with low level of sterilization [117]. To overcome this, the researchers in [117] introduced a polymer-based pulse oximetry sensor as a disposable sensor. It is a lightweight, flexible, robust, and recyclable sensor to minimize the chances of infections among patients with lower cost than thoroughly decontaminating procedure. Researchers in [118] presented a design and an implementation of a finger ring sensor. The developed sensor is embedded in a ring that fits any finger, which provides comfortable wearing in addition to perfect results for sleep monitoring. It detects the sleep apnea syndrome (SAS) successfully and helps in enhancing sleep quality [118]. Researchers in [119] presented a prototype of the adhesive patch sensor. They developed a multisensory

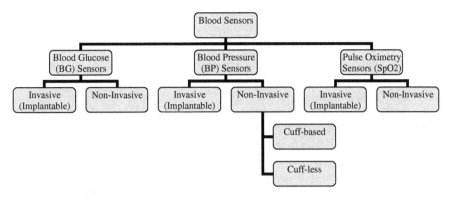

Fig. 5 Blood sensors classification and types

chip embedded in the adhesive patch for measuring temperature and the pulse oximetry parameters.

In addition, many research show how the pulse oximetry sensor can be used to measure oxygen saturations from many positions on the body such as using it at the sternum [120, 121], the esophagus [122]. Other medical applications use pulse oximetry for ill babies and children in emergency cases [123]. This sensor is also used for nonmedical applications such as using it for fingerprint anti-spoofing [124]. Figure 5 shows the different types under each blood sensor.

3   Biofeedback-Based Healthcare Systems

This section presents some examples of existing systems and classifies them in light of the biofeedback classification as the clinical or ubiquitous biofeedback. Reviewing the literature shows that the existing systems can be classified according to their usage as clinical or well-being usage. Figure 6 shows the suggested classification of biofeedback healthcare systems.

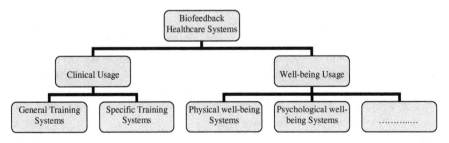

Fig. 6 Suggested classification of biofeedback healthcare systems

Under clinical usage, systems can be classified as general training systems or specific for chronic diseases. Under well-being usage, systems can be classified as systems for physical or psychological well-being. These two classes represent 2 out of the 11 fundamental dimensions used to define wellness [125]. Therefore, more classes can be added to represent systems developed under the remaining dimensions, as illustrated in Fig. 2.

General training systems under clinical usage are the early developed biofeedback-based healthcare systems such as [15]. Some of them are patented systems such as [126] and [127]. Many specific training systems have been developed for chronic diseases management or treatment. Some examples are systems developed for respiratory training such as [12, 128–130], migraine and headache such as [19, 25], addiction [21], heart and brain diseases [130, 131], psychiatric rehabilitation and mental health therapy [132, 133], fibromyalgia [43], autism [134], evaluating medication response [135], and cerebral palsied [136]. Training or treating the stress-related disorders is one of the most areas where biofeedback training used extensively. Urinary incontinence, which is treated by pelvic floor muscle (PFM) training [137], psoriasis [138], posttraumatic stress disorder [133], and stress in obese patients [139] are examples of these disorders.

Systems under well-being usage refer to the biofeedback-based healthcare systems developed for personal use and not for clinical. They are example of personal healthcare systems used to increase individuals' awareness about their health statuses [140]. They aim to motivate their users to improve their well-being by providing real-time results often combined with advices and recommendations. Such systems rely on wearable sensory technologies to perform their functions and represent a promising solution for healthcare [141]. Authentication is an important feature in these systems and has been considered by several research and patents [142].

According to [125], physical wellness refers to the active and continued effort to maintain an optimum level of physical activity, focus on diet, and make healthy lifestyle choices including self-care. This definition determines the four main factors of physical wellness or well-being, which are physical activity, nutrition, self-care, and healthy lifestyle actions. The physical well-being literature could be classified in accordance with these factors.

Many systems have been developed to track the physical activity level of their users such as adults, elderly people, and athletes. Several patents have been registered to support these systems such as [143], [144], and [13]. Some examples of recent research are for athletes [145], adults [8], and elderly people [146]. A collection of systems developed to track and improve physical activity levels in addition to promote healthy lifestyles are presented in Table 2. They aim to increase users' awareness of their activity level or provide them with advice to increase their physical activity level. For each system, Table 2 shows the targeted users, source of input, the type of output, and feedback type.

Examples of systems developed under other physical well-being factors are the diet advisory system for children in [11] as an example of nutrition factor, the

Table 2 Examples of biofeedback-based healthcare systems under physical well-being class

System	Target			Source of input		Type of output		Feedback type		
	Adult	Elder	Athlete	Sensors	Manual	Personalized	General	Visual	Audible	Haptic
Intelligent knee sleeve [147]	✓		✓	✓		✓			✓	
StepUp [148]				✓			✓	✓		
Flowie [149]		✓		✓			✓	✓	✓	
CAMMInA [150]		✓			✓		✓	✓		
Motivate [151]	✓				✓	✓		✓		
Ice hockey skating [152]			✓	✓		✓		✓		
CAB [8]	✓			✓		✓		✓	✓	✓
Kickboxing [153]			✓	✓		✓		✓		
Vertical jump [154]			✓	✓		✓				✓

research in [155, 156] as examples of self-care, and the biofeedback systems in [157–161] as examples of healthy lifestyle actions.

Most of the biofeedback healthcare systems under psychological well-being usage focus on stress management, and related issues such as anxiety and depression. One of the early research [162] discussed the role of biofeedback training in the treatment of functional disorders including anxiety and depression. Another research shows how the EEG sensors can be utilized in the biofeedback treatment of anxiety disorders [22].

These biofeedback-based systems aim to increase users' awareness about their psychological status toward minimizing stress level [158] and enhancing emotional feelings [163, 164] and mood [165]. Many researchers developed games to achieve this goal such as the biofeedback serious game for stress management in general [7], or during gameplay [166]. Also, biofeedback games have been utilized in stressful tasks [167] and critical decision-making situations [168].

Many researches discuss the role of biofeedback systems in stress management for various age groups and from different perspectives such as the research in [30] that discuss utilizing biofeedback to address anxiety and depression in children and adolescents. Different sensors have been utilized to monitor stress such as using EMG to recognize facial gesture for stress monitoring [169] and PPG sensors to assess stress level in a real-time manner. VR biofeedback system in [170] and the respiratory biofeedback app in [171] are examples of using PPG sensors. Also, biofeedback systems have been used to manage stress while performing professional tasks such as teaching [172]. Currently, many researches consider predicting stress as a proactive procedure to minimize stress effects such as research in [173].

4   Challenges and Future Directions

Reviewing the literature emphasizes many issues and challenges facing the utilization of biofeedback in healthcare. Most of the research highlighted the issues and challenges facing the clinical biofeedback while limited number of studies tackled the U-Biofeedback challenges.

For the clinical biofeedback, some studies discussed the challenges in general while others investigated them for specific diseases. The research in [174] is one of the early studies that discussed the clinical biofeedback in general. It presents the theoretical and practical issues for utilizing biofeedback as a therapy. It shows that patient motivation is one of the main challenges because the commitment to the biofeedback treatment sessions is critical for their success. A combined behavioral-biological model is proposed in this research to predict if the intended biofeedback training will be clinically significant for a given patient. This study proves that the biofeedback training works effectively for patients having acute organ damage. It also highlights the importance of using cognitive and somatic mediators to support self-regulation. The research in [175] is another example of studies that discussed the issues of therapeutic biofeedback in general.

Many studies discussed the challenges in biofeedback applications for specific diseases such epilepsy [176], recurrent headache [177, 178], cardiovascular disorders [179], cerebral palsy [180], dysphonia [181], and chronic pain [20]. In addition, some studies highlight the issues associated with a specific population such as the study in [182] that presents the issues of utilizing clinical biofeedback training with children, and specific biofeedback training such as EEG alpha feedback training [183]. Also, a recent study [184] discusses the challenges of utilizing Group Biofeedback (GBF) beside its advantages for chronic diseases management. Another recent study presents healthcare professionals opinions about the benefits and challenges of using biofeedback and wearable technology for orthopaedic rehabilitation [185].

Although the U-Biofeedback overcomes several challenges of clinical biofeedback such as patient commitment for the training sessions, clinical setup, and coach presence, reviewing the literature pointed out some issues and challenges face its utilization. The technical issues of biofeedback sensors such as battery life and communication quality are some of the major challenges in U-Biofeedback applications. The accuracy of collected data and application's ease of use are other examples of these challenges. Recent studies [186, 187] discussed these challenges in sport biofeedback applications. Researchers in [186] explained the challenges related to sensors, processing, communication technologies, and devices, whereas researchers in [187] focused on communication and processing as the main issues toward developing high-performance real-time biofeedback systems. Another study discussed the challenges in real-time biofeedback motion tracking and processing [188].

Thus, the challenges-related research in U-Biofeedback shows the interest of effective utilization of biofeedback technology in sport, which opens doors for further studies in this area. It also highlights the need to discuss the challenges that face the U-Biofeedback applications for personal well-being such as weight management and quit smoking.

5 Conclusion

This chapter discussed utilizing biofeedback technology in the healthcare field. It started with a brief history of this technology including both types clinical and ubiquities biofeedback, followed by a list of previous reviews. Then, it presented the various types of biosensors including their types, features, and functions. A classification of biofeedback-based healthcare systems according to their usage is proposed as clinical and well-being systems. A wide range of existing systems of both classes is presented. Finally, the challenges and issues facing the deployment of biofeedback-based healthcare systems are discussed. Challenges of using biofeedback applications in sports are addressed recently in the literature.

References

1. H. Al Osman, M. Eid, A. El Saddik, U-biofeedback: A multimedia-based reference model for ubiquitous biofeedback systems. Multimed. Tools Appl. **72**(3), 3143–3168 (2014)
2. Mayo Clinic, *Biofeedback* (Mayo Clinic, 2019), [Online] https://www.mayoclinic.org/tests-procedures/biofeedback/about/pac-20384664. Accessed 26 Mar 2019
3. D.W. Shearn, Operant analysis in psychophysiology, in *Handbook of Psychophysiology*, ed. by N.S. Greenfield, R.A. Sternbach (Holt, Rinehart, Winston, New York, 1972)
4. K.R. Pelletier, Theory and applications of clinical biofeedback. J. Contemp. Psychother. **7**(1), 29–34 (1975)
5. J. Basmajian, Introduction: Principles and background. Biofeedback Princ. Pract. Clin., 1–4 (1989)
6. J. Kamiya, Operant control of the EEG alpha rhythm and some of its reported effects on consciousness, in *Altered States Consciousness* (Wiley, New York, 1969), pp. 489–501
7. H. Al Osman, H. Dong, A. El Saddik, Ubiquitous biofeedback serious game for stress management. IEEE Access **4**, 1274–1286 (2016)
8. H.F. Badawi, H. Dong, A. El Saddik, Mobile cloud-based physical activity advisory system using biofeedback sensors. Futur. Gener. Comput. Syst. **66**, 59–70 (2017)
9. Z. Zhang, H. Wu, W. Wang, B. Wang, A smartphone based respiratory biofeedback system, in *Proceedings – 2010 3rd International Conference on Biomedical Engineering and Informatics, BMEI 2010*, vol. 2 (2010), pp. 717–720
10. S. Hamdan, H. Al Osman, M. Eid, A. El Saddik, A biofeedback system for sleep management, in *2012 IEEE International Symposium on Robotic and Sensors Environments, ROSE 2012 – Proceedings* (2012), pp. 133–137
11. H. Badawi, M. Eid, A. El Saddik, Diet advisory system for children using biofeedback sensor, in *MeMeA 2012 – 2012 IEEE Symposium on Medical Measurements and Applications, Proceedings* (2012)
12. D. Hillsman, Respiratory biofeedback and performance evaluation system, US3991304A, 1976
13. A.G. Hock, Biofeedback system for sensing body motion and flexure, US6032530A, 2000
14. J. M. J. F. F. M. Horton, Modular biofeedback training system, US4110918A, 1976
15. E.B. Blanchard, L.D. Young, Clinical applications of biofeedback training: a review of evidence. Arch. Gen. Psychiatry **30**(5), 573–589 (1974)
16. F. Butler, *Biofeedback: A Survey of the Literature* (1978)
17. T.J. Teyler, Biofeedback: a survey of the literature. Psyccritiques **24**(1), 75 (1979)
18. G.D. Zimet, Locus of control and biofeedback: a review of the literature. Percept. Mot. Skills **49**(3), 871–877 (1979)
19. J. Johansson, L.-G. Öst, Self-control procedures in biofeedback: a review of temperature biofeedback in the treatment of migraine. Biofeedback Self. Regul. **7**(4), 435–442 (1982)
20. J.A. Turner, C.R. Chapman, Psychological interventions for chronic pain: a critical review. II. Operant conditioning, hypnosis, and cognitive-behavioral therapy. Pain **12**(1), 23–46 (1982)
21. D.L. Trudeau, The treatment of addictive disorders by brain wave biofeedback: a review and suggestions for future research. Clin. EEG Neurosci. **31**(1), 13–22 (2000)
22. N.C. Moore, A review of EEG biofeedback treatment of anxiety disorders. Clin. EEG Neurosci. **31**(1), 1–6 (2000)
23. M.S. Medlicott, S.R. Harris, A systematic review of the effectiveness of exercise, manual therapy, electrotherapy, relaxation training, and biofeedback in the management of temporomandibular disorder. Phys. Ther. **86**(7), 955–973 (2006)
24. C. Imperatori, M. Mancini, G. Della Marca, E.M. Valenti, B. Farina, Feedback-based treatments for eating disorders and related symptoms: a systematic review of the literature. Nutrients **10**(11) (2018)
25. Y. Nestoriuc, A. Martin, W. Rief, F. Andrasik, Biofeedback treatment for headache disorders: a comprehensive efficacy review. Appl. Psychophysiol. Biofeedback **33**(3), 125–140 (2008)

26. A. Tremback-Ball, E. Gherghel, A. Hegge, K. Kindig, H. Marsico, R. Scanlon, The effectiveness of biofeedback therapy in managing Bladder Bowel Dysfunction in children: a systematic review. J. Pediatr. Rehabil. Med. **11**(3), 161–173 (2018)

27. D.M. Thompson, D.A. Hall, D.-M. Walker, D.J. Hoare, Psychological therapy for people with tinnitus: a scoping review of treatment components. Ear Hear. **38**(2), 149–158 (2017)

28. D. Bega, P. Gonzalez-Latapi, C. Zadikoff, T. Simuni, A review of the clinical evidence for complementary and alternative therapies in Parkinson's disease. Curr. Treat. Options Neurol. **16**(10) (2014)

29. G. Chiarioni, Biofeedback treatment of chronic constipation: myths and misconceptions. Tech. Coloproctol. **20**(9), 611–618 (2016)

30. H. Thabrew, P. Ruppeldt, J.J. Sollers, Systematic review of biofeedback interventions for addressing anxiety and depression in children and adolescents with long-term physical conditions. Appl. Psychophysiol. Biofeedback **43**(3), 179–192 (2018)

31. *Scopus*, [Online] https://www.scopus.com/. Accessed 28 Nov 2018

32. A. Stubberud, M. Linde, Digital technology and mobile health in behavioral migraine therapy: a narrative review. Curr. Pain Headache Rep. **22**(10) (2018)

33. K. Bodner et al., A cross-sectional review of the prevalence of integrative medicine in pediatric pain clinics across the United States. Complement. Ther. Med. **38**, 79–84 (2018)

34. T. Rose, C.S. Nam, K.B. Chen, Immersion of virtual reality for rehabilitation – Review. Appl. Ergon. **69**, 153–161 (2018)

35. G.J. Macfarlane et al., EULAR revised recommendations for the management of fibromyalgia. Ann. Rheum. Dis. **76**(2), 318–328 (2017)

36. D. Vadas, L. Kalichman, Post-stroke hip fracture in older people: a narrative review. Int. J. Ther. Rehabil. **23**(2), 58–63 (2016)

37. M.D. Fejka, Fecal incontinence: a review of current treatment options. J. Am. Acad. Physician Assist. **29**(9), 27–30 (2016)

38. J. Lake, The integrative management of PTSD: a review of conventional and CAM approaches used to prevent and treat PTSD with emphasis on military personnel. Adv. Integr. Med. **2**(1), 13–23 (2015)

39. C.A. Anderson, M.I. Omar, S.E. Campbell, K.F. Hunter, J.D. Cody, C.M.A. Glazener, Conservative management for postprostatectomy urinary incontinence. Cochrane Database Syst. Rev. **2015**(1) (2015)

40. J.T. Olin et al., Inducible laryngeal obstruction during exercise: moving beyond vocal cords with new insights. Phys. Sportsmed. **43**(1), 13–21 (2015)

41. R.A. Adam, P.A. Norton, Non-surgical treatment of urinary incontinence, in *Clinical Gynecology*, 2nd edn. (2015), pp. 410–416

42. A. Snaith, D. Wade, Dystonia. BMJ Clin. Evid. **2014** (2014)

43. M. Santoro, T. Cronan, A systematic review of neurofeedback as a treatment for fibromyalgia syndrome symptoms. J. Musculoskelet. Pain **22**(3), 286–300 (2014)

44. E. Collins, F. Hibberts, M. Lyons, A.B. Williams, A.M.P. Schizas, Outcomes in non-surgical management for bowel dysfunction. Br. J. Nurs. **23**(14), 776–780 (2014)

45. M. Feretis, M. Chapman, The role of anorectal investigations in predicting the outcome of biofeedback in the treatment of faecal incontinence. Scand. J. Gastroenterol. **48**(11), 1265–1271 (2013)

46. G.K. Kristofersson, M.J. Kaas, Stress management techniques in the prison setting. J. Forensic Nurs. **9**(2), 111–119 (2013)

47. M. Hashefi, J.D. Katz, M.C. Reid, Nonpharmacologic, complementary, and alternative interventions for managing chronic pain in older adults. Clin. Geriatr. **21**(3), 18–27 (2013)

48. R. Bize, B. Burnand, Y. Mueller, M. Rège-Walther, J.Y. Camain, J. Cornuz, Biomedical risk assessment as an aid for smoking cessation. Cochrane Database Syst. Rev. **12** (2012)

49. T. Pelton, P. van Vliet, K. Hollands, Interventions for improving coordination of reach to grasp following stroke: a systematic review. Int. J. Evid. Based. Healthc. **10**(2), 89–102 (2012)

50. A. El Saddik, Digital twins: the convergence of multimedia technologies. IEEE Multimed. **25**(2), 87–92 (2018)

51. J.S. Wilson, *Sensor Technology Handbook* (Elsevier, 2004)
52. G. Roberts-Grey, *PHILIPS – Sleep Apnea -Sleep Better, Save More Money* (PHILIPS, 2019), [Online] https://www.usa.philips.com/c-e/hs/better-sleep-breathing-blog/better-sleep/sleep-better-save-more-money.html. Accessed 28 Mar 2019
53. *GE Healthcare Life Sciences – Sensor Chips* [Online] https://www.gelifesciences.com/en/ro/shop/protein-analysis/spr-label-free-analysis/sensor-chips. Accessed 28 Mar 2019
54. *GARMIN* [Online] https://www.garmin.com/en-CA/. Accessed 28 Mar 2019
55. *Fitbit* [Online] https://www.fitbit.com/en-ca/home. Accessed 28 Mar 2019
56. *OURA* [Online] https://ouraring.com/. Accessed 28 Mar 2019
57. M. Thompson, L. Thompson, *The Neurofeedback Book: An Introduction to Basic Concepts in Applied Psychophysiology* (Association for Applied Psychophysiology and Biofeedback, Wheat Ridge, CO, 2003)
58. R. Merletti, Standards for reporting EMG data. J. Electromyogr. Kinesiol. **9**(1), 3–4 (1999)
59. K. Iniewski, *Biological and Medical Sensor Technologies* (CRC Press, 2017)
60. M. Chen, S. Gonzalez, A. Vasilakos, H. Cao, V.C.M. Leung, Body area networks: a survey. Mob. Netw. Appl. **16**(2), 171–193 (2011)
61. T. O'Donovan, J. O'Donoghue, C. Sreenan, D. Sammon, P. O'Reilly, K.A. O'Connor, A context aware wireless Body Area Network (BAN), in *3rd International Conference on Pervasive Computing Technologies for Healthcare – Pervasive Health 2009, PCTHealth 2009* (2009)
62. G. Yang, Y. Cao, J. Chen, H. Tenhunen, L.-R. Zheng, An Active-Cable connected ECG monitoring system for ubiquitous healthcare, in *Proceedings – 3rd International Conference on Convergence and Hybrid Information Technology, ICCIT 2008*, vol. 1 (2008), pp. 392–397
63. V. Shnayder, B. Chen, K. Lorincz, T.R.F. Fulford-Jones, M. Welsh, *Sensor Networks for Medical Care* (2005)
64. C. Park, P.H. Chou, Y. Bai, R. Matthews, A. Hibbs, An ultra-wearable, wireless, low power ECG monitoring system, in *IEEE 2006 Biomedical Circuits and Systems Conference Healthcare Technology, BioCAS 2006* (2006), pp. 241–244
65. J. Liang, Y. Wu, Wireless ECG monitoring system based on OMAP, in *Proceedings – 12th IEEE International Conference on Computational Science and Engineering, CSE 2009*, vol. 2 (2009), pp. 1002–1006
66. C.J. Deepu, X.Y. Xu, X.D. Zou, L.B. Yao, Y. Lian, An ECG-on-chip for wearable cardiac monitoring devices, in *Proceedings – 5th IEEE International Symposium on Electronic Design, Test and Applications, DELTA 2010* (2010), pp. 225–228
67. *PHILIPS- Products and Services* [Online] https://www.usa.philips.com/healthcare/medical-products. Accessed 28 Mar 2019
68. V. Galetic et al., Ericsson mobile health solution overview, in *MIPRO 2010 – 33rd International Convention on Information and Communication Technology, Electronics and Microelectronics, Proceedings* (2010), pp. 350–354
69. SCHILLER-MEDILOG®AR
70. *GE Healthcare* [Online] https://www.gehealthcare.com/en/global-gateway. Accessed 28 Mar 2019
71. *NOKIA-Healthcare* [Online] https://networks.nokia.com/industries/healthcare. Accessed 28 Mar 2019
72. J. Welch, F. Guilak, S.D. Baker, A wireless ECG smart sensor for broad application in life threatening event detection, in *Annual International Conference of the IEEE Engineering in Medicine and Biology – Proceedings*, vol. 26 V (2004), pp. 3447–3449
73. R. Fensli, E. Gunnarson, O. Hejlesen, A wireless ECG system for continuous event recording and communication to a clinical alarm station, in *Annual International Conference of the IEEE Engineering in Medicine and Biology – Proceedings*, vol. 26 III (2004), pp. 2208–2211
74. R. Fensli, E. Gunnarson, T. Gundersen, A wearable ECG-recording system for continuous arrhythmia monitoring in a wireless tele-home-care situation, in *Proceedings – IEEE Symposium on Computer-Based Medical Systems* (2005), pp. 407–412

75. J. Proulx, R. Clifford, S. Sorensen, D.-J. Lee, J. Archibald, Development and evaluation of a bluetooth EKG monitoring sensor, in *Proceedings – IEEE Symposium on Computer-Based Medical Systems*, vol. 2006 (2006), pp. 507–511

76. P. Hamilton, Open source ECG analysis. Comput. Cardiol. **29**, 101–104 (2002)

77. F. Chiarugi, P.J. Lees, C.E. Chronaki, M. Tsiknakis, S.C. Orphanoudakis, Developing manufacturer-independent components for ECG viewing and for data exchange with ECG devices: can the SCP-ECG standard help? Comput. Cardiol. **28**, 185–188 (2001)

78. A. Searle, L. Kirkup, A direct comparison of wet, dry and insulating bioelectric recording electrodes. Physiol. Meas. **21**(2), 271–283 (2000)

79. T.S. Poo, K. Sundaraj, Design and development of low cost biceps tendonitis monitoring system using EMG sensor, in *Proceedings – CSPA 2010: 2010 6th International Colloquium on Signal Processing and Its Applications* (2010)

80. R. Merletti, H. Hermens, R. Kadefors, European community projects on surface electromyography. Annu. Int. Conf. IEEE Eng. Med. Biol. **2**, 1119–1122 (2001)

81. J. Sipilä, A. Tolvanen, P. Taelman, *sEMG measuring by garments* (2007)

82. W. Youn, J. Kim, Development of a compact-size and wireless surface EMG measurement system, in *ICCAS-SICE 2009 – ICROS-SICE International Joint Conference 2009, Proceedings* (2009), pp. 1625–1628

83. Y. Makino, S. Ogawa, H. Shinoda, EMG sensor integration based on two dimensional communication, in *Proceedings of INSS 2008 – 5th International Conference on Networked Sensing Systems* (2008), p. 257

84. Y.-H. Liu, H.-P. Huang, Towards a high-stability EMG recognition system for prosthesis control: a one-class classification based non-target EMG pattern filtering scheme, in *Conference Proceedings – IEEE International Conference on Systems, Man and Cybernetics* (2009), pp. 4752–4757

85. Q. Wang, X. Zhang, X. Chen, R. Chen, W. Chen, Y. Chen, A novel pedestrian dead reckoning algorithm using wearable EMG sensors to measure walking strides, in *2010 Ubiquitous Positioning Indoor Navigation and Location Based Service, UPINLBS 2010* (2010)

86. Y. Makino, S. Ogawa, H. Shinoda, Flexible EMG sensor array for haptic interface, in *Proceedings of the SICE Annual Conference* (2008), pp. 1468–1473

87. B.D. Farnsworth, D.M. Talyor, R.J. Triolo, D.J. Young, Wireless in vivo EMG sensor for intelligent prosthetic control, in *TRANSDUCERS 2009 – 15th International Conference on Solid-State Sensors, Actuators and Microsystems* (2009), pp. 358–361

88. T. Ebrahimi, J.-M. Vesin, G. Garcia, Brain-computer interface in multimedia communication. IEEE Signal Process. Mag. **20**(1), 14–24 (2003)

89. E. Waterhouse, New horizons in ambulatory electroencephalography. IEEE Eng. Med. Biol. Mag. **22**(3), 74–80 (2003)

90. A.J. Casson, E. Rodriguez-Villegas, Data reduction techniques to facilitate wireless and long term AEEG epilepsy monitoring, in *Proceedings of the 3rd International IEEE EMBS Conference on Neural Engineering* (2007), pp. 298–301

91. A.J. Casson, E. Rodriguez-Villegas, Toward online data reduction for portable electroencephalography systems in epilepsy. IEEE Trans. Biomed. Eng. **56**(12), 2816–2825 (2009)

92. A.J. Casson, L. Logesparan, E. Rodriguez-Villegas, An introduction to future truly wearable medical devices-from application to ASIC, in *2010 Annual International Conference of the IEEE Engineering in Medicine and Biology Society, EMBC'10* (2010), pp. 3430–3431

93. U. Barcaro et al., A decision support system for the acquisition and elaboration of EEG signals: the AmI-GRID environment, in *Annual International Conference of the IEEE Engineering in Medicine and Biology – Proceedings* (2007), pp. 4331–4334

94. S. Saini, S. Kaur, K. Das, V. Saini, Using the first drop of blood for monitoring blood glucose values in critically ill patients: an observational study. Indian J. Crit. Care Med. **20**(11), 658–661 (2016)

95. A. Trabelsi, M. Boukadoum, C. Fayomi, E. M. Aboulhamid, Blood glucose sensor implant using NIR spectroscopy: preliminary design study, in *Proceedings of the International Conference on Microelectronics, ICM* (2010), pp. 176–179

96. A. Tura, A. Maran, G. Pacini, Non-invasive glucose monitoring: assessment of technologies and devices according to quantitative criteria. Diabetes Res. Clin. Pract. **77**(1), 16–40 (2007)
97. T. Karacolak, A.Z. Hood, E. Topsakal, Design of a dual-band implantable antenna and development of skin mimicking gels for continuous glucose monitoring. IEEE Trans. Microw. Theory Tech. **56**(4), 1001–1008 (2008)
98. B. Freer, J. Venkataraman, Feasibility study for non-invasive blood glucose monitoring, in *2010 IEEE International Symposium on Antennas and Propagation and CNC-USNC/URSI Radio Science Meeting – Leading the Wave, AP-S/URSI 2010* (2010)
99. B.R. Jean, E.C. Green, M.J. McClung, A microwave frequency sensor for non-invasive blood-glucose measurement, in *2008 IEEE Sensors Applications Symposium, SAS-2008 – Proceedings* (2008), pp. 4–7
100. T. Yilmaz, Y. Hao, Electrical property characterization of blood glucose for on-body sensors, in *Proceedings of the 5th European Conference on Antennas and Propagation, EUCAP 2011* (2011), pp. 3659–3662
101. M. Stemmann, F. Ståhl, J. Lallemand, E. Renard, R. Johansson, Sensor calibration models for a non-invasive blood glucose measurement sensor, in *2010 Annual International Conference of the IEEE Engineering in Medicine and Biology Society, EMBC'10* (2010), pp. 4979–4982
102. H.M. Saraoğlu, M. Koçan, Determination of blood glucose level-based breath analysis by a quartz crystal microbalance sensor array. IEEE Sens. J. **10**(1), 104–109 (2010)
103. F. Ravariu, C. Ravariu, O. Nedelcu, The modeling of a sensor for the human blood pressure. Proc. Int. Semiconductor Conf., CAS **1**, 67–70 (2002)
104. R. Melamud et al., Development of an SU-8 Fabry-Perot blood pressure sensor, in *Proceedings of the IEEE International Conference on Micro Electro Mechanical Systems (MEMS)* (2005), pp. 810–813
105. P.A. Shaltis, A. Reisner, H.H. Asada, Wearable, cuff-less PPG-based blood pressure monitor with novel height sensor, in *Annual International Conference of the IEEE Engineering in Medicine and Biology – Proceedings* (2006), pp. 908–911
106. K.-C. Park, H. Kang, Y. Huh, K.C. Kim, Cuffless and noninvasive measurement of systolic blood pressure, diastolic blood pressure, mean arterial pressure and pulse pressure using radial artery tonometry pressure sensor with concept of Korean traditional medicine, in *29th Annual International Conference of the IEEE Engineering in Medicine and Biology Society* (2007), pp. 3597–3600
107. J. Muehlsteff, X.A. Aubert, G. Morren, Continuous cuff-less blood pressure monitoring based on the pulse arrival time approach: the impact of posture, in *Proceedings of the 30th Annual International Conference of the IEEE Engineering in Medicine and Biology Society, EMBS'08 – "Personalized Healthcare through Technology"* (2008), pp. 1691–1694
108. L. Lading, F. Nyboe, D. Nilsson, H. Pranov, T.W. Hansen, Sensor for vascular compliance and blood pressure, in *Proceedings of IEEE Sensors* (2009), pp. 181–184
109. H. Fassbender et al., Fully implantable blood pressure sensor for hypertonic patients, in *Proceedings of IEEE Sensors* (2008), pp. 1226–1229
110. J. Fiala et al., Implantable sensor for blood pressure determination via pulse transit time, in *Proceedings of IEEE Sensors* (2010), pp. 1226–1229
111. K.-U. Kirstein, J. Sedivy, T. Salo, C. Hagleitner, T. Vancura, A. Hierlemann, A CMOS-based tactile sensor for continuous blood pressure monitoring, in *Proceedings – Design, Automation and Test in Europe, DATE '05*, vol. 2005 (2005), pp. 210–214
112. E. Kaniusas et al., Method for continuous nondisturbing monitoring of blood pressure by magnetoelastic skin curvature sensor and ECG. IEEE Sens. J. **6**(3), 819–828 (2006)
113. J.P. Buschmann, J. Huang, New ear sensor for mobile, continuous and long term pulse oximetry, in *2010 Annual International Conference of the IEEE Engineering in Medicine and Biology Society, EMBC'10* (2010), pp. 5780–5783
114. S. Reichelt et al., Development of an implantable pulse oximeter. IEEE Trans. Biomed. Eng. **55**(2), 581–588 (2008)
115. N. Watthanawisuth, T. Lomas, A. Wisitsoraat, A. Tuantranont, Wireless wearable pulse oximeter for health monitoring using ZigBee wireless sensor network, in *ECTI-CON 2010 –*

The 2010 ECTI International Conference on Electrical Engineering/Electronics, Computer, Telecommunications and Information Technology (2010), pp. 575–579

116. S.-J. Jung, Y.-D. Lee, Y.-S. Seo, W.-Y. Chung, Design of a low-power consumption wearable reflectance pulse oximetry for ubiquitous healthcare system, in *2008 International Conference on Control, Automation and Systems, ICCAS 2008* (2008), pp. 526–528

117. Y. Chuo, B. Omrane, C. Landrock, J.N. Patel, B. Kaminska, Platform for all-polymer-based pulse-oximetry sensor, in *Proceedings of IEEE Sensors* (2010), pp. 155–159

118. J. Solà et al., SpO2 sensor embedded in a finger ring: design and implementation, in *Annual International Conference of the IEEE Engineering in Medicine and Biology – Proceedings* (2006), pp. 4295–4298

119. S.B. Duun, R.G. Haahr, K. Birkelund, E.V. Thomsen, A ring-shaped photodiode designed for use in a reflectance pulse oximetry sensor in wireless health monitoring applications. IEEE Sens. J. **10**(2), 261–268 (2010)

120. C. Schreiner, P. Catherwood, J. Anderson, J. McLaughlin, Blood oxygen level measurement with a chest-based Pulse Oximetry prototype System. Comput. Cardiol. **37**, 537–540 (2010)

121. J. Solà, O. Chételat, J. Krauss, On the reliability of pulse oximetry at the sternum, in *Annual International Conference of the IEEE Engineering in Medicine and Biology – Proceedings* (2007), p. 1537

122. J.P. Phillips, R.M Langford, S.H Chang, K. Maney, P.A Kyriacou, D.P Jones, Evaluation of a fiber-optic esophageal pulse oximeter, in *Proceedings of the 31st Annual International Conference of the IEEE Engineering in Medicine and Biology Society: Engineering the Future of Biomedicine, EMBC 2009* (2009), pp. 1509–1512

123. H. Bezuidenhout, D. Woods, J. Wyatt, J. Lawn, Are you blue yet? Developing low cost, alternative powered pulse oximetry for ill babies and children. IET Seminar Digest **2006**(11370), 83–87 (2006)

124. P. Venkata Reddy, A. Kumar, S.M.K. Rahman, T.S. Mundra, A new method for fingerprint antispoofing using pulse oxiometry, in *IEEE Conference on Biometrics: Theory, Applications and Systems, BTAS'07* (2007)

125. L.T. Foster, C.P. Keller, B. McKee, A. Ostry, *British Columbia Atlas of Wellness*, 2nd edn. (Western Geographical Press, 2011)

126. M.J. James, J.F. Fee, R.M. Horton, Modular biofeedback training system, US Patent 4,110,918, 1978

127. T.W. Glynn, M.J. James, Biofeedback training method and system, US Patent 3,942,516, 1976

128. D. Hillsman, Metered dose inhaler biofeedback training and evaluation system, US4984158A, 1991

129. D. Kilis, C.J. Matson, Inhalation device training system, US5167506A, 1992

130. T.L. Zucker, K.W. Samuelson, F. Muench, M.A. Greenberg, R.N. Gevirtz, The effects of respiratory sinus arrhythmia biofeedback on heart rate variability and posttraumatic stress disorder symptoms: A pilot study. Appl. Psychophysiol. Biofeedback **34**(2), 135–143 (2009)

131. M.B. Sterman, L.R. Macdonald, R.K. Stone, Biofeedback training of the sensorimotor electroencephalogram rhythm in man: effects on epilepsy. Epilepsia **15**(3), 395–416 (1974)

132. R. Markiewicz, The use of EEG biofeedback/neurofeedback in psychiatric rehabilitation. Psychiatr. Pol. **51**(6), 1095–1106 (2017)

133. S.R. Criswell, R. Sherman, S. Krippner, Cognitive behavioral therapy with heart rate variability biofeedback for adults with persistent noncombat-related posttraumatic stress disorder. Perm. J. **22** (2018)

134. B.G. Travers et al., Biofeedback-based, videogame balance training in autism. J. Autism Dev. Disord. **48**(1), 163–175 (2018)

135. Y.-Z. Lai, C.-H. Tai, Y.-S. Chang, K.-H. Chung, A mobile cloud-based biofeedback platform for evaluating medication response, in *Proceedings – 2017 IEEE 7th International Symposium on Cloud and Service Computing, SC2 2017*, vol. 2018 (2018), pp. 183–188

136. C.P. Wooldridge, G. Russell, Head position training with the cerebral palsied child: an application of biofeedback techniques. Arch. Phys. Med. Rehabil. **57**(9), 407–414 (1976)

137. H. Hasegawa, T. Tanaka, T. Wakaiki, K. Shimatani, Y. Kurita, *Biofeedback for Training Pelvic Floor Muscles with EMG Signals of Synergistic Muscles*, vol. 789 (2019)

138. L. Rousset, B. Halioua, Stress and psoriasis. Int. J. Dermatol. **57**(10), 1165–1172 (2018)

139. P.-W. Meyer, H.-C. Friederich, A. Zastrow, Breathe to ease – respiratory biofeedback to improve heart rate variability and coping with stress in obese patients: a pilot study. Ment. Heal. Prev. **11**, 41–46 (2018)

140. H. Badawi, F. Laamarti, F. Arafsha, A. El Saddik, Standardizing a shoe insole based on ISO/IEEE 11073 Personal Health Device (X73-PHD) standards. Adv. Intell. Syst. Comput. **918**, 764–778 (2019)

141. T. Zhang, J. Lu, F. Hu, Q. Hao, Bluetooth low energy for wearable sensor-based healthcare systems, in *2014 IEEE Healthcare Innovation Conference, HIC 2014* (2014), pp. 251–254

142. B.M. Dugan, S.M. Santisi, J.P. Latrille, Systems and methods for providing authenticated biofeedback information to a mobile device and for using such information, US20090270743A1, 2009

143. H.S. Merki, R.-R.C. Dries, Apparatus for the biofeedback control of body functions, US5002055A, 1991

144. L.M. Nashner, D.F. Goldstein, Apparatus and method for assessment and biofeedback training of body coordination skills critical and ball-strike power and accuracy during athletic activities, US5697791A, 1997

145. F. Lamaarti, F. Arafsha, B. Hafidh, A. El Saddik, Automated Athlete Haptic Training System for Soccer Sprinting, in *Proceedings - 2nd International Conference on Multimedia Information Processing and Retrieval, MIPR 2019*, 2019, pp. 303–309

146. M. Owlia, C. Ng, K. Ledda, M. Kamachi, A. Longfield, T. Dutta, Preventing back injury in caregivers using real-time posture-based feedback. Adv. Intell. Syst. Comput. **820**, 750–758 (2019)

147. B.J. Munro, T.E. Campbell, G.G. Wallace, J.R. Steele, The intelligent knee sleeve: a wearable biofeedback device. Sensors Actuators, B Chem. **131**(2), 541–547 (2008)

148. A. Khalil, S. Glal, StepUp: a step counter mobile application to promote healthy lifestyle, in *Proceedings of the 2009 International Conference on the Current Trends in Information Technology, CTIT 2009* (2009), pp. 208–212

149. I.M. Albaina, T. Visser, C.A. Van Der Mast, M.H. Vastenburg, Flowie: a persuasive virtual coach to motivate elderly individuals to walk, in *2009 3rd International Conference on Pervasive Computing Technologies for Healthcare – Pervasive Health 2009, PCTHealth 2009* (2009)

150. M.D. Rodríguez, J.R. Roa, A.L. Morán, S. Nava-Muñoz, CAMMInA: a mobile ambient information system to motivate elders to exercise. Pers. Ubiquitous Comput. **17**(6), 1127–1134 (2013)

151. Y. Lin, J. Jessurun, B. De Vries, H. Timmermans, in *Motivate: Context Aware Mobile Application for Activity Recommendation*. Lecture Notes in Computer Science (including subseries Lecture Notes in Artificial Intelligence and Lecture Notes in Bioinformatics), LNCS, vol. 7040 (2011), pp. 210–214

152. E. Buckeridge, M.C. LeVangie, B. Stetter, S.R. Nigg, B.M. Nigg, An on-ice measurement approach to analyse the biomechanics of ice hockey skating. PLoS One **10**(5), e0127324 (2015)

153. A. Isaev, Y. Romanov, V. Erlikh, Integrative activity of the kickboxer's body within modern sport training using biofeedback. Gazz. Medica Ital. Arch. Per Le Sci. Mediche **177**(3), 43–55 (2018)

154. S.M.N. Arosha Senanayake, A.G. Naim, Smart sensing and biofeedback for vertical jump in sports. Smart Sensors Measur. Instrum. **29**, 63–81 (2019)

155. A. Riposan-Taylor, I.J. Taylor, Personal connected devices for healthcare, in *The Internet of Things for Smart Urban Ecosystems* (2019), pp. 333–361

156. R. Elsaadi, M. Shafik, Deployment of assisted living technology using intelligent body sensors platform for elderly people health monitoring. Adv. Transdiscip. Eng. **3**, 219–224 (2016)

157. H. Badawi, A. El Saddik, Towards a context-aware biofeedback activity recommendation mobile application for healthy lifestyle, in *Procedia Computer Science*, vol. 21 (2013)

158. A. Rinaldi, C. Becchimanzi, F. Tosi, *Wearable Devices and Smart Garments for Stress Management*, vol. 824 (2019)

159. G. Kolev, N. Smykova, M. Selivanova, Wi-FIT project: self-learning medical expert system for lifestyle enhancement, in *IET Conference on Assisted Living 2009* (2009)

160. A. Danesh, F. Laamarti, A. El Saddik, in *HAVAS: The Haptic Audio Visual Sleep Alarm System*. Lecture Notes in Computer Science (including subseries Lecture Notes in Artificial Intelligence and Lecture Notes in Bioinformatics), vol. 9194 (2015), pp. 247–256

161. R.-X. Yu et al., Spectroscopic biofeedback on cutaneous carotenoids as part of a prevention program could be effective to raise health awareness in adolescents. J. Biophotonics **7**(11–12), 926–937 (2014)

162. G.B. Whatmore, D.R. Kohli, *The Physiopathology and Treatment of Functional Disorders; Including Anxiety States and Depression and the Role of Biofeedback Training* (1974)

163. A. Albraikan, B. Hafidh, A. El Saddik, IAware: a real-time emotional biofeedback system based on physiological signals. IEEE Access **6**, 78780–78789 (2018)

164. N. Peira, M. Fredrikson, G. Pourtois, Controlling the emotional heart: heart rate biofeedback improves cardiac control during emotional reactions. Int. J. Psychophysiol. **91**(3), 225–231 (2014)

165. Y. Ma, B. Xu, Y. Bai, G. Sun, R. Zhu, Daily mood assessment based on mobile phone sensing, in *Proceedings – BSN 2012: 9th International Workshop on Wearable and Implantable Body Sensor Networks* (2012), pp. 142–147

166. R. Al Rihawi, B. Ahmed, R. Gutierrez-Osuna, Dodging stress with a personalized biofeedback game, in *CHI PLAY 2014 – Proceedings of the 2014 Annual Symposium on Computer-Human Interaction in Play* (2014), pp. 399–400

167. O. Hilborn, H. Cederholm, J. Eriksson, C. Lindley, in *A Biofeedback Game for Training Arousal Regulation During a Stressful Task: The Space Investor*. Lecture Notes in Computer Science (including subseries Lecture Notes in Artificial Intelligence and Lecture Notes in Bioinformatics), LNCS, vol. 8008, no. PART 5 (2013), pp. 403–410

168. P. Jerčić et al., A serious game using physiological interfaces for emotion regulation training in the context of financial decision-making, in *ECIS 2012 – Proceedings of the 20th European Conference on Information Systems* (2012)

169. S. Orguc, H.S. Khurana, K.M. Stankovic, H.S. Leel, A.P. Chandrakasan, EMG-based real time facial gesture recognition for stress monitoring, in *Proceedings of the Annual International Conference of the IEEE Engineering in Medicine and Biology Society, EMBS*, vol. 2018 (2018), pp. 2651–2654

170. U. Chauhan, N. Reithinger, J.R. MacKey, Real-time stress assessment through PPG sensor for VR biofeedback, in *Proceedings of the 20th International Conference on Multimodal Interaction, ICMI 2018* (2018)

171. B. Choi, Breathing information extraction algorithm from PPG signal for the development of respiratory biofeedback app. Trans. Korean Inst. Electr. Eng. **67**(6), 794–798 (2018)

172. K. Horgan, S. Howard, F. Gardiner-Hyland, Pre-service teachers and stress during microteaching: an experimental investigation of the effectiveness of relaxation training with biofeedback on psychological and physiological indices of stress. Appl. Psychophysiol. Biofeedback **43**(3), 217–225 (2018)

173. R. Alharthi, R. Alharthi, B. Guthier, A. El Saddik, CASP: context-aware stress prediction system. Multimed. Tools Appl. **78**, 9011–9031 (2017)

174. G.E. Schwartz, Biofeedback as therapy. Some theoretical and practical issues. Am. Psychol. **28**(8), 666–673 (1973)

175. N.E. Miller, B.R. Dworkin, Critical issues in therapeutic applications of biofeedback. Biofeedback Theory Res., 129–161 (1977)

176. R.J. Quy, S.J. Hutt, S. Forrest, Sensorimotor rhythm feedback training and epilepsy: some methodological and conceptual issues. Biol. Psychol. **9**(2), 129–149 (1979)
177. F. Andrasik, E.B. Blanchard, J.G. Arena, N.L. Saunders, K.D. Barron, Psychophysiology of recurrent headache: methodological issues and new empirical findings. Behav. Ther. **13**(4), 407–429 (1982)
178. H.E. Adams, P.J. Brantley, J.K. Thompson, Biofeedback and headache: methodological issues. Clin. Biofeedback Effic. Mech. 358–367 (1982)
179. A.H. Black, J. Brener, L.V. DiCara, P.A. Obrist, *Cardiovascular Psychophysiology: Current Issues in Response Mechanisms, Biofeedback and Methodology* (Routledge, 2017)
180. E. Swinnen, Future challenges in functional gait training for children and young adults with cerebral palsy. Dev. Med. Child Neurol. **60**(9), 852 (2018)
181. G.O.D. Amorim, P.M.M. Balata, L.G. Vieira, T. Moura, H.J.D. Silva, Biofeedback in dysphonia – progress and challenges. Braz. J. Otorhinolaryngol. **84**(2), 240–248 (2018)
182. V. Attanasio, F. Andrasik, E.J. Burke, Clinical issues in utilizing biofeedback with children. Clin. Biofeedback Heal. **8**(2), 134–141 (1985)
183. S. Ancoli, J. Kamiya, Methodological issues in alpha biofeedback training. Biofeedback Self. Regul. **3**(2), 159–183 (1978)
184. C.J. Fisher, C.S. Moravec, L. Khorshid, The 'how and why' of group biofeedback for chronic disease management. Appl. Psychophysiol. Biofeedback **43**(4), 333–340 (2018)
185. R. Argent, P. Slevin, A. Bevilacqua, M. Neligan, A. Daly, B. Caulfield, Clinician perceptions of a prototype wearable exercise biofeedback system for orthopaedic rehabilitation: a qualitative exploration. BMJ Open **8**(10) (2018)
186. A. Kos, V. Milutinović, A. Umek, Challenges in wireless communication for connected sensors and wearable devices used in sport biofeedback applications. Futur. Gener. Comput. Syst. **92**, 582–592 (2019)
187. A. Umek, A. Kos, The role of high performance computing and communication for real-time biofeedback in sport. Math. Probl. Eng. **2016** (2016)
188. A. Kos, A. Umek, S. Tomazic, Biofeedback in sport: challenges in real-time motion tracking and processing, in *2015 IEEE 15th International Conference on Bioinformatics and Bioengineering, BIBE 2015* (2015)

Health 4.0: Digital Twins for Health and Well-Being

Namrata Bagaria, Fedwa Laamarti, Hawazin Faiz Badawi, Amani Albraikan, Roberto Alejandro Martinez Velazquez, and Abdulmotaleb El Saddik

Abstract With the increasing prevalence in the use of wearables, social media, smart living, and personalized recommender systems for consumer health, it becomes imperative to converge these technologies to provide personalized, context driven, proactive, and preventive care in real time. Digital Twins are a convergence technology and involve making a digital replica of any living or nonliving entity. At present, Digital Twins are extensively used in Industry 4.0 where Digital Twins help in optimizing the performance of machines by proactive and predictive maintenance. This chapter gives an overview of the existing literature and aims to provide an overview of existing literature on Digital Twins for personal health and well-being— key terminologies, key applications, and key gaps.

Keywords Digital Twins · Personal health · Well-being · Convergence · Wellness · Artificial intelligence

1 Introduction

Industry 4.0 is the current trend of automating manufacturing using sensors, actuators, intelligent prediction softwares, and data visualization. The hallmark of Industry 4.0 is data visualization using advanced 3D modelling and predictive analytics, using data from the sensors, providing proactive information on the health of a machine. Digital Twins is the technology at the heart of industry 4.0 and El Saddik has defined Digital Twins as "a convergence technology, which promises to bridge the gap between real and virtual" [1]. Another feature of the Digital Twins is value creation for the customer through product life cycle management once the product is out of the factory, thus pushing the manufacturing industry

N. Bagaria · F. Laamarti · H. F. Badawi · A. Albraikan · R. A. M. Martinez Velazquez · A. El Saddik (✉)
University of Ottawa, Ottawa, ON, Canada
e-mail: nbagaria@uottawa.ca; flaamart@uottawa.ca; hbada049@uottawa.ca; aalbr012@uottawa.ca; rmart121@uottawa.ca; elsaddik@uottawa.ca

© Springer Nature Switzerland AG 2020   143
A. El Saddik et al. (eds.), *Connected Health in Smart Cities*,
https://doi.org/10.1007/978-3-030-27844-1_7

from a mass to customized manufacturing mindset. This essentially means industry 4.0 is making manufacturing personal, customized, and putting the customer at the heart of production. This very shift, from mass manufacturing to consumer-centric manufacturing is what Health 4.0 can learn from. At present, there is no consensus on the definition of Health 4.0. However, drawing from the principles of Industry 4.0, Health 4.0 can be defined as shift from mass and reactive healthcare to personalized and proactive healthcare. Therefore, the Digital Twins becomes the technology, which holds the promise to deliver Health 4.0.

1.1   Health and Well-Being Definitions

There is no one universal definition of health. In fact, there are four main schools of thought on the definition of health:

1. Medical Model of Health Definition: Popular around the 1920s, health is defined as a "A state characterized by anatomic, physiologic and psychologic integrity; ability to perform personally valued family, work and community roles; ability to deal with physical, biologic, psychological and social stress" [2].
2. Holistic Model of Health Definition: In 1946, World Health Organization (WHO) definition, "A state of complete physical, mental and social well-being and not merely the absence of disease or infirmity" is the most commonly used definition of health [3].
3. Wellness Model of Health Definition: Promoted by the WHO definition was "The extent to which an individual or group is able to realize aspirations and satisfy needs, and to change or cope with the environment. Health is a resource for everyday life, not the objective of living; it is a positive concept, emphasizing social and personal resources, as well as physical capacities" [4]. For the purpose of this chapter, the wellness definition of health is used as a reference.
4. Ecological Definition of Health: In the mid-1990s, there was a push toward an ecological definition of health and an ecological definition is "A state in which humans and other living creatures with which they interact can coexist indefinitely" [5].

In addition, it is relevant to this chapter to also mention the definitions of well-being and wellness.

1. Well-being: "A good or satisfactory condition of existence; a state characterized by health, happiness, and prosperity; welfare" [6].
2. Wellness: The state of being in good health, especially as an actively pursued goal [7]. Wellness is hence an active process through which people become aware of, and make choices toward, a more successful existence [8]. The National Wellness Institute promotes six dimensions of wellness: emotional, occupational, physical, social, intellectual, and spiritual [8].

1.2 Parameters for Health and Well-Being

As we can see that there is a wide range of definitions on health which cover the different aspects of health and health is multidimensional. We curated a comprehensive list of parameters which help in determining the health and well-being of a person. This list is made using the four definitions of health, and consists of physical, lifestyle, mental, socioeconomic, and contextual factors, which determine the health and well-being of a person. World Health Organization [9], Ottawa Charter of Health Promotion [10], and Wikipedia [11–13] were used to populate this list. The purpose of this list is to showcase the complexity of individual health and well-being. This list is for informational purpose only and should be used for any form of diagnostic or prognostic purpose by individuals or organizations.

1. Physical health parameters: Generics, history of illness or diseases (past or present or family), vital signs—heart rate, temperature, blood pressure, respiratory rate, laboratory profile (blood, urine, stool tests), radiology and imaging (X-rays, scans), etc.
2. Lifestyle parameters: Diet, sleep, exercise, stress, quality of life, sexual health.
3. Mental and psychological health parameters: Consciousness, orientation (in time, place, and person), personality, attitude, emotions, mood, mental health illness, addictions, emotional intelligence, decision-making skills, resilience, relationships (personal and professional), job satisfaction, meaningful life, thought patterns, beliefs, and motivation.
4. Socioeconomic parameters—Education, income, housing, employment, and workplace conditions.
5. Gender parameters—Gender identity and sexual orientation.
6. Contextual parameters—Location (home, work), leisure and entertainment preferences, hobbies, environment quality (air, water, noise, radioactivity, built), neighborhood (walkability, safety, access to grocery), access to health system, life expectancy in the country of residence, peace and security in the country of residence, well-being index, quality of life index, social justice, and equity.
7. Cultural parameters—Religion, language, gender roles, and culturally distinct traditions.

1.3 Digital Transformation in Health

Personal health or consumer health informatics is a subdomain of biomedical and health informatics and is defined as "the study, development, and implementation of computer and telecommunications applications and interfaces designed to be used by health consumers" [14, 15]. The field of consumer health informatics started 25 years ago with the vision that one day, the end users or the patients will be in charge of their own health [15]. Scientific information in the field of consumer health informatics has grown significantly over the past 25 years and there has

Table 1 Summarizing the digital transformation of web, industry, and health

Version	Web	Industry	Health
1.0	Read only web [16]	Mechanization, water power, and steam power [17]	Printed health information
2.0	The writing and participating web [16]	Mass production, assembly line, and electricity [17]	Online communities, social media, patient-generated content, and wearables [18]
3.0	The semantic executing web [16]	Computer and automation [17]	Personalized health-related information [19]
4.0	Mobile web—Connects all devices in the real and virtual world in real time [16]	Cyber physical systems and Digital Twins [17]	Virtualization and personalization [20]

Table 2 Design principles for Health 4.0 [21, 22]

Sr. No.	Health 4.0
Principle 1	Interoperability
Principle 2	Virtualization
Principle 3	Decentralization
Principle 4	Real-time capability
Principle 5	Service orientation
Principle 6	Modularity
Principle 7	Safety, security, and resilience

been an evolution of consumer health with the evolution of the World Wide Web. The evolution of World Wide Web from 1.0 to 4.0 has brought about evolution of industry from Industry 1.0 to 4.0 and now this effect is spilling over to Health and we are seeing a momentum toward Health 4.0. Table 1 provides a synopsis of this digital transformation.

In the book, "Health 4.0: How Virtualization and Big Data are Revolutionizing Healthcare," the authors have laid the design principles of Health 4.0 and these are heavily borrowed from the principles of Industry 4.0 [21, 22]. They defined Health 4.0 as "Health 4.0 is progressive virtualization in order to enable the personalization of health and care next to real time for patients, professionals and formal and informal carers." Table 2 summarizes the design principles for Health 4.0.

2 Digital Twins

2.1 Defining Digital Twins

In a white paper by Deloitte, "Industry 4.0 and the Digital Twins technology," the authors have identified Digital Twins as the anchoring technology for

Industry 4.0 [23]. In his paper, "Digital Twins: A Convergence of Multimedia Technologies, El Saddik has defined Digital Twins as "Digital replications of living as well as non-living entities that enable data to be seamlessly transmitted between the physical and virtual worlds." According to El Saddik, "Digital Twins facilitate the means to monitor, understand, and optimize the functions of all physical entities and for humans provide continuous feedback to improve quality of life and well-being" [1]. The concept of Digital Twins in depicted in Figure 1.

2.2   Digital Twins for Health and Well-Being

Digital Twins (DT) technology plays a fundamental role in shaping the future of healthcare. Personal Digital Twins is a data-driven technology that reflects the health status of individuals inferred from the continuously collected data. It represents a priceless source that can be utilized in a triangular fashion: preventive healthcare, medical healthcare, and effective communication between DTs.

DT for preventive healthcare will enhance people's awareness about their health through the biofeedback features, and help them take the right action by means of personalized recommendations among others. Medical healthcare is also enhanced by the DT concept in terms of enabling health institutions and health-related organization to provide smart health services and telemedicine. Figure 1 illustrates the convergence of technologies to bring about the realization of the DT concept.

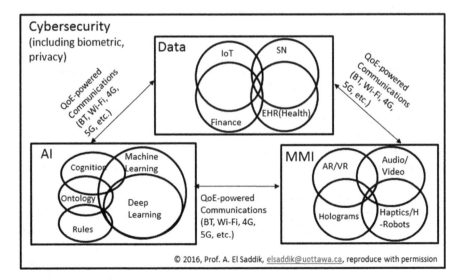

Fig. 1 Digital Twins Multimedia Ecosystem for health and well-being

2.3 Digital Twins Characteristics

The following Digital Twins characteristics are derived from [1]:

1. Unique Identifier: To communicate with its twin
2. Sensors: To replicate the senses of the real twin, i.e., sight, hearing, taste, smell, and touch
3. Artificial Intelligence: To make fast and intelligent decisions on behalf of the real twin
4. Communication: To interact in near real-time with the environment, real twins, and/or other Digital Twins
5. Representation: To interact with real twin or other twins, virtual representation can be in the form of 3D avatar, hologram, or even a humanoid social robots
6. Trust: To carry out sensitive tasks and decision-making of the real twin
7. Privacy and Security: To protect the identity of its twin as well as its privacy

3 Health Through Digital Twins

In Sect. 1 of this chapter, we had mentioned the different parameters for health and well-being and these different parameters for health can be considered as different pieces of the puzzle, which help construct the entire story of a person's health and well-being. The physical and mental parameters of a person's health help assess the current status of an individual's body and mind whereas the lifestyle parameters are contributing factors to a person's current health status. The lifestyle parameters are influenced by social, cultural, economic status, and context of an individual and thus there exist interdependencies of multiple parameters, which determine the health of a single individual. Therefore, we cannot simply tell an individual to make a health behavior change or resolve a health condition without understanding the completely understanding all the parameters of health. Since these many parameters are measured through different methods (such as wearables, social media, and laboratory tests), there becomes a need to converge the different data points of a person in one place. Apart from converging the data in one place, it also becomes imperative to help a user make use of the data and thus comes in the need for analytics and feedback for health and well-being.

Apart from this based on the geography of a person, the Digital Twins can help in grocery shopping, consumption of fresh fruits and vegetables, help increase walking in the neighborhood based on walkability and temperature of neighborhood and also suggest walking groups through different social media or group activity platforms. Thus, the Digital Twins not only used body parameters to help make a decision for behavioral change but also considers the social and contextual factors.

Thus, a Digital Twins is made from the convergence of multimedia technologies involving big data, predictive analytics, visualization techniques, cybersecurity, and communications. The Digital Twins can be as simple as one sensor or one body parameter or can be as complex as a complete human body from genomic to gross body level. Since human beings are not just their biological bodies but also their physical and social environments, contextual factors become very important in designing a Digital Twins for health and well-being. Once the anatomy of a Digital Twins is understood, it is important to understand its physiology or functionality. The main function of the Digital Twins is to communicate with its real twin or with other Digital Twins (which may be possible in the near future) and help make the best decisions based on the complete set of parameters. We have illustrated this concept through three different case studies.

4 Case Studies

4.1 DT for Heart Care

Most heart-related diseases can be avoided only by leading a healthy life. There are risk factors associated with these diseases, alcohol consumption, obesity, smoking, sedentary lifestyle, and poor diet are the main factors. By reducing these risk factors or even suppressing them, the individual can significantly reduce the chances of being affected by any of these diseases.

With Digital Twins you can promote a healthy lifestyle as a strategy to prevent heart diseases. Digital Twins collects data from different BAN type of sensors, for example, an accelerometer, GPS, or a smartwatch that monitors heart rate and galvanic response. The AI module can use machine learning to estimate the level of physical activity for the real twin on a daily basis. From this estimation, the real twin receives recommendations on different activities outdoors or indoors to participate according to personal preferences or physical condition in the real twin.

Digital Twins knows everything about its real counterpart, based on caloric consumption, weight, clinical data, and/or biological signals obtained from different sensors, it can also detect situations related to obesity, alcohol, or tobacco consumption for which it can help the real twin to reduce or suppress effectively based on your personal preferences. This is how Digital Twins can also act as a persuasive system that supports the user to reduce or even eliminate the risk factors associated with heart disease and ultimately, prevent them. Take obesity, for example, since the Digital Twins knows about food consumption preferences, what the real twin likes or dislikes it can recommend the best meal plan that is best suited for the real twin along with a set of exercises and activities that are more adequate to the physical state of the real twin.

4.2   DT and Emotions

Digital Twins is the enabling technology that facilitates the means to monitor, understand, and provides continuous feedback to improve quality of life and well-being. Thus, a Digital Twins can consider a solution to enhance mood to enhance the quality of life and emotional well-being. The Digital Twins for emotional well-being system is a closed loop feedback system in which information taken from the human body is translated into a language perceivable by any of the human senses. The loop begins with human sensory information from the body. The physiological signals are then interpreted and converted to a recognizable emotion state. Feedback is provided to the individual through recommendations while monitoring the user behavior and action tendency. If the quality of service is not satisfied, then the system will loop back to the matching process to recalculate the feedback. Once the biofeedback information is consumed by the human brain, a change in the mental state will occur, which will cause a change in the human physiological state. The cycle then starts again.

The primary goal of Digital Twins system for emotional well-being should include tracking, assist, remind, intervene, and reinforce learning. A biofeedback loop can allow users to see their bodily reactions in real time, and assist users in finding both the positive and the negative stressful patterns in their behavior. While opportune moment detection helps provide just-in-time interventions as needed. Then, reinforce learning helps to learn the user preferences.

4.3   DT for Sport

The Digital Twins has many applications related to health and well-being, among which is sport. Indeed, Digital Twins can help improve tremendously the quality of sport both by giving the athletes access to automated training as well as by giving them the benefit of personalized feedback during and after the training.

Indeed, the DT can allow athletes to work out even in the absence of the coach but following his/her recommendations. We suggest here an application of the DT in sport, where we show that how athletes can benefit from it. We used sensors as the DT data source and actuators as DT representation to give feedback to the real twin who is here the athlete. The DT replaces temporarily the coach by helping the athlete follow his/her recommendations without the coach's presence.

We studied the case of training for soccer sprinting. As sensors, we used the smart insoles [24] in order to collect pressure point data and send it to the DT storage. The DT was configured by the coach for each athlete following their level, then the DT sends notifications to the athletes to inform them of the availability of a new training set for them. The athlete can start their sprint training at their own preferred time, during which the DT accompanies them with tracking and feedback. The feedback is delivered through haptic armbands that signal to the athlete when to start sprinting and when to switch to periods of recovery for the duration recommended by the coach. After the training is completed, the DT makes it available to the coach (and the athlete) by means of visualizations in the form of graphs and feet heatmaps showing the results of the training that the coach can analyze and provide the next training recommendation based on the athlete performance. We performed a pilot study with three soccer athletes who reported that the DT for sport proved very useful for them. They rated it at an efficiency of eight out of ten and declared that they would adopt it to facilitate their sprint training.

The Digital Twins system can also automate the performance analysis using artificial intelligence, and act as a coach assistant, providing him/her with suggested athlete recommendations and waiting for the coach's approval before notifying the athlete of the training outcome and next steps.

5 Conclusion

Digital Twins bring about the promise to help improve the health and well-being of individuals, provided they are able to get their trust and provide data privacy. Some challenges exist among which delivering a high degree of personalization, which is context aware, culturally apt, matching user's lifestyle, and preferences. Our current interest is the study of role of incentives to self-health behaviors and links them to create a well-being economy or to initiate dialogue for a well-being economy. In the end, we need consumer evangelism and participation in use and scale of digital technologies for personal health and well-being.

References

1. A. El Saddik, Digital twins: the convergence of multimedia technologies. IEEE MultiMedia **25**(2), 87–92 (2018). https://doi.org/10.1109/MMUL.2018.023121167
2. J. Stokes, J. Noren, S. Shindell, Definition of terms and concepts applicable to clinical preventive medicine. J. Community Health **8**(1), 33–41 (1928). http://www.ncbi.nlm.nih.gov/pubmed/676
3. J. Stokes, J. Noren, S. Shindell, *Constitution of the World Health Organization* (1982), https://www.who.int/governance/eb/who_constitution_en.pdf. Accessed 15 Mar 2019
4. World Health Organization. Regional Office for Europe, *Health Promotion: A Discussion Document on the Concept and Principles*. Summary report of the Working Group on Concept and Principles of Health Promotion, Copenhagen, 9–13 July 1984 (WHO Regional Office for Europe, Copenhagen, 1984), http://www.who.int/iris/handle/10665/107835. http://apps.who.int/iris/bitstream/handle/10665/107835/E90607.pdf?sequence=1&isAllowed=y. Accessed 15 Mar 2019
5. J.M. Last, J.H. Abramson, International Epidemiological Association, *A Dictionary of Epidemiology* (Oxford University Press, 1995)
6. https://www.dictionary.com/browse/well-being. Accessed 15 Mar 2019
7. https://en.oxforddictionaries.com/definition/wellness. Accessed 15 Mar 2019
8. https://www.nationalwellness.org/page/AboutWellness. Accessed 15 Mar 2019

9. World Health Organisation, https://www.who.int/social_determinants/en/. Accessed 15 Mar 2019
10. Ottawa Charter for Health Promotion, https://www.who.int/healthpromotion/conferences/previous/ottawa/en/. Accessed 15 Mar 2019
11. Wikipedia, https://en.wikipedia.org/wiki/Health. Accessed 15 Mar 2019
12. Wikipedia, https://en.wikipedia.org/wiki/Health_indicator. Accessed 15 Mar 2019
13. Wikipedia, https://en.wikipedia.org/wiki/Vital_signs. Accessed 15 Mar 2019
14. *The Ferguson Report: The Newsletter of Consumer Health Informatics and Online Health.* Ferguson Report (1999), http://www.fergusonreport.com/articles/tfr07-03.htm
15. G. Demiris, Consumer health informatics: past, present, and future of a rapidly evolving domain. Yearb. Med. Inform. **Suppl 1**, S42–S47 (2016). https://doi.org/10.15265/IYS-2016-s005
16. T. Fleerackers, M. Meyvis, *Web 1.0 vs Web 2.0 vs Web 3.0 vs Web 4.0 vs Web 5.0 – A Bird's Eye on the Evolution and Definition*, https://flatworldbusiness.wordpress.com/flat-education/previously/web-1-0-vs-web-2-0-vs-web-3-0-a-bird-eye-on-the-definition/. Accessed 15 Mar 2019
17. C. Roser, *Illustration of Industry 4.0, Showing the Four "Industrial Revolutions" with a Brief English Description*, AllAboutLean.com. Accessed 15 Mar 2019
18. Wikipedia, https://en.wikipedia.org/wiki/Health_2.0. Accessed 15 Mar 2019
19. Wikipedia, https://en.wikipedia.org/wiki/Health_3.0. Accessed 15 Mar 2019
20. C. Thuemmler, The Case for Health 4.0, in *Health 4.0: How Virtualization and Big Data are Revolutionizing Healthcare*, (Springer International Publishing, Cham, 2017), pp. 1–22
21. M. Hermann, T. Pentek, B. Otto, Design principles for Industrie 4.0 scenarios, in *2016 49th Hawaii International Conference on System Sciences (HICSS)* (IEEE), pp. 3928–3937. https://doi.org/10.1109/HICSS.2016.488
22. C. Thuemmler, C. Bai (eds.), *Health 4.0: How Virtualization and Big Data are Revolutionizing Healthcare* (Springer International Publishing, Cham, 2017)., https://doi.org/10.1007/978-3-319-47617-9
23. A. Parrott, L. Warshaw, No Title, (2017), https://www2.deloitte.com/insights/us/en/focus/industry-4-0/digital-twin-technology-smart-factory.html. Accessed 15 Mar 2019
24. H. Badawi, F. Laamarti, F. Arafsha, A. El Saddik, Standardizing a shoe insole based on ISO/IEEE 11073 personal health device (X73-PHD) standards, in *Proceedings of the International Conference on Information Technology & Systems (ICIT)* (2019)

Incorporating Artificial Intelligence into Medical Cyber Physical Systems: A Survey

Omid Rajabi Shishvan, Daphney-Stavroula Zois, and Tolga Soyata

Abstract Medical Cyber Physical Systems (MCPSs) prescribe a platform in which patient health information is acquired by the emerging Internet of Things (IoT) sensors, pre-processed locally, and processed via advanced machine intelligence algorithms in the cloud. The emergence of MCPSs holds the promise to revolutionize remote patient healthcare monitoring, accelerate the development of new drugs or treatments, and improve the quality-of-life for patients who are suffering from various medical conditions among other various applications. The amount of raw medical data gathered through the IoT sensors in an MCPS provides a rich platform that artificial intelligence algorithms can use to provide decision support for either medical experts or patients. In this paper, we provide an overview of MCPSs and the data flow through these systems. This includes how raw physiological signals are converted into features and are used by machine intelligence algorithms, the types of algorithms available for the healthcare domain, how the data and the decision support output are presented to the end user, and how all of these steps are completed in a secure fashion to preserve the privacy of the users.

Keywords IoT · Cloud computing · Sensors · Physiological signals · Machine learning · Cyber-physical systems

1 Introduction

The rapid emergence of IoT devices in conjunction with advances in computational capabilities have led to a growing interest of MCPSs in both research and commercial fields [1]. With applications spanning from general areas such as fitness tracking and personal health [2] to more technical fields such as remote health monitoring and medical decision support systems [3, 4], MCPSs have emerged as an

O. R. Shishvan · D.-S. Zois · T. Soyata (✉)
University at Albany, SUNY, Albany, NY, USA
e-mail: orajabishishvan@albany.edu; dzois@albany.edu; tsoyata@albany.edu

© Springer Nature Switzerland AG 2020   153
A. El Saddik et al. (eds.), *Connected Health in Smart Cities*,
https://doi.org/10.1007/978-3-030-27844-1_8

effective technology that can not only improve general medical practice [5] but also create new business opportunities [6]. These systems consist of a network of sensors worn on the body of patients and gather physiological and environmental signals; these signals are first pre-processed at a location that is close to the acquisition source, and transmitted to either a private or public cloud. A private cloud is owned directly by a Healthcare Organization (HCO), while a public cloud is rented from cloud service providers, such as Amazon EC2. The primary purpose of the cloud is to execute a set of machine intelligence algorithms and provide decision support to healthcare professionals (e.g., doctors and nurses). In addition to the previously gathered corpus of relevant information, MCPSs use the acquired data to train machine intelligence algorithms and make inferences regarding the potential medical conditions of a patient based on his/her physiological data.

These aforementioned emerging clinical and personal healthcare applications both benefit from devices that acquire medical data and process them with varying degrees of intelligence; in this way, an MCPS is not limited to IoT devices, but any sensory device, coupled with a platform that can run the decision support algorithms.

Given the sensitive nature of the personal medical information, measures must be taken within the MCPS to remain in compliance with confidentiality laws that protect personal health information. For example, Health Information Privacy and Accountability Act (HIPAA) laws in the USA [7] have strict restrictions requiring that medical information can only be released to authorized users. This privacy issue is especially important if the HCO uses public infrastructures as a computation platform where the hardware is shared with multiple unknown users.

In this chapter, an overview of an MCPS and the artificial intelligence algorithms that are used in it are presented. Specifically, in Sect. 2, the general structure of an MCPS is described. In Sect. 3, the data acquisition component of the MCPS is described. Details of the decision support process are presented in Sect. 4, in which the algorithms are studied based on their goals. Sections 4.1 through 4.4 describe these goals, including knowledge discovery, classification, regression, and sequential decision-making, respectively. Section 5 is where visualization is elaborated on, which is an important stage of the decision support process. Issues surrounding data privacy and security are discussed in Sect. 6. Section 7 discusses the challenges and open issues in incorporating artificial intelligence in MCPSs, and summary and concluding remarks are provided in Sect. 8.

2   Medical Cyber-Physical Systems

One of the most promising applications for an MCPS is real-time, long-term health monitoring [6, 8]. The general structure of an MCPS consists of multiple components as shown in Fig. 1. The data acquisition, aggregation, and pre-processing layer gathers all relevant and necessary information through wearable sensors in a Wireless Body Area Network (WBAN), environmental sensors, and other external

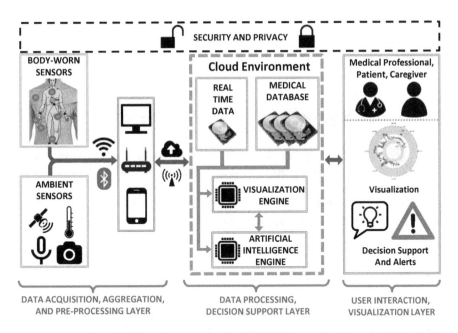

Fig. 1 An overview of different components of a MCPS. The raw data is acquired from body-worn sensors. After a pre-processing phase, the signals are aggregated and transferred to the cloud, where they are processed by machine intelligence algorithms. The outcomes of the algorithms are then presented to the users in the form of visualization, decision support suggestions, or alerts. All of these steps are subject to security measures to ensure that the data is kept secure and private

sources of data such as the Internet. This data is then aggregated, and features are extracted and transmitted to the cloud for use by machine intelligence algorithms. These algorithms yield outcomes that can be then used for decision support or visualization purposes. All of these components are subject to privacy guidelines to ensure the security and privacy of the data that is traveling within the MCPS. We discuss these layers in more detail in the sections to follow.

2.1 Data Acquisition, Aggregation, and Pre-processing

Data acquisition is the first component of an MCPS, which gathers physiological and ambient signals, primarily through WBAN sensors but also sensors deployed in the environment. This component also aggregates the data, performs the necessary pre-processing, and transmits the resulting data to the cloud. This transmission is usually done through conventional communication links such as 3G, 4G, or 5G networks [9, 10] or other emerging communication links such as the communication links provided by Low Power Wide Area Network (LoRaWAN) protocol [11]. Note that this data can either be in raw format (cf. Sect. 3.1) or represented by a set of features that is extracted from it (cf. Sect. 3.2). The format of the data depends on many factors, such as the application, the bandwidth of the data connection, or the system's power supply limits. We will discuss this component further in Sect. 3.

2.2 Decision Support Using Machine Intelligence

The decision support component of an MCPS is responsible for the analysis of the data to detect informative patterns. Depending on the application, the goal of this layer may be to find novel patterns in the input data (Sect. 4.1), classify the input data into a limited number of *classes* (Sect. 4.2), provide an estimate for given input data (Sect. 4.3), or provide a suggestion for a decision-making task (Sect. 4.4).

2.3 Data Visualization

It is vital that data is reported in a format comprehensible to both medical professionals and patients. This includes all acquired data, decision support suggestions, and emergency alerts. Medical data gathered through sensors is typically too voluminous for the human brain to process [12], which in turn necessitates the generation of informative summaries. It is essential that these summaries highlight sections of data that require attention without sacrificing accuracy; this can significantly reduce human errors and ensure efficient diagnosis. Section 5 discusses data visualization in depth.

2.4 Data Privacy

All personal medical data in the USA is protected under the HIPAA regulations [7]. Through its transition between the components of an MCPS, personal medical data should be treated in such a way that its integrity remains intact without compromising the patient's privacy. This requires special provisions during the design of an MCPS, such as encrypting data and enforcing restricted access to personnel. Section 6 provides detailed explanation on data privacy and security.

3 Data Acquisition, Aggregation, and Pre-processing

Machine intelligence algorithms are used by MCPSs to generate desired outcomes based on a variety of different data. In this section, the different stages of the data acquisition, aggregation, and pre-processing process are discussed along with the different types of data used.

3.1 Raw Data

WBAN sensors collect and communicate (through wireless protocols such as IEEE 802.11ah [13], WirelessHART [14], Bluetooth Low Energy (BLE) [15, 16], and ZigBee [17]) a variety of raw medical data including but not limited to data from respiration sensors, heart-rate monitors, blood pressure, glucose, and oxygen saturation monitoring sensors, and muscle activity sensors [1]. Note that other ambient sensors such as environmental temperature, location, and sound may be useful for some applications. These signals are usually gathered with relatively high sampling frequency and are prone to environmental noise, whether induced by patients' movements or by other electrical devices in the vicinity [18]. As a result, redundant information is included in the raw data that can be omitted without losing any valuable information. Thus, direct transmission of raw data to the next layer of the system can not only waste valuable bandwidth, but also expend battery resources in mobile devices that operate under severe energy constraints. To address both drawbacks, *features* are extracted from raw data to retain information that is useful for decision support and visualization.

3.2 Features

The process during which *features* are extracted from raw data is studied in Sect. 3.3. These features are presented as variables, which are used as an input to machine intelligence algorithms or the visualization system. Section 3.4 studies generic (application-independent) features (such as the average of the signal), which can be used in almost any application, although application-specific features (such as certain time intervals of an electrocardiogram (ECG)), as studied in Sect. 3.5, can have a much better representative power.

3.3 Feature Extraction

Feature extraction [19] can be accomplished via different dimensionality reduction techniques that extract the most statistically significant information from raw data. Common feature extraction methods include

- **Principal Component Analysis (PCA)** is a technique for dimensionality reduction that transforms a collection of correlated data to a collection of uncorrelated data points. PCA is widely used in the literature; for example, authors in [20] detect sensorineural hearing loss in Magnetic Resonance Imaging (MRI) images by transforming these images into features through wavelet decomposition and dimensionality reduction via PCA.

- **Kernel PCA (KPCA)** is based on PCA and uses pre-defined kernel functions, such as polynomial or Gaussian functions, to perform non-linear data transformation. For example, authors in [21] use kernel PCA to reduce 700 features to only 5 features, which are then used to assess depressive symptoms in different individuals.
- **Canonical Correlation Analysis (CCA)** is a method for analyzing the correlation between two different multivariate inputs. In [22], authors develop a hybrid brain-computer interface smart glass that is used for controlling electronic devices. They use CCA as part of their system to find the most similar Electroencephalograph (EEG) recordings and classify the user's action based on that.
- **Multidimensional Scaling (MDS)** is a dimensionality reduction method that transforms data points into a lower dimension, while maintaining the Euclidean distance between the data points. For example, authors in [23] use MDS as part of their process for daily activity recognition among subjects in which the data is presented as a matrix and MDS is used to convert them to a lower dimensional space that makes classifying the activity matrix easier.
- **Artificial Neural Networks (ANNs)** can be structured in such a way that they are able to extract features from the raw data. For example, autoencoders are a type of ANNs that take a high-dimensional signal as an input, convert them to a signal with lower dimension, and reconstruct the original signal from the converted signal. This lower dimensional data provides efficient feature reduction [24]. An example application of ANNs is presented in [25], where the authors use deep belief networks in an emotion recognition scheme in which the network extracts features from high dimensional audio and video input signals. Another application is discussed in [26], where authors build a fall detection system that utilizes frequency modulated radars. They use an autoencoder to extract features from the data and show that it improves the performance as compared to conventional methods such as PCA.

3.4 Application-Independent Features

In many applications, features extracted from raw data are very generic and do not depend on the application of interest. As a result, they can be extracted from a variety of medical data and should be interpreted based on the context of the application. The features can be categorized as: *temporal*, *spectral*, and *cepstral*. Temporal and spectral features are extracted from the time and frequency domain of a signal respectively, while cepstral features are extracted based on the changes in a signal's spectral bands.

3.4.1   Temporal Features

Statistical information of data, ranging from its mean and median to kurtosis and different percentiles, are typical examples of temporal features that may reveal useful information. Frequently, temporal features on their own are sufficient to accurately summarize a variety of data. For example, in [27], temporal features such as the mean of maxima and the mean of minima from acceleration and heart rhythm signals can adequately and accurately detect the patients' physical activity. Another application is presented in [28], where the median frequency among other temporal features is extracted from skin conductance, ECG, and electromyogram (EMG) signals and used to detect mental stress among people. More complex temporal features (e.g., Lempel-Ziv complexity, Hermite polynomial expansion (HPE) coefficients, central tendency measure) can be extracted from the data by applying advanced processing algorithms. For example, authors in [29] use both central tendency measure and Lempel-Ziv complexity of SpO^2 signals for real-time detection of sleep apnea.

3.4.2   Spectral Features

In addition to temporal features, analyzing the signals in the frequency domain can also provide useful information about their characteristics. Some of the features in this domain include power of the signal in various frequency bands, phase angle, and the spectral entropy. An example application of spectral features is discussed in [30], where EEG signals are analyzed. By using features such as dominant frequency and normalized spectral entropy, an epilepsy application is developed.

3.4.3   Cepstral Features

Cepstral features have proven to be useful for removing disturbance in the data induced by uncontrollable parameters such as sensor displacement. The cepstrum of a signal is the inverse Fourier transform of the logarithm of the spectrum of the signal. Cepstral features have been used for respiration problems detection from breath sound recordings [31], detecting heart rhythm arrhythmia from ECG recordings [32], and sound signal classification for assistive technologies for hearing impaired patients [33].

3.5   *Application-Specific Features*

Each biomarker signal has its own unique characteristics that can be extracted as features with high information content. For example, in an ECG recording (depicted in Fig. 2), some specific features with high information content are the RR interval and the QT interval [34]. Furthermore, it is sometimes useful to *fuse* together

Fig. 2 A simplified example
of an ECG waveform
showing two consecutive
heartbeats. The QT and RR
intervals are indicated in the
plot

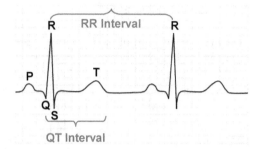

simple features such as the RR and QT intervals in order to create more informative features. For instance, a corrected form of QT values is calculated by normalizing it with respect to the RR value:

$$QTcB = \frac{QT}{\sqrt{RR}} \tag{1}$$

Another example of an application-specific feature is the power of an EEG signal in different bandwidths such as between 0.5 and 4 Hz (Delta wave) and 7.5 and 12.5 Hz (Alpha wave).

3.6 Feature Selection

Even though a large set of features can be extracted, not all of them are necessarily useful for machine intelligence algorithms. In practice, features must bear useful information and low redundancy, while at the same time, they need to be fast to process, to avoid burdening system performance [35]. Feature selection techniques can be used to select only the subset of features that contribute the most to the success of the entire system. Some feature selection methods that are commonly used are

- **Sequential Backward Selection (SBS)** starts by using all available features and sequentially eliminates the features that have minimal impact on system performance (e.g., accuracy). In [36], authors use SBS to select the most important features from all available time-domain and frequency-domain features to enable accurate sleep apnea detection using pulse oximeters.
- **Sequential Forward Selection (SFS)**, unlike SBS, starts with an empty set of features and incorporates the features that have the maximum effect on the system performance in every step. An example application of SFS is provided in [37], where the authors develop a wearable glove system to detect stress events in drivers. They use SFS to select only the features that achieve satisfactory level of accuracy in proposed system.

- **Sequential Forward Floating Selection (SFFS)** combines SBS and SFS techniques; at each step, it dynamically adds or removes a variable number of features. This approach starts with forward selection and then employs backward selection. An example application of SFFS is discussed in [38], where authors use SFFS to select the features for their proposed cognitive ability evaluation scheme. They use SFFS on a set of 33 features and show that it selects certain features more frequently while it completely ignores some other features.
- **Correlation-Based Feature Selection (CFS)** selects the subset of features that have the highest correlation with the output classes, yet they are not correlated to each other. In [39], authors detect epileptic seizures using EEG signals and use an improved version of CFS to select the best features from different domains including time and frequency. They show that CFS is able to maintain accuracy with a reduced number of features.
- **Genetic Algorithms (GA)** optimize a problem by searching among possible solutions using natural selection-based techniques. An initial set of solutions is identified, from which the best options are selected. These selections are then modified through *mutations*, converging to the optimal solution. An example application of using GA for feature selection is discussed in [40], where evolution-based algorithms select the best features from EEG signals for emotion recognition. Another example is provided in [41], where authors use GA to select ECG features for cardiac disease classification.

4   Decision Support

One of the most important functions of an MCPS is to provide decision support to aid in clinical diagnosis or personal health monitoring. Decision support systems transform the results of machine intelligence algorithms (i.e., output values) into appropriate formats that facilitate the understanding of patients and medical experts. There are various types of decision support including but not limited to providing an alert (e.g., warning for low blood sugar), estimating the likelihood of a disease (e.g., a developing arrhythmia), or displaying an intuitive visualization of the acquired signals over a long-term observation period (e.g., Holter ECG monitoring).

Decision support systems can be categorized by their respective goals as follows:

- **Knowledge discovery**: Knowledge discovery algorithms aim to identify previously unknown relations in data. Applications such as data clustering and anomaly detection fall under this category. We will elaborate on this category in Sect. 4.1.
- **Classification**: Classification algorithms work with datasets with known input-output relations and their output can be categorized into a limited number of classes. We will provide more details on this category in Sect. 4.2.

- **Regression**: Regression algorithms work with continuous outputs, as we will study in Sect. 4.3.
- **Sequential decision-making**: Sequential decision-making algorithms are used when a task requires automated decisions to be made over time in order to improve performance; we will provide more details on this category in Sect. 4.4.

4.1 Knowledge Discovery

Algorithms in this category aim to discover relations in a dataset with *unlabeled* data, i.e., data points with no previously known input/output relationships. Clustering and anomaly detection are typical and most common tasks related to knowledge discovery. Clustering involves grouping similar data points together, using techniques such as K-means, hierarchical clustering, and probabilistic clustering models also known as mixture models. On the other hand, anomaly detection focuses on identifying data points that do not conform to expected patterns when compared to other data points in a dataset. It is important to note that many anomaly detection algorithms are based on clustering algorithms that identify data points which do not belong to any major cluster.

Clustering and anomaly detection have been applied to a variety of healthcare applications including but not limited to healthcare insurance fraud, discovering unknown drug interactions, tracking epidemics, and estimating survival rates. In [42], authors employ outlier detection techniques to detect insurance frauds in health insurance claims. Specifically, they calculate the proportion of claims of fraudulent versus non-fraudulent providers, and show that fraudulent providers tend to file claims related to certain health issues more often. In [43], authors use mixture models to cluster patients into different mortality rate groups based on their physiological data gathered in Intensive Care Units (ICUs). Clustering techniques are also successful in producing trajectories of physiological data over time based on patients' individual clusters. For instance, the authors in [44] use an hierarchical clustering algorithm to detect the severity of three disease types (i.e., Crohn's disease, cystic fibrosis, down syndrome) based on lab test results. Even though patients diagnosed with Crohn's disease and cystic fibrosis can be successfully clustered based on the severity of their disease, this is not the case for down syndrome patients. The last observation is attributed to limited quantity of data. A similar application is discussed in [45], where K-means is employed on medical and mood data collected from chronic obstructive pulmonary disease (COPD) patients to track their symptoms over time and monitor the progression of their disease.

Association rule mining is another typical example of knowledge discovery, where the goal is to identify relations between variables in a dataset. For example, authors in [46] employ association rule mining on the FDA adverse event reporting system database to detect drug pairs that are associated with increased blood glucose

Table 1 Confusion matrix

	Predicted condition	
Actual condition	Positive	Negative
Positive	True positive (TP)	False negative (FN)
Negative	False positive (FP)	True negative (TN)

levels. They are able to show that a potential candidate for elevated blood glucose levels is a (previously unknown) drug combination of Paroxetine and Pravastatin, and a clinical trial verifies their findings.

4.2 Classification

In many datasets, the output values have a limited number of possibilities (i.e., *classes*), which implies that the output values are already divided into subgroups. A classification algorithm determines which subpopulation (class) each input value belongs to. The results of classification algorithms, specially the ones with binary outputs, can be presented in a confusion matrix as shown in Table 1. Based on these definitions, other metrics such as accuracy, F1-score, and the Area under receiver operating characteristic curve (AUC) are defined and used to describe the performance of classifiers. For example, accuracy is defined by Eq. (2) and F1-score is defined by Eq. (3) while AUC is defined by plotting the graph of true positive rate vs. false positive rate and calculating the area under its curve. For all of these metrics, the closer their value to "1", the better the classifier.

$$\text{Accuracy} = \frac{TP + TN}{TP + FP + FN + TN} \tag{2}$$

$$\text{F1-score} = \frac{2TP}{2TP + FP + FN} \tag{3}$$

An example classification application is described in [47], where the authors classify patients into one of two sub-populations, (i) patients with sleep apnea, and (ii) without apnea. Such a classification, in which there are only two possible output values is termed *binary classification*. Their classification scheme is a linear integer model that takes input features such as age, sex, smoking condition, and snoring during sleep. The authors report an AUC value of 0.785. Another classification application is presented in [48], where the authors take the ECG recordings of patients and detect whether they have long QT syndrome [34, 49] or not. They extract features such as the heart rate from the ECG data and feed them into multiple classification algorithms such as Support Vector Machines (SVMs), k-nearest neighbors, and AdaBoost. They are able to achieve accuracies higher than 70% using SVMs with radial basis function.

In [50], authors take histopathological images and classify gliomas (a type of cancer) into two classes: (i) low-grade glioma and (ii) high-grade glioma. They process the images and divide them into separate segments, where for each segment a cell-count profile is created. A decision tree algorithm is then applied to the cell-count profiles, which identifies the glioma as a low-grade or a high-grade one with 80% accuracy. Another work in [51] uses retinal images to detect Retinopathy of prematurity, a cause of blindness among children. They manually prepare a mask for the vessels in the images, fit splines into these masks, and extract feature from these splines. SVM classifiers are used to classify these vessel features into healthy and abnormal cases, where they achieve ≈95% accuracy in this task.

The work presented in [52] uses data gathered through smartphones for the purpose of remote health monitoring and physical activity classification. Authors take smartphone accelerometer data and extract features such as mean, standard deviation, and the peaks of the measurements from the signal. By using these features in a decision tree algorithm, they are able to classify multiple physical activities of the subjects, including {sitting, walking, going up or down the stairs, cycling}, with more than 80% accuracy. Authors in [27] also investigate activity recognition with an SVM classifier. They gather ECG and accelerometer data and extract time and cepstral features from these two signals. By fusing these two sets of features, they are able to distinguish nine physical activities with accuracies as high as 97.3%.

A study that uses mobile phone data in addition to wearable sensors is conducted in [28], where authors recognize stress among the participants in the study. Data for the study is gathered through a wrist sensor that has an accelerometer and measures skin conductance and mobile phone usage. They combine this information with a user survey that includes information about their mood, tiredness, and alcoholic and caffeinated beverage intake. Authors classify subjects as {stressed and not-stressed} with accuracy as high as 87.5%.

In [53], authors build a sleep apnea monitoring system that classifies the subjects based on their ECG signals. Participants undergo a sleep study, in which their ECG measurements are recorded; they are able to detect respiratory movements from these recordings in addition to extracting both time-based features and spectral features from the signals. By using an SVM classifier, they are able to achieve accuracies between 85% and 90% in sleep apnea detection. Authors in [54] build a non-intrusive mental-health tracker system. The system gathers features such as subject's head movement, heart rate, eye blinks, pupil radius, and facial expressions through a webcam and records other features that include the interactions of the subject with the computer and the content that the user views. Using this input data, they are able to classify subjects' emotion as positive, neutral, and negative with an AUC of 0.95.

Some classification applications include a large amount of data with high complexity, causing traditional feature extraction and classification techniques to fail providing acceptable results. Deep neural networks (DNNs), such as convolutional neural networks (CNNs) or recurrent neural networks (RNNs), have shown to be successful in classifying these cases. For example, in [25], authors use stacked autoencoders for feature extraction in an emotion recognition application. Since the input data includes video and audio data, authors use both conventional features and features extracted via deep belief networks to classify the emotion through an SVM classifier. They show that features extracted automatically through a DNN improve the classification accuracy of the SVM.

CNNs are one of the most commonly used DNNs for classification, due to their structure being able to capture both local and global features in multimedia inputs such as images or videos. Authors in [55] use CNNs to detect mitosis in breast cancer histology images. Their network is able to label image pixels as mitosis or non-mitosis, which results in a classification with an F1-score of 0.8. In [56], authors propose a CNN for gland segmentation in histology images. This work is able to detect benign and malignant glands; they report that under their segmentation scheme, extracted glands have less than 50 pixels of Hausdorff distance to the real ones. Another work that uses image inputs is presented in [57], where authors detect damage to retina due to diabetes in retinal fundus photographs. Their work is able to achieve an AUC of 0.99 in its classification task.

In [58], authors use a CNN with 1 dimensional input to classify different types of heart beat arrhythmia in ECG recordings. They develop a network that takes 5 min of each person's ECG in addition to multiple general heartbeat samples and train a personalized CNN to detect 5 types of arrhythmia. The network shows successful performance with accuracies as high as 99% in certain tasks. The work presented in [59] uses both CNNs and RNNs to annotate chest X-ray images with proper description. The CNN part of the paper is responsible to analyze the X-ray images and detect abnormalities in them. The output of the CNN is then fed to the RNN to produce appropriate annotations for the images to describe them, such as "normal" or "cadiomegaly/light." They show their work is able to annotate the images within acceptable range.

4.3   Regression/Estimation

In many applications, output data can take any value in a continuous range, rather than belonging to discrete groups or classes. In this case, the application is formulated as a regression or estimation problem, where the goal is to generate a continuous–valued output (contrary to a discrete output as done in classification discussed in Sect. 4.2) based on a set of input data.

An example regression application is discussed in [60], in which a robust heart rhythm estimation algorithm is proposed to combat false alarms in ICU caused by noise induced by the environment. The authors develop an estimation approach based on the Kalman filter [61, 62] that estimates the heart rate of an ICU patient from ECG and arterial blood pressure sensors and show that the proposed approach works well even when more noise is artificially added to the data. In [63], a disease trajectory prediction system is designed to predict the course of a disease in the future based on some initial patient medical data. The authors show that the proposed system can provide accurate prognosis at a personal level. The authors in [64] study the problem of prognosis of a disease in patients by focusing on the course of diabetes in diabetic patients. Their goal is to predict the possibility of a patient needing emergency care in the future. To this end, they consider lab tests, the list of the drugs that the patient uses, diagnoses, and other input features that are processed and selected by techniques such as filtering or PCA. They report the probability of a patient needing an emergency care in the future in addition to predicting their future lab test results. They show that their techniques are effective by reporting concordance indexes as high as 0.67.

A regression problem that focuses on drug discovery is discussed in [65]. The authors use DNNs with various inputs, including molecule structures of different drugs, that output on-target or off-target activities. They compare the performance of DNNs with other methods such as random forests with respect to the prediction of activities, and show that the former methods outperform the latter ones by improving the squared Pearson's correlation coefficient between the predicted activities and the observed ones from 0.42 to 0.5. In [66], the authors focus on the problem of estimating user fatigue through DNNs. They collect data from muscle and heart activity sensors, accelerometers, and a brain–computer interface that collects EEG signals. These signals are then provided as input to a DNN, which estimates the physical load of the participants and their physical fatigue.

4.4 Sequential Decision-Making

Sequential Decision-Making (SDM) models are typically used in medical applications to monitor and/or improve the medical process by estimating the task of interest as well as controlling any related variables. Example of sequential decision-making models are Markov Decision Processes (MDPs), Partially Observable Markov Decision Processes (POMDPs), and Multi Armed Bandits (MABs).

An example application of such models is discussed in [67, 68], where a WBAN [68] consisting of sensors such as accelerometers and ECGs, in addition to a mobile phone, is used for physical activity recognition. The system uses a POMDP model to select the best sensing strategy to achieve two different goals: (i) infer the physical activity of the individual accurately, and (ii) prolong mobile phone battery lifetime. The authors are able to show that the POMDP approach can lead to up 64% energy savings while losing only 10^{-4} in activity detection accuracy. Another application of sequential decision-making models is described in [69], where a video camera tracks the movements of patients with dementia to assist them with a handwashing task. To estimate the severity of dementia in patients and provide assistance in this task, a POMDP formulation is adopted, which decides when to intervene in the handwashing task. The model can do nothing and let the individual finish their task, provide cues such as task description to the individual, or call the caregiver.

In [70], a stress reduction system is introduced that uses a contextual MAB formulation to detect the relationship among different interventions to cope with stress and their outcome on different individuals for a given context. The data for the model comes from different sensors such as GPS, accelerometer, calendar, etc. in addition to other information gathered from the individual including personality traits and self-reports. The system evaluation shows that the participants in the study show lower symptoms related to depression. Another study that uses MAB approaches is presented in [71], where a personalized physical activity recommendation system is modeled as a MAB problem, which monitors the activities of individuals and provides suggestions to the users at different times for a healthier lifestyle. In [72], the authors develop a drug sensitivity prediction system that considers expert inputs to improve the efficacy of prescribed drugs for a given individual. The prediction refers to the effect of different drugs on patients with blood cancer and the features come from the genomic features of the cancer cells. To enhance the prediction, an expert provides an opinion to the prediction algorithm based on the genomic features, but the sheer number of features limits the feasibility of this input as the expert cannot provide an opinion on thousands of features. To address this issue, the authors use a MAB formulation to learn from the expert inputs and take their opinion only on the features that are considered the most important. This scheme improves the prediction accuracy by 8%.

5 Visualization

A vital part of a decision support system is presenting the important and necessary information to the users of the system in an intuitive format. A highly-effective way of achieving this goal is through data visualization that shows all relevant information in addition to machine-intelligence-based annotations for parts of data that require extra attention from the users. Visualization techniques vary based on both the application and the target users; for example, to provide feedback to medical experts, a system may need to include higher precision data with all the relevant medical information, while a lower level of technicality is sufficient for visualizing data for patients.

Despite the importance of proper data visualization and the benefits that it provides for the users, existing visualization techniques in the medical scientific disciplines are somewhat limited [73]. To date, several medical data visualization techniques have been introduced, which vary in complexity ranging from simple tables or bar graphs to advanced interactive multidimensional plotting systems. The focus of these techniques has been mostly on the data that are gathered through clinical visits. Visualization for MCPS data is more challenging due to the long duration of data acquisition and high dimensionality.

Traditional visualization techniques include lists, tables, graphs, charts, tress, pictograms, and formats to show spatial data [74] and causal relations within data elements. These formats present all information without removing any essential part

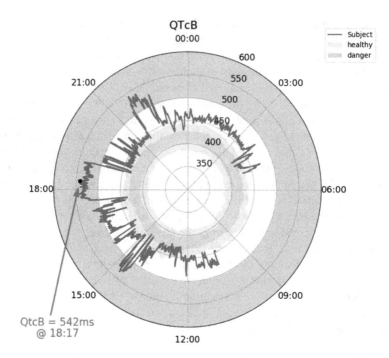

Fig. 3 A sample QTcB clock showing the calculated QTcB values of subject s30771 in [75] available in the PhysioBank database [76]. The plot shows the QTcB value for the entire recording duration and the highest value of QTcB is shown on the graph

and highlight the most important parts of the data. For example, the case shown in Fig. 3 is a 24-h visualization of a patient's ECG data [34, 49], where a "clock" shows the QTcB (Eq. (1)) value of a patient throughout the recording period. This visualization technique is designed to designate the top of the clock as midnight (00:00) and the bottom of it as noon (12:00) to visualize the entire 24-h recoding of the patient's ECG by using a single clock. The radial dimension of the clock (i.e., from the inside to the outside) represents the values of QTcB at a given time; the inner entries are colored green and represent "healthy" QTcB values (300–420 ms), whereas the values closer to the outer edges are colored red and represent "abnormal" QTcB values (500–600 ms). This visualization allows a cardiologist to view a patient's entire 24-h ECG recording period at a quick glance, which allows them to view 20–30 patient's Holter recordings within a negligible amount of time and identify the health conditions of each patient rapidly; this eliminates the need to search through traditional ECG recordings, which are printed on paper.

Multiple other techniques are proposed for plotting ECG data for different purposes. For example, authors in [77] develop an interactive ECG visualization system built on top of the research presented in [34], where multiple panels allow the medical professionals to plot different parts of the data with higher precision or show various statistical distributions related to the data. Another study that targets long-term ECG recordings is presented in [78], where heartbeats are shown in different clusters and the clusters with fewer members represent the heart beats with arrhythmia.

One of the main categories of visualization techniques involves presenting data to individuals who are self-tracking their health, physical fitness, and lifestyle. A rich body of work depends on self-logged information from users in addition to physical tracking devices to provide a visual feedback to them [79–82]. Many novel approaches are used for the feedback mechanism such as making data sculptures form the information [83], displaying them through abstract art [84], or even feedback for self-monitoring through edible chocolate [85].

Many of the proposed visualization schemes treat professional medical personnel as audience too. For example, hGraph [86] and its dependent programming libraries (like the one introduced in [87]) depict a summary of user activity, blood pressure, sleep, and in-clinic data and are dedicated to medical data visualization. Other systems such as Open mHealth [88] provide visualization as part of their overall architecture. Some other frameworks such as TimeLine [89] focus on visualizing only electronic health records and do not incorporate data from user activity in their figures. OpenICE [90] is another open platform for MCPS, which incorporates data visualization for vital signs of patients; it color-codes the vitals as being normal, not normal, and severely out of range.

PhysioEx is introduced in [91], which analyzes the streams of medical data and plots the duration, frequency, and trajectory of different events in the stream through a temporal intensity map. In the study presented in [92], a tele-rehabilitation system is designed that gathers patient activity through mobile sensors and visualizes them remotely for the care-giver for a better understanding of whether the patients adhere to their rehabilitation program or not and how their rehabilitation is progressing through time. A system that is implemented in ICU settings is proposed in [93], where all ICU data is shown and are accompanied by some notifications such as empty medication. Testing of this system shows that task completion times for nurses is significantly decreased and their situational awareness is increased.

There are many available tools that are used for creating these visualizations which are created by different companies. Plotly[1] provides different visualization tool libraries that are compatible with programming languages such as R, Python, and Java. AnyChart[2] also provides a data visualization platform that can create various forms of charts as well as real-time data streams. Tableau[3] is another tool that is widely used for creating visualizations. IBM Watson analytics[4] also provides a visualization kit for healthcare that can be used in R and Python programming languages through APIs. Some other widely used tools include software provided

---

[1]https://plot.ly/.

[2]https://www.anychart.com/.

[3]https://www.tableau.com/.

[4]https://www.ibm.com/watson/uk-en/health/.

by Sisense,[5] Microsoft Power BI,[6] Qlikview,[7] and SAP Lumira.[8] Note that these tools are not necessarily limited to healthcare applications and can be used to create visualizations in various industries.

6 Privacy

In the US, Health Insurance Portability and Accountability Act (HIPAA) [7] mandates the assurance of medical data privacy at every component of an MCPS. Security of an MCPS, whether concerning the general security of the system [8] or security of its specific components, has been addressed in the literature extensively and is an ongoing developing research topic.

Attacks on an MCPS can be categorized as either active or passive. *Active* attacks aim at accessing secret information by deviating from the security protocols, while a *passive* adversaries follow the security protocols, yet are able to access restricted information. The security layer of an MCPS should ensure that both of these types of threats are made ineffective in all layers of the system [8]. A general modeling of threats is presented in [94], where authors categorize the stakeholders in an MCPS and build trust and threat models based on them throughout the system. They categorize different potential threats such as confidentiality, integrity, and availability of data in different sections of the system such as the communication links and the software/hardware platform and list the possible remedies that may prevent these threats from inflicting damage on the system.

The study in [95] investigates the idea of integrating forensic principles into the design of an MCPS, which gives the HCO a means to investigate the intruders in case its MCPS is compromised. Their idea does not necessarily stop adversaries from intruding the system, but provides a means for detecting them after their attack. The authors discuss a forensic-by-design framework for an MCPS by breaking it down into different components such as risk assessment, forensic readiness principles, security and privacy requirements, relevant legislations and regulations, medical and safety requirements, and software and hardware requirements in addition to providing forensic-readiness testing criteria.

In addition to conventional privacy measures, there has been a growing interest in using machine intelligence algorithms to ensure the security of an MCSP. For example, authors in [96] develop an ANN-based intrusion detection system for an MCPS. The idea behind their system is to find anomalies in data access patterns and potentially deny access to a user request with an anomalous request for data. Based on this idea, the authors develop an evolving ANN that decides if an incoming

---

[5]https://www.sisense.com/.

[6]https://powerbi.microsoft.com/en-us/.

[7]https://www.qlik.com/us/.

[8]https://saplumira.com/.

request is normal or an attack; if it is classified as an attack, the request is sent to another ANN to classify the specific type of the attack. Another study presented in [97] uses machine learning algorithms for unusual behavior detection within a healthcare organization network. Their system monitors data access patterns in a computer network and detects anomalous behavior and is able to enhance system performance through feedback given to it by security analysts. Their work includes a visualization phase that helps identify the most valuable nodes for a potential attacker.

7 Future Directions, Open Issues, and Challenges

Incorporating Artificial Intelligence (AI) in MCPSs is still in its infancy with numerous possibilities for further advances in this area. As the amount of accumulated medical data increases, concurrently with the increasing computing power and storage capability of cloud platforms, AI-powered MCPSs will undoubtedly influence the medical field increasingly. While the rich datasets will help improve the accuracy of AI-based algorithms, it will facilitate the collection of much larger quantities of data. This positive feedback cycle will eventually allow the testing of more sophisticated—and data-hungry—algorithms that were not feasible to test previously.

Personalization of the algorithms is also another topic of interest. As the deployment of MCPSs becomes more mainstream, each individual will have a more detailed personal medical history. Designing AI algorithms that are adaptable to a given individual and providing their analysis based on specifics of one's medical history is an open issue which has to be studied further.

Security of an MCPS and keeping medical records private during the processing of medical data is one of the most important challenges that should be considered in all layers of an MCPS. This may lead into the emergence of AI algorithms that can be coupled with advanced encryption schemes, such as homomorphic encryption to keep the medical data secure at all times, even if the algorithm is executed on a public cloud server.

Another challenge associated with MCPSs is the power consumption of the sensors in the data acquisition layer. Although power consumption of the layers that are connected to the grid are minimally affected from this constraint, layers that operate on batteries impose severe limits to the design of an MCPS. This power consumption constraint manifests itself both in the first layer, where the battery-operated sensors acquire the data, and the battery-operated pre-processing layer, where the nodes process data at the local nodes and all of the local and even long-range communication links are powered by batteries. Designing a system that maximizes the battery life is crucial in an MCPS.

Adaptability of algorithms with newer types of data is another aspect that can be studied. As newer sensors are developed and novel methods of sensing are introduced that can be used in everyday situations, the acquired signal from these new sensors may be different than the traditional signals. Making the algorithms adapt to newer—and more advanced—sensors is another topic of interest.

8 Summary and Concluding Remarks

In this paper, we review different aspects of MCPSs and elaborate on incorporating artificial intelligence into them. We outline the general structure of an MCPS, which consists of multiple components. These components are (i) data acquisition, aggregation, and preprocessing, (ii) data processing and decision support, and (iii) visualization and user interaction.

Component (i) is responsible for acquiring patient data, extracting features from this data, aggregating it, and preparing it for transmission into the cloud. We provide a set of algorithms that enable the extraction of features from raw data. Table 2 provides a list of this set of algorithms.

Component (ii) includes the machine intelligence algorithms that process the summarized data from the previous component to prepare it for presentation to the end user. We discuss a rich set of machine intelligence algorithms that reside in this component and categorize them based on their goal. These goals are categorized into knowledge discovery, classification, regression, and sequential decision-making. Examples of algorithms falling into each of these categories are also presented. A summarized list of these algorithms is shown in Table 3.

The final component (iii) is the interface between the machine intelligence and healthcare professionals. We discuss different techniques on providing feedback to the users through data visualization with example applications. We also study the issues that relate to the privacy and security of the personal medical data that is being processed by the MCPS; we provide information about system-level and crypto-level mechanisms that ensure data security and privacy.

Table 2 Algorithms used in data acquisition, aggregation, and pre-processing components

Component stage	Algorithms, methods, and mechanisms
Feature extraction	Principal Component Analysis (PCA)
	Kernel PCA (KPCA)
	Canonical Correlation Analysis (CCA)
	Multidimensional Scaling (MDS)
	Artificial Neural Networks (ANNs)
Feature selection	Sequential Backward Selection (SBS)
	Sequential Forward Selection (SFS)
	Sequential Forward Floating Selection (SFFS)
	Correlation-based Feature Selection (CFS)
	Genetic Algorithms (GA)

Table 3 Algorithms used in the decision support component, broken down by goal

Algorithmic goal	Algorithms, methods, and mechanisms
Knowledge discovery	K-Means
	Hierarchical Clustering
	Probabilistic Clustering
Classification	Support Vector Machines (SVM)
	k-Nearest Neighbor
	Decision Tree
	AdaBoost
	Convolutional Neural Networks (CNNs)
	Recurrent Neural Networks (RNNs)
Regression/estimation	Kalman Filters
	Linear/Nonlinear Regression
	Deep Neural Networks (DNNs)
Sequential decision-making	Markov Decision Processes (MDPs)
	Partially Observable MDPs (POMDPs)
	Multi Armed Bandits (MABs)

References

1. M. Hassanalieragh, A. Page, T. Soyata, G. Sharma, M.K. Aktas, G. Mateos, B. Kantarci, S. Andreescu, Health monitoring and management using Internet-of-Things (IoT) sensing with cloud-based processing: opportunities and challenges, in *2015 IEEE International Conference on Services Computing (SCC)*, New York (June 2015), pp. 285–292
2. X. Chen, Z. Zhu, M. Chen, Y. Li, Large-scale mobile fitness app usage analysis for smart health. IEEE Commun. Mag. **56**(4), 46–52 (2018)
3. P. Wu, M.Y. Nam, J. Choi, A. Kirlik, L. Sha, R.B. Berlin, Supporting emergency medical care teams with an integrated status display providing real-time access to medical best practices, workflow tracking, and patient data. J. Med. Syst. **41**(12), 186 (2017)
4. J. Jezewski, A. Pawlak, K. Horoba, J. Wrobel, R. Czabanski, M. Jezewski, Selected design issues of the medical cyber-physical system for telemonitoring pregnancy at home. Microprocess. Microsyst. **46**, 35–43 (2016)
5. G. Honan, A. Page, O. Kocabas, T. Soyata, B. Kantarci, Internet-of-everything oriented implementation of secure Digital Health (D-Health) systems, in *Proceedings of the 2016 IEEE Symposium on Computers and Communications (ISCC)*, Messina (Jun 2016), pp. 718–725
6. A. Page, S. Hijazi, D. Askan, B. Kantarci, T. Soyata, Research directions in cloud-based decision support systems for health monitoring using Internet-of-Things driven data acquisition. Int. J. Serv. Comput. **4**(4), 18–34 (2016)
7. 104th Congress Public Law 191, Health Insurance Portability and Accountability Act of 1996 (1996). https://www.gpo.gov/fdsys/pkg/PLAW-104publ191/html/PLAW-104publ191.htm. Accessed 28 July 2017
8. O. Kocabas, T. Soyata, M.K. Aktas, Emerging security mechanisms for medical cyber physical systems. IEEE/ACM Trans. Comput. Biol. Bioinform. **13**(3), 401–416 (2016)

9. G. Yang, L. Xie, M. Mäntysalo, X. Zhou, Z. Pang, L. Da Xu, S. Kao-Walter, Q. Chen, L.R. Zheng, A health-IoT platform based on the integration of intelligent packaging, unobtrusive bio-sensor, and intelligent medicine box. IEEE Trans. Ind. Inf. **10**(4), 2180–2191 (2014)

10. D.M. West, How 5G technology enables the health internet of things. Brookings Center for Technology Innovation **3**, 1–20 (2016)

11. A. Mdhaffar, T. Chaari, K. Larbi, M. Jmaiel, B. Freisleben, IoT-based health monitoring via lorawan, in *IEEE EUROCON 2017-17th International Conference on Smart Technologies* (IEEE, Piscataway, 2017), pp. 519–524

12. A. Page, T. Soyata, J. Couderc, M. Aktas, B. Kantarci, S. Andreescu, Visualization of health monitoring data acquired from distributed sensors for multiple patients, in *IEEE Global Telecommunications Conference (GLOBECOM)*, San Diego (Dec 2015), pp. 1–7

13. S. Aust, R.V. Prasad, I.G. Niemegeers, IEEE 802.11ah: advantages in standards and further challenges for sub 1 GHz Wi-Fi, in *2012 IEEE International Conference on Communications (ICC)* (IEEE, Piscataway, 2012), pp. 6885–6889

14. S. Han, Y.H. Wei, A.K. Mok, D. Chen, M. Nixon, E. Rotvold, Building wireless embedded internet for industrial automation, in *IECON 2013-39th Annual Conference of the IEEE Industrial Electronics Society* (IEEE, Piscataway, 2013), pp. 5582–5587

15. G. Mokhtari, Q. Zhang, G. Nourbakhsh, S. Ball, M. Karunanithi, Bluesound: a new resident identification sensor—using ultrasound array and BLE technology for smart home platform. IEEE Sens. J. **17**(5), 1503–1512 (2017)

16. W.L. Chen, L.B. Chen, W.J. Chang, J.J. Tang, An IoT-based elderly behavioral difference warning system, in *2018 IEEE International Conference on Applied System Invention (ICASI)* (IEEE, Piscataway, 2018), pp. 308–309

17. Y. Li, Z. Chi, X. Liu, T. Zhu, Passive-ZigBee: enabling ZigBee communication in IoT networks with 1000x+ less power consumption, in *Proceedings of the 16th ACM Conference on Embedded Networked Sensor Systems* (ACM, New York, 2018), pp. 159–171

18. A.M. Rahmani, T.N. Gia, B. Negash, A. Anzanpour, I. Azimi, M. Jiang, P. Liljeberg, Exploiting smart e-health gateways at the edge of healthcare Internet-of-Things: a fog computing approach. Futur. Gener. Comput. Syst. **78**, 641–658 (2018)

19. M.L. Raymer, W.F. Punch, E.D. Goodman, L.A. Kuhn, A.K. Jain, Dimensionality reduction using genetic algorithms. IEEE Trans. Evol. Comput. **4**(2), 164–171 (2000)

20. Y. Chen, M. Yang, X. Chen, B. Liu, H. Wang, S. Wang, Sensorineural hearing loss detection via discrete wavelet transform and principal component analysis combined with generalized eigenvalue proximal support vector machine and Tikhonov regularization. Multimed. Tools Appl. **77**(3), 3775–3793 (2018)

21. A. Ghandeharioun, S. Fedor, L. Sangermano, D. Ionescu, J. Alpert, C. Dale, D. Sontag, R. Picard, Objective assessment of depressive symptoms with machine learning and wearable sensors data, in *Proceedings of the International Conference on Affective Computing and Intelligent Interaction (ACII)*, San Antonio (2017)

22. Y. Kim, N. Kaongoen, S. Jo, Hybrid-BCI smart glasses for controlling electrical devices, in *2015 54th Annual Conference of the Society of Instrument and Control Engineers of Japan (SICE)* (IEEE, Piscataway, 2015), pp. 1162–1166

23. C. Li, W.K. Cheung, J. Liu, J.K. Ng, Bayesian nominal matrix factorization for mining daily activity patterns, in *2016 IEEE/WIC/ACM International Conference on Web Intelligence (WI)* (IEEE, Piscataway, 2016), pp. 335–342

24. G.E. Hinton, R.R. Salakhutdinov, Reducing the dimensionality of data with neural networks. Science **313**(5786), 504–507 (2006)

25. Y. Kim, H. Lee, E.M. Provost, Deep learning for robust feature generation in audiovisual emotion recognition, in *2013 IEEE International Conference on Acoustics, Speech and Signal Processing* (IEEE, Piscataway, 2013), pp. 3687–3691

26. B., Jokanović, M. Amin, Fall detection using deep learning in range-Doppler radars. IEEE Trans. Aerosp. Electron. Syst. **54**(1), 180–189 (2018)

27. M. Li, V. Rozgic, G. Thatte, S. Lee, A. Emken, M. Annavaram, U. Mitra, D. Spruijt-Metz, S. Narayanan, Multimodal physical activity recognition by fusing temporal and cepstral information. IEEE Trans. Neural Syst. Rehabil. Eng. **18**(4), 369–380 (Aug 2010)

28. A. Sano, R.W. Picard, Stress recognition using wearable sensors and mobile phones, in *IEEE Humane Association Conference on Affective Computing and Intelligent Interaction (ACII)* (2013), pp. 671–676

29. B. Xie, H. Minn, Real-time sleep apnea detection by classifier combination. IEEE Trans. Inf. Technol. Biomed. **16**(3), 469–477 (2012)

30. V. Srinivasan, C. Eswaran, N. Sriraam, Artificial neural network based epileptic detection using time-domain and frequency-domain features. J. Med. Syst. **29**(6), 647–660 (2005)

31. B. Lei, S.A. Rahman, I. Song, Content-based classification of breath sound with enhanced features. Neurocomputing **141**, 139–147 (2014)

32. D. Sow, A. Biem, M. Blount, M. Ebling, O. Verscheure, Body sensor data processing using stream computing, in *Proceedings of the International Conference on Multimedia Information Retrieval* (ACM, New York, 2010), pp. 449–458

33. S. Souli, Z. Lachiri, Audio sounds classification using scattering features and support vectors machines for medical surveillance. Appl. Acoust. **130**, 270–282 (2018)

34. A. Page, T. Soyata, J. Couderc, M.K. Aktas, An open source ECG clock generator for visualization of long-term cardiac monitoring data. IEEE Access **3**, 2704–2714 (2015)

35. C.M. Bishop, *Pattern Recognition and Machine Learning (Information Science and Statistics)* (Springer, New York, 2006)

36. D. Sánchez-Morillo, M. López-Gordo, A. León, Novel multiclass classification for home-based diagnosis of sleep apnea hypopnea syndrome. Expert Syst. Appl. **41**(4), 1654–1662 (2014)

37. D.S. Lee, T.W. Chong, B.G. Lee, Stress events detection of driver by wearable glove system. IEEE Sens. J. **17**(1), 194–204 (2017)

38. W.H. Wang, Y.L. Hsu, P.C. Chung, M.C. Pai, Predictive models for evaluating cognitive ability in dementia diagnosis applications based on inertia-and gait-related parameters. IEEE Sens. J. **18**(8), 3338–3350 (2018)

39. M. Mursalin, Y. Zhang, Y. Chen, N.V. Chawla, Automated epileptic seizure detection using improved correlation-based feature selection with random forest classifier. Neurocomputing **241**, 204–214 (2017)

40. B. Nakisa, M.N. Rastgoo, D. Tjondronegoro, V. Chandran, Evolutionary computation algorithms for feature selection of EEG-based emotion recognition using mobile sensors. Expert Syst. Appl. **93**, 143–155 (2017)

41. H. Li, D. Yuan, X. Ma, D. Cui, L. Cao, Genetic algorithm for the optimization of features and neural networks in ECG signals classification. Sci. Rep. **7**, 41011 (2017)

42. V. Chandola, S.R. Sukumar, J.C. Schryver, Knowledge discovery from massive healthcare claims data, in *Proceedings of the 19th ACM SIGKDD International Conference on Knowledge Discovery and Data Mining* (ACM, New York, 2013), pp. 1312–1320

43. B.M. Marlin, D.C. Kale, R.G. Khemani, R.C. Wetzel, Unsupervised pattern discovery in electronic health care data using probabilistic clustering models, in *Proceedings of the 2nd ACM SIGHIT International Health Informatics Symposium* (ACM, New York, 2012), pp. 389–398

44. D.P. Chen, S.C. Weber, P.S. Constantinou, T.A. Ferris, H.J. Lowe, A.J. Butte, Clinical arrays of laboratory measures, or "clinarrays", built from an electronic health record enable disease subtyping by severity, in *AMIA* (2007)

45. D. Sanchez-Morillo, M.A. Fernandez-Granero, A.L. Jiménez, Detecting COPD exacerbations early using daily telemonitoring of symptoms and k-means clustering: a pilot study. Med. Biol. Eng. Comput. **53**(5), 441–451 (2015)

46. N.P. Tatonetti, J.C. Denny, S.N. Murphy, G.H. Fernald, G. Krishnan, V. Castro, P. Yue, P.S. Tsau, I. Kohane, D.M. Roden, et al., Detecting drug interactions from adverse-event reports: interaction between paroxetine and pravastatin increases blood glucose levels. Clin. Pharmacol. Ther. **90**(1), 133 (2011)

47. B. Ustun, M.B. Westover, C. Rudin, M.T. Bianchi, Clinical prediction models for sleep apnea: the importance of medical history over symptoms. J. Clin. Sleep Med. Off. Publ. Am. Acad. Sleep Med. **12**(2), 161–168 (2016)
48. S. Hijazi, A. Page, B. Kantarci, T. Soyata, Machine learning in cardiac health monitoring and decision support. IEEE Comput. Mag. **49**(11), 38–48 (2016)
49. A. Page, M.K. Aktas, T. Soyata, W. Zareba, J. Couderc, "QT Clock" to improve detection of QT prolongation in long QT syndrome patients. Heart Rhythm **13**(1), 190–198 (2016)
50. H.S. Mousavi, V. Monga, G. Rao, A.U.K. Rao, et al., Automated discrimination of lower and higher grade gliomas based on histopathological image analysis. J. Pathol. Inform. **6**(1), 15 (2015)
51. E. Ataer-Cansizoglu, V. Bolon-Canedo, J.P. Campbell, A. Bozkurt, D. Erdogmus, J. Kalpathy-Cramer, S. Patel, K. Jonas, R.V.P. Chan, S. Ostmo, et al., Computer-based image analysis for plus disease diagnosis in retinopathy of prematurity: performance of the "i-ROP" system and image features associated with expert diagnosis. Transl. Vis. Sci. Technol. **4**(6), 5–5 (2015)
52. I. Bisio, F. Lavagetto, M. Marchese, A. Sciarrone, A smartphone-centric platform for remote health monitoring of heart failure. Int. J. Commun. Syst. **28**(11), 1753–1771 (2015)
53. M. Bsoul, H. Minn, L. Tamil, Apnea MedAssist: real-time sleep apnea monitor using single-lead ECG. IEEE Trans. Inf. Technol. Biomed. **15**(3), 416–427 (2011)
54. D. Zhou, J. Luo, V.M.B. Silenzio, Y. Zhou, J. Hu, G. Currier, H.A. Kautz, Tackling mental health by integrating unobtrusive multimodal sensing, in *AAAI*, 1401–1409 (2015)
55. D.C. Cireşan, A. Giusti, L.M. Gambardella, J. Schmidhuber, Mitosis detection in breast cancer histology images with deep neural networks, in *International Conference on Medical Image Computing and Computer-assisted Intervention* (Springer, Berlin, 2013), pp. 411–418
56. H. Chen, X. Qi, L. Yu, P.A. Heng, DCAN: deep contour-aware networks for accurate gland segmentation (2016). Preprint arXiv:1604.02677
57. V. Gulshan, L. Peng, M. Coram, M.C. Stumpe, D. Wu, A. Narayanaswamy, S. Venugopalan, K. Widner, T. Madams, J. Cuadros, et al., Development and validation of a deep learning algorithm for detection of diabetic retinopathy in retinal fundus photographs. JAMA **316**(22), 2402–2410 (2016)
58. S. Kiranyaz, T. Ince, M. Gabbouj, Real-time patient-specific ECG classification by 1-D convolutional neural networks. IEEE Trans. Biomed. Eng. **63**(3), 664–675 (2016)
59. H.C. Shin, K. Roberts, L. Lu, D. Demner-Fushman, J. Yao, R.M. Summers, Learning to read chest X-rays: recurrent neural cascade model for automated image annotation (2016). Preprint arXiv:1603.08486
60. Q. Li, R.G. Mark, G.D. Clifford, Robust heart rate estimation from multiple asynchronous noisy sources using signal quality indices and a Kalman filter. Physiol. Meas. **29**(1), 15 (2007)
61. R.E. Kalman, A new approach to linear filtering and prediction problems. J. Basic Eng. **82**(1), 35–45 (1960)
62. R.E. Kalman, R.S. Bucy, New results in linear filtering and prediction theory. J. Basic Eng. **83**(1), 95–108 (1961)
63. P. Schulam, S. Saria, A framework for individualizing predictions of disease trajectories by exploiting multi-resolution structure, in *Advances in Neural Information Processing Systems* (2015), pp. 748–756
64. H. Neuvirth, M. Ozery-Flato, J. Hu, J. Laserson, M.S. Kohn, S. Ebadollahi, M. Rosen-Zvi, Toward personalized care management of patients at risk: the diabetes case study, in *Proceedings of the 17th ACM SIGKDD International Conference on Knowledge Discovery and Data Mining* (ACM, New York, 2011), pp. 395–403
65. J. Ma, R.P. Sheridan, A. Liaw, G.E. Dahl, V. Svetnik, Deep neural nets as a method for quantitative structure–activity relationships. J. Chem. Inf. Model. **55**(2), 263–274 (2015)
66. Y. Gordienko, S. Stirenko, Y. Kochura, O. Alienin, M. Novotarskiy, N. Gordienko, Deep learning for fatigue estimation on the basis of multimodal human-machine interactions (2017). Preprint arXiv:1801.06048

67. D.S. Zois, M. Levorato, U. Mitra, Energy-efficient, heterogeneous sensor selection for physical activity detection in wireless body area networks. IEEE Trans. Signal Process. **61**(7), 1581–1594 (2013)
68. U. Mitra, B.A. Emken, S. Lee, M. Li, V. Rozgic, G. Thatte, H. Vathsangam, D.S. Zois, M. Annavaram, S. Narayanan, M. Levorato, D. Spruijt-Metz, G. Sukhatme, KNOWME: a case study in wireless body area sensor network design. IEEE Commun. Mag. **50**(5), 116–125 (2012)
69. J. Hoey, C. Boutilier, P. Poupart, P. Olivier, A. Monk, A. Mihailidis, People, sensors, decisions: customizable and adaptive technologies for assistance in healthcare. ACM Trans. Interactive Intell. Syst. **2**(4), 1–36 (2012)
70. P. Paredes, R. Gilad-Bachrach, M. Czerwinski, A. Roseway, K. Rowan, J. Hernandez, PopTherapy: coping with stress through pop-culture, in *Proceedings of the 8th International Conference on Pervasive Computing Technologies for Healthcare (PervasiveHealth)* (2014), pp. 109–117
71. M. Rabbi, M.H. Aung, T. Choudhury, Towards health recommendation systems: an approach for providing automated personalized health feedback from mobile data, in *Mobile Health* (Springer, Berlin, 2017), pp. 519–542
72. I. Sundin, T. Peltola, M.M. Majumder, P. Daee, M. Soare, H. Afrabandpey, C. Heckman, S. Kaski, P. Marttinen, Improving drug sensitivity predictions in precision medicine through active expert knowledge elicitation (2017). Preprint arXiv:1705.03290
73. D. Chou, Health it and patient safety: building safer systems for better care. JAMA **308**(21), 2282–2282 (2012)
74. A.A. Bui, W. Hsu, Medical data visualization: toward integrated clinical workstations, in *Medical Imaging Informatics* (Springer, Berlin, 2010), pp. 139–193
75. F. Jager, A. Taddei, G.B. Moody, M. Emdin, G. Antolič, R. Dorn, A. Smrdel, C. Marchesi, R.G. Mark, Long-term ST database: a reference for the development and evaluation of automated ischaemia detectors and for the study of the dynamics of myocardial ischaemia. Med. Biol. Eng. Comput. **41**(2), 172–182 (2003)
76. A. Golberger, L. Amaral, L. Glass, J.M. Hausdorff, P.C. Ivanov, R. Mark, J. Mietus, G. Moody, P. Chung-Kan, H. Stenley, Physiobank, physiotoolkit, and physionet: component of a new research resource for complex physiologic signals. Circulation **101**(23), e215–e220 (2000)
77. K. Xu, S. Guo, N. Cao, D. Gotz, A. Xu, H. Qu, Z. Yao, Y. Chen, ECGLens: interactive visual exploration of large scale ECG data for arrhythmia detection, in *Proceedings of the 2018 CHI Conference on Human Factors in Computing Systems (CHI '18)* (ACM, New York, 2018), Paper 663, 12 pp. https://doi.org/10.1145/3173574.3174237
78. C.A. Christmann, G. Zolynski, A. Hoffmann, G. Bleser, Effective visualization of long term health data to support behavior change, in *Digital Human Modeling. Applications in Health, Safety, Ergonomics, and Risk Management: Health and Safety. DHM 2017*, ed. by V. Duffy. Lecture Notes in Computer Science, vol. 10287 (Springer, Cham, 2017)
79. C.A. Christmann, G. Zolynski, A. Hoffmann, G. Bleser, Effective visualization of long term health data to support behavior change, in *International Conference on Digital Human Modeling and Applications in Health, Safety, Ergonomics and Risk Management* (Springer, Berlin, 2017), pp. 237–247
80. A. Cuttone, M.K. Petersen, J.E. Larsen, Four data visualization heuristics to facilitate reflection in personal informatics, in *International Conference on Universal Access in Human-Computer Interaction* (Springer, Berlin, 2014), pp. 541–552
81. S. Theis, P. Rasche, C. Bröhl, M. Wille, A. Mertens, User-driven semantic classification for the analysis of abstract health and visualization tasks, in *International Conference on Digital Human Modeling and Applications in Health, Safety, Ergonomics and Risk Management* (Springer, Berlin, 2017), pp. 297–305
82. K. Tollmar, F. Bentley, C. Viedma, Mobile health mashups: making sense of multiple streams of wellbeing and contextual data for presentation on a mobile device, in *2012 6th International Conference on Pervasive Computing Technologies for Healthcare (PervasiveHealth)* (IEEE, Piscataway, 2012), pp. 65–72

83. S. Stusak, A. Tabard, F. Sauka, R.A. Khot, A. Butz, Activity sculptures: exploring the impact of physical visualizations on running activity. IEEE Trans. Vis. Comput. Graph. **20**(12), 2201–2210 (2014)

84. C. Fan, J. Forlizzi, A.K. Dey, A spark of activity: exploring informative art as visualization for physical activity, in *Proceedings of the 2012 ACM Conference on Ubiquitous Computing* (ACM, New York, 2012), pp. 81–84

85. R.A. Khot, D. Aggarwal, R. Pennings, L. Hjorth, F. Mueller, Edipulse: investigating a playful approach to self-monitoring through 3D printed chocolate treats, in *Proceedings of the 2017 CHI Conference on Human Factors in Computing Systems* (ACM, New York, 2017), pp. 6593–6607

86. F. Jonathan, J. Sonin, hGraph: an open system for visualizing personal health metrics. Involution Studios, Arlington, Tech. Rep. (April 2012)

87. A. Ledesma, M. Al-Musawi, H. Nieminen, Health figures: an open source javascript library for health data visualization. BMC Med. Inform. Decis. Mak. **16**(1), 38 (2016)

88. D. Estrin, I. Sim, Open mHealth architecture: an engine for health care innovation. Science **330**(6005), 759–760 (2010)

89. A.A. Bui, D.R. Aberle, H. Kangarloo, Timeline: visualizing integrated patient records. IEEE Trans. Inf. Technol. Biomed. **11**(4), 462–473 (2007)

90. J. Plourde, D. Arney, J.M. Goldman, OpenICE: an open, interoperable platform for medical cyber-physical systems, in *2014 ACM/IEEE International Conference on Cyber-Physical Systems (ICCPS)* (IEEE, Piscataway, 2014), pp. 221–221

91. R. Kamaleswaran, C. Collins, A. James, C. McGregor, PhysioEx: visual analysis of physiological event streams, in *Computer Graphics Forum*, vol. 35 (Wiley Online Library, 2016), pp. 331–340

92. B. Maradani, H. Levkowitz, The role of visualization in tele-rehabilitation: a case study, in *2017 7th International Conference on Cloud Computing, Data Science & Engineering-Confluence* (IEEE, Piscataway, 2017), pp. 643–648

93. S.H. Koch, C. Weir, D. Westenskow, M. Gondan, J. Agutter, M. Haar, D. Liu, M. Görges, N. Staggers, Evaluation of the effect of information integration in displays for ICU nurses on situation awareness and task completion time: a prospective randomized controlled study. Int. J. Med. Inform. **82**(8), 665–675 (2013)

94. H. Almohri, L. Cheng, D. Yao, H. Alemzadeh, On threat modeling and mitigation of medical cyber-physical systems, in *2017 IEEE/ACM International Conference on Connected Health: Applications, Systems and Engineering Technologies (CHASE)* (IEEE, Piscataway, 2017), pp. 114–119

95. G. Grispos, W.B. Glisson, K.K.R. Choo, Medical cyber-physical systems development: a forensics-driven approach, in *2017 IEEE/ACM International Conference on Connected Health: Applications, Systems and Engineering Technologies (CHASE)* (IEEE, Piscataway, 2017), pp. 108–113

96. N. Mowla, I. Doh, K. Chae, Evolving neural network intrusion detection system for MCPS, in *2017 19th International Conference on Advanced Communication Technology (ICACT)* (IEEE, Piscataway, 2017), pp. 183–187

97. A. Boddy, W. Hurst, M. Mackay, A. El Rhalibi, A study into data analysis and visualisation to increase the cyber-resilience of healthcare infrastructures, in *Proceedings of the 1st International Conference on Internet of Things and Machine Learning (IML '17)* (ACM, New York, 2017), Article 32, 7 pp. https://doi.org/10.1145/3109761.3109793

Health Promotion Technology and the Aging Population

Ophelia John and Pascal Fallavollita

Abstract In an effort to improve the quality of care for any population, technology is integrated into the healthcare system. Different types of technologies can aid in health promotion through prevention, education, and monitoring techniques. Prevention methods are becoming more common with older adults to assist with their activities of daily living as well as to support them in learning and remembering healthy behaviors. The willingness to adopt a new technology is key to successfully modifying behavior and what hinder the outcome are issues of competency as well as access.

The purpose of this book chapter is to use empirical studies to review the types of health technology used with the older population, as well as the overall level of success on their behaviors. Once the research question was defined, an inclusion and exclusion criterion was used to select the peer-reviewed articles. Various studies that fulfilled the predefined criteria were used. Data was extracted from 39 articles for the evaluation of the different health technologies and their uses.

mHealth and phones are the most popular type used for health promotion, as it is present in 36% of the articles evaluated. Other successful and popular types of technology used were websites and modules (26%), as well as monitoring technology (23%). In all of the studies, the elderly population was able to successfully use the technology, indicating that the adoption of new technology is possible at any age. Technology can be used to affect the elderly population to integrate healthier habits into their lives. The variety of accessible technologies allows individuals to use it in conjunction for their desired outcomes.

Keywords Aging population · Mobile health · Assistive technology · Serious games

O. John · P. Fallavollita (✉)
Faculty of Health Sciences, Interdisciplinary School of Health Sciences, University of Ottawa, Ottawa, ON, Canada
e-mail: Ojohn@uottawa.ca; pfallavo@uottawa.ca

© Springer Nature Switzerland AG 2020   179
A. El Saddik et al. (eds.), *Connected Health in Smart Cities*,
https://doi.org/10.1007/978-3-030-27844-1_9

1   Introduction

In the USA, with similar projections for Canada, it is estimated that approximately 21% of the population will be 65 years or older by the year 2040 [1]. This growing population will require formal or informal continuing care to combat frailty, chronic conditions, and other outcomes associated with aging [2]. A longitudinal study on elderly people in Manitoba found that those who are institutionalized or cohabiting with individuals, other than their spouse, are less likely to be healthy [3]. The populations that are living independently are able to better manage their own health, yet the dependent populations require additional resources to make healthcare more comprehensive and accessible to them [3]. At the present state, there are inadequate healthcare workers trained to care for the complex care that is required for the older adults [1].

In Canada, there are healthcare policy initiatives that focus on the prevention of chronic disorders and the promotion of healthy aging. These initiatives help with reducing the healthcare costs associated with treatment [4]. The cost of poor health affects both the government and the ill individual. If the elderly population does not have adequate funding, the demand for prescription drugs decreases and as a result the demand for physician visits increases [5]. Financial stability is required during retirement since poor health is more frequent among seniors who lack financial security [6]. The cost of treating health conditions can be a financial burden on the elderly. As such, an emphasis on health promotion is required to aid in the prevention of chronic diseases. Web-based wellness programs may decrease healthcare costs and encourage the use of preventative services [7].

The increased use of health promotion technology on the elderly population is a solution to the growing need for support from this age group. The 10 different types of technologies identified in the literature review are mHealth/phones, website/modules, monitoring technology, health games/computer, internet, text messaging, assistive technology, virtual coaching, exercise simulations, and tablets. The most popular types of technology from the papers included mHealth/phones (14), website/modules (10), and monitoring technology (9).

The types of technologies used vary greatly, as some are not intended solely for health promotion. For example, the use of a Smartphone is incorporated in many of the studies but the cell phone's primary use is not for health promotion. Alternatively, "exergames," exercise-simulation games, are an example of technology that is exclusive to health promotion [8]. Exercise simulations make adults more likely to participate in physical activity [8]. The technology used was selected to accommodate the senior population, therefore, there was no need to personalize any of the technology. Another popular type of universal technology is the use of reminders and messaging to motivate adults to increase physical activity [9]. The messages were successful whether or not they were personalized for the participant's needs [9]. As long as the participant finds the technology or the information it is delivering interesting, the use of universal technology is able to modify their behavior [10].

2   Method

Major databases were searched for peer-reviewed articles from 2007 to 2017. Of the articles found, the 39 that fulfilled the inclusion criteria were evaluated for the types of technology and their success at modifying behavior in seniors. The objective was to find different types of health promotion technology.

2.1   Inclusion and Exclusion Criteria

Key terms were used in the initial search to identify articles surrounding the topics of "health promotion," "technology," and "behaviour." Articles were used if they identified a specific type of health technology as well as if the technology was tailored for the elderly population. In this systematic review, a senior is defined as over the age of 50 years.

3   Results

The systematic review of 39 peer-reviewed articles demonstrated the 10 different types of technology used for health promotion.

3.1   Assistive Technology

Assistive technology in the form of tools, aids the senior by modifying an activity to suit the extent of their mobility or cognitive skills. Devices that record messages, sensors, and tracking devices are all examples of assistive technology used to promote health in individuals with dementia. In men and women with dementia, memory aids are useful at helping them maintain their independence [11]. Automated pill dispensers that beep when it is time to take a pill and recorded messages for appointments are successful examples used to maintain the health of older adults and increase their quality of life [11].

3.2   Exercise Simulations

Exercise simulations encourage movement and muscular stress in a controlled area. These technologies allow for fun workouts in the home independent of a large space or the weather [12]. This technology can promote activity through the interaction of monitoring technologies, including balance boards and game consoles, and the applications/games. This technology can include the use of virtual reality to immerse the participant in the game. Virtual reality is successful at promoting healthy habits by engaging seniors in an interactive exercise regime. These exercise simulations are not limited to the location of an individual and can provide a safe and entertaining option for physical activity [8] (Fig. 1).

3.3   Health Games/Computer Applications

Health Games/Computer Applications encourage activity through the education or entertainment of an individual. Participants are able to keep track of their level of activity and therefore make conscious decisions to increase it. A recurring barrier to the use of this technology is the attitude of others and the assumption that the seniors do not know how to use the technology [14]. Accepting that the technology is usable to the senior population will increase the frequency of use for this population [14]. These games and applications provide an interactive experience for the user allowing them to learn comfortably at their desired pace [15].

3.4   Internet

Internet access is used as a supporting technology. Access to the Internet provides the seniors with the ability to do their own health research independent of a caregiver. The benefits of Internet access extended to both seniors and their caregivers. Caregivers to seniors with Internet access had improved mental health compared the caregivers to seniors without Internet access [16]. Participants in a study were taught about healthy aging and interventions that would impact their future [17]. This method followed a social-cognitive model and after an online assessment the web-based tool provided information as well as skills and motivation to make lasting changes [17]. It is estimated that more than 50% of the American seniors 65 and older use the Internet or email so [11]. The increasing popularity and accessibility of the Internet present an opportunity to engage the senior population in new health promotion tactics.

3.5   mHealth and Phone Lines

mHealth and phone lines allow seniors to use their cell phone to access different health promotion initiatives, including health reminders. It also includes automated telephone chats to encourage and regulate health behavior. Typically, mHealth is developed for individuals with symptoms of chronic diseases, however, a study in

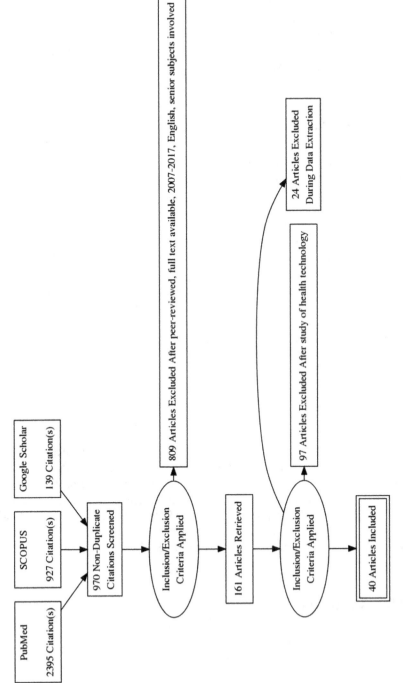

Fig. 1 PRISMA flow diagram [13]

2014 used the technology in a novel way as a method of reducing risk factors for lifestyle-related chronic conditions [18]. The new method was used, in conjunction with exercise, to prescribe changes to a sedentary lifestyle [18]. A limitation of implementing mHealth was the associated cost by providing the participants with the technology [18]. When this technology is partnered with monitoring technology it increases physical activity [18].

3.6 Monitoring Technology

Monitoring technology includes Smartphone, blood pressure monitors, glucometers, sensors for movement, and pedometers [18]. These technologies will feedback information to an application or individual to help them make informed health-related decisions. The importance of monitoring technology was a significant factor for modifying behaviors in seniors [19]. This was highlighted when trying to change the behavior of seniors aged 65–95 years with the use of cholesterol tests [19]. Qualitative data demonstrated that the role of a health condition motivates older adults to improve their diet and exercise patterns. Monitoring technology can illustrate the degree of severity of their condition as well as reveal the results their lifestyle changes have made to their condition [19]. Both gradual and abrupt changes can be tracked using monitoring technology. The most common form of monitoring technology was the pedometer. It was used to track everyday physical activity and promote an increase in walking.

3.7 Tablets

Tablets facilitate teaching by providing access to modules and internet-based applications. Additionally, this form of technology provides a platform for virtual coaching [20]. Tablets are used as a supplementary tool alongside other types of technology. This electronic device is favored over laptops or desktops due to the convenience of its ease of transport. Tablets assist in teaching the senior population [20]. A barrier to its increased use is the assumption that the senior population cannot incorporate this technology into their lifestyles [15].

3.8 Text Messaging

Text messaging is an effective way to quickly and consistently send fixed reminders to the patients to encourage them to exercise or follow a certain diet. A study in 2016 demonstrated that the effectiveness of this intervention was not based on an interactive component as there was no requirement to reply to daily text messages

[21]. Several unique messages were developed for the intervention that always contained an instruction to exercise and a statement of praise [21]. The frequency in weekly exercise was higher in individuals who received SMS texting than those who did not and the effects of the text messaging lasted 12 weeks after it ceased [21].

3.9 Virtual Coaching

Virtual coaching can be either automated or in person. Having a motivational coach increases participation in physical activity. A study in 2013 used a pedometer to track the physical activity of sedentary older adults who received an Embodied Conversational Agent (ECA) and a control [20]. After participating in the ECA intervention, the participants walked significantly more than the control group [20]. The ECA intervention uses a tablet to simulate a face-to-face conversation with an animated character [20]. The daily session varied each time but always included a greeting, social chat, a check-in, and a tip [20]. The use of a virtual coach provides the same level of success in behavior modification as an in-person coach without requiring the financial investment of training.

3.10 Websites/Modules

Websites/modules have specific learning objectives that are universally presented to the audience. These modules can be used as a means to educate the elderly population on either new technologies or behavior modification [22]. The use of this type of technology is dependent on the use of an electronic device, such as a tablet or computer, and access to the Internet. In seniors aged 65–75 years, the use of modules required self-regulation and without adequate participation, changes in physical activity would be affected [23] (Table 1).

4 Discussion

Health technology has the potential to promote a healthy lifestyle for seniors. These types of technology save on costs as they do not require a trained individual to administer the education. The helpfulness of person-to-person interactions is overestimated as the impact does not always warrant the investment of training the health professional. For instance, heart failure patients in Finland were assigned more follow-up visits in addition to telephone checkups but there was no significance

Table 1 The frequency of technologies in reviewed articles

Type of technology	Articles	Total
mHealth/phones	[14, 18, 21, 24–34]	14
Website/modules	[20, 22, 23, 25, 27, 33, 35–38]	10
Monitoring technology	[18–20, 23, 26, 39–41]	9
Health games/computer	[14, 15, 31, 42, 43]	5
Internet	[16, 17, 29, 37, 44]	5
Text messaging	[21, 38, 45–47]	5
Assistive technology	[10, 11, 26, 48]	4
Exercise simulation	[8, 12, 40]	3
Virtual coaching	[20, 29, 49]	3
Tablet	[10, 20]	2

Source: Developed for this study

in the improvement of health post-surgery compared to those without additional follow-ups [24]. Automated telephone counseling has the same effect in motivating the elderly population as counseling by trained educators [49]. In a study with 218 adults, automated telephone chats were as effective as the human-delivered interventions [34].

Another benefit to using technology for health behavior modification is that their benefits can be seen when using more than one type at a time. In the majority of studies, multiple technologies are incorporated into a method instead of using a single-type technology. The impact of technology can be enhanced with the use of more than one form per intervention. When a senior use monitoring technology to keep track of their level of physical activity throughout the day, the amount of activity can be increased with targeted text messaging or virtual coaching via the Internet or their phones to encourage them to do more [21].

5 Conclusion

Approximately 47% of seniors in the USA have access to the Internet [50]. A basic set of skills are required to get the full use of technology, including accessing the Internet and the ability to run applications on different software [26]. In order to accommodate the senior population and ensure different types of technology are being used properly for health promotion they need to be modified to the age group.

Further research is required on the success of the long-term effects of newly adopted health technology.

Study Highlights

What was already known on the topic:

- Health technology can be used for primary prevention of disease by promoting healthy behaviors.

What the study added to our knowledge:

- There are 10 effective categories of health technology that can be used in health promotion to modify senior's behaviors.
- The different categories can be used successfully in combination or as a standalone.

References

1. L.A. Charles, B.M. Dobbs, R.M. Mckay, O. Babenko, J.A. Triscott, Training of specialized geriatric physicians to meet the needs of an aging population-a unique Care of the Elderly Physician Program in Canada. J. Am. Geriatr. Soc. **62**(7), 1390–1392 (2014). https://doi.org/10.1111/jgs.12907
2. B.A. Meisner, Aging in Canada. Can. J. Public Health **105**(5), 399 (2014)
3. S. Sarma, W. Simpson, A panel multinomial logit analysis of elderly living arrangements: Evidence from aging in Manitoba longitudinal data, Canada. Soc. Sci. Med. **65**(12), 2539–2552 (2007). https://doi.org/10.1016/j.socscimed.2007.07.012
4. D. Cohen, D.G. Manuel, P. Tugwell, C. Sanmartin, T. Ramsay, Direct healthcare costs of acute myocardial infarction in Canada's elderly across the continuum of care. J. Econ. Ageing. **3**, 44–49 (2014). https://doi.org/10.1016/j.jeoa.2014.05.002
5. X. Li, D. Guh, D. Lacaille, J. Esdaile, A.H. Anis, The impact of cost sharing of prescription drug expenditures on health care utilization by the elderly: Own- and cross-price elasticities. Health Policy **82**(3), 340–347 (2007). https://doi.org/10.1016/j.healthpol.2006.11.002
6. V. Preston, A. Kim, S. Hudyma, N. Mandell, M. Luxton, J. Hemphill, Gender, race, and immigration: Aging and economic security in Canada. Can. Rev. Soc. Policy **68**, 90 (2013)
7. L.C. Williams, B.T. Day, Medical cost Savings for web-Based Wellness Program Participants from employers engaged in health promotion activities. Am. J. Health Promot. **25**(4), 272–280 (2011). https://doi.org/10.4278/ajhp.100415-quan-119
8. M.-L. Bird, B. Clark, J. Millar, S. Whetton, S. Smith, Exposure to "Exergames" increases older adults' perception of the usefulness of Technology for Improving Health and Physical Activity: A pilot study. JMIR Serious Games. **3**(2), e8 (2015). https://doi.org/10.2196/games.4275
9. Y. Lu, Y. Chang, Investigation of the internet adoption on senior farmers. Eng. Comput. **33**(6), 1853–1864 (2016). https://doi.org/10.1108/ec-08-2015-0259
10. R. Oosterom-Calo, T.A. Abma, M.A. Visse, W. Stut, S.J. Velde, J. Brug, An interactive-technology health behavior promotion program for heart failure patients: A pilot study of experiences and needs of patients and nurses in the hospital setting. JMIR Res. Protoc. **3**(2), e32 (2014)
11. P.R. Cangelosi, J.M. Sorrell, Use of technology to enhance mental health for older adults. J. Psychosoc. Nurs. Ment. Health Serv. **52**(9), 17–20 (2014). https://doi.org/10.3928/02793695-20140721-01

12. M. Albu, L. Atack, I. Srivastava, Simulation and gaming to promote health education: Results of a usability test. Health Educ. J. **74**(2), 244–254 (2014). https://doi.org/10.1177/0017896914532623

13. PRISMA, in *Transparent Reporting of Systematic Reviews and Meta-analyses, 2009* (cited 17 October 2015). http://www.prisma-statement.org/

14. J. Lee, A.L. Nguyen, J. Berg, A. Amin, M. Bachman, Y. Guo, L. Evangelista, Attitudes and preferences on the use of Mobile health technology and health games for self-management: Interviews with older adults on anticoagulation therapy. JMIR Mhealth Uhealth **2**(3), e32 (2014). https://doi.org/10.2196/mhealth.3196

15. R. Young, E. Willis, G. Cameron, M. Geana, "Willing but unwilling": Attitudinal barriers to adoption of home-based health information technology among older adults. Health Informatics J. **20**(2), 127–135 (2013). https://doi.org/10.1177/1460458213486906

16. K. Goodall, P. Ward, L. Newman, Use of information and communication technology to provide health information: What do older migrants know, and what do they need to know? Qual. Prim. Care **18**, 27–32 (2010)

17. R.F. Cook, R.K. Hersch, D. Schlossberg, S.L. Leaf, A web-based health promotion program for older workers: Randomized controlled trial. J. Med. Internet Res. **17**(3), e82 (2015). https://doi.org/10.2196/jmir.3399

18. E. Knight, M.I. Stuckey, R.J. Petrella, Health promotion through primary care: Enhancing self-management with activity prescription and mHealth. Phys. Sportsmed. **42**(3), 90–99 (2014). https://doi.org/10.3810/psm.2014.09.2080

19. B. Shoshana, N. Schoenberg, B. Howell, What motivates older adults to improve diet and exercise patterns? The Gerontologist **55**, 681–681 (2015). https://doi.org/10.1093/geront/gnv350.06

20. T.W. Bickmore, R.A. Silliman, K. Nelson, D.M. Cheng, M. Winter, L. Henault, M.K. Paasche-Orlow, A randomized controlled trial of an automated exercise coach for older adults. J. Am. Geriatr. Soc. **61**(10), 1676–1683 (2013). https://doi.org/10.1111/jgs.12449

21. A.M. Müller, S. Khoo, T. Morris, Text messaging for exercise promotion in older adults from an upper-middle-income country: Randomized controlled trial. J. Med. Internet Res. **18**(1), e5 (2016). https://doi.org/10.2196/jmir.5235

22. L.V. Velsen, M. Illario, S. Jansen-Kosterink, C. Crola, C.D. Somma, A. Colao, M. Vollenbroek-Hutten, A community-based, technology-supported health Service for Detecting and Preventing Frailty among older adults: A participatory design development process. J Aging Res. **2015**, 1–9 (2015). https://doi.org/10.1155/2015/216084

23. S. Muellmann, I. Bragina, C. Voelcker-Rehage, E. Rost, S. Lippke, J. Meyer, J. Schnauber, M. Wasmann, M. Toborg, F. Koppelin, T. Brand, H. Zeeb, C.R. Pischke, Development and evaluation of two web-based interventions for the promotion of physical activity in older adults: Study protocol for a community-based controlled intervention trial. BMC Public Health **17**(1), 512 (2017). https://doi.org/10.1186/s12889-017-4446-x

24. A.L. Vuorinen, J. Leppänen, H. Kaijanranta, M. Kulju, T. Heliö, M. van Gils, J. Lähteenmäki, Use of home Telemonitoring to support multidisciplinary Care of Heart Failure Patients in Finland: Randomized controlled trial. J. Med. Internet Res. **16**(2), e282 (2014)

25. F. Lattanzio, A.M. Abbatecola, R. Bevilacqua, C. Chiatti, A. Corsonello, L. Rossi, S. Bustacchini, R. Bernabei, Advanced technology care innovation for older people in Italy: Necessity and opportunity to promote health and wellbeing. J. Am. Med. Dir. Assoc. **15**(7), 457–466 (2014). https://doi.org/10.1016/j.jamda.2014.04.003

26. A. Barakat, R.D. Woolrych, A. Sixsmith, W.D. Kearns, H.S. Kort, EHealth technology competencies for health professionals working in home care to support older adults to age in place: Outcomes of a two-day collaborative workshop. Med. 2.0 **2**(2), e10 (2013). https://doi.org/10.2196/med20.2711

27. K. Pangbourne, P. Aditjandra, J. Nelson, New technology and quality of life for older people: Exploring health and transport dimensions in the UK context. IET Intell. Transp. Syst. **4**(4), 318 (2010). https://doi.org/10.1049/iet-its.2009.0106

28. A. King, B. Hekler, L. Grieco, S. Winter, J. Sheats, M. Buman, B. Banerjee, T. Robinson, J. Cirimele, Effects of three motivationally targeted Mobile device applications on initial physical activity and sedentary behavior change in midlife and older adults: A randomized trial. PLoS One **11**(7), e0156370 (2016). https://doi.org/10.1371/journal.pone.0160113

29. A. Voukelatos, D. Merom, C. Rissel, C. Sherrington, W. Watson, K. Waller, The effect of walking on falls in older people: The easy steps to health randomized controlled trial study protocol. BMC Public Health **11**(1), 888 (2011). https://doi.org/10.1186/1471-2458-11-888

30. K. Sahlen, H. Johansson, L. Nyström, L. Lindholm, Health coaching to promote healthier lifestyle among older people at moderate risk for cardiovascular diseases, diabetes and depression: A study protocol for a randomized controlled trial in Sweden. BMC Public Health **13**(1), 199 (2013). https://doi.org/10.1186/1471-2458-13-199

31. S. Nikou, Mobile technology and forgotten consumers: The young-elderly. Int. J. Consum. Stud. **39**(4), 294–304 (2015). https://doi.org/10.1111/ijcs.12187

32. M. Bowen, Beyond repair: Literacy, technology, and a curriculum of aging. Coll. Eng. **75**(5), 437–457 (2012)

33. D. Kutz, K. Shankar, K. Connelly, Making sense of mobile- and web-based wellness information technology: Cross-generational study. J. Med. Internet Res. **15**(5), e83 (2013). https://doi.org/10.2196/jmir.2124

34. E.B. Hekler, M.P. Buman, J. Otten, C.M. Castro, L. Grieco, B. Marcus, R.H. Friedman, M.A. Napolitano, A.C. King, Determining who responds better to a computer- vs. human-delivered physical activity intervention: Results from the community health advice by telephone (CHAT) trial. Int. J. Behav. Nutr. Phys. Act. **10**(1), 109 (2013). https://doi.org/10.1186/1479-5868-10-109

35. R. Oosterom-Calo, t.S.J. Velde, W. Stut, J. Brug, Development of Motivate4Change using the intervention mapping protocol: An interactive technology physical activity and medication adherence promotion program for hospitalized heart failure patients. JMIR Res. Protoc. **4**(3), e88 (2015)

36. D.E. Wall, C. Least, J. Gromis, B. Lohse, Nutrition education intervention improves vegetable-related attitude, self-efficacy, preference, and knowledge of fourth-grade students. J. Sch. Health **82**(1), 37–43 (2011)

37. S.J. Robroek, D.E. Lindeboom, A. Burdorf, Initial and sustained participation in an internet-delivered long-term worksite health promotion program on physical activity and nutrition. J. Med. Internet Res. **14**(2), e43 (2012). https://doi.org/10.2196/jmir.1788

38. B.C. Bock, K.E. Heron, E.G. Jennings, J.C. Magee, K.M. Morrow, User preferences for a text message–based smoking cessation intervention. Health Educ. Behav. **40**(2), 152–159 (2012). https://doi.org/10.1177/1090198112463020

39. M.J. Rantz, M. Skubic, M. Popescu, C. Galambos, R.J. Koopman, G.L. Alexander, L.J. Phillips, K. Musterman, J. Back, S.J. Miller, A new paradigm of technology-enabled 'vital signs' for early detection of health change for older adults. Gerontology **61**, 281–290 (2015)

40. T. Tsai, A.M. Wong, C. Hsu, K.C. Tseng, Research on a community-based platform for promoting health and physical fitness in the elderly community. PLoS One **8**(2), e57452 (2013). https://doi.org/10.1371/journal.pone.0057452

41. L. Powell, J. Parker, M.M. St-James, S. Mawson, The effectiveness of lower-limb wearable Technology for Improving Activity and Participation in adult stroke survivors: A systematic review. J. Med. Internet Res. **18**(10), e259 (2016). https://doi.org/10.2196/jmir.5891

42. S. Yusif, J. Soar, A. Hafeez-Baig, Older people, assistive technologies, and the barriers to adoption: A systematic review. Int. J. Med. Inform. **94**, 112–116 (2016). https://doi.org/10.1016/j.ijmedinf.2016.07.004

43. H. Eyles, R. Mclean, B. Neal, R.N. Doughty, Y. Jiang, C.N. Mhurchu, Using mobile technology to support lower-salt food choices for people with cardiovascular disease: Protocol for the SaltSwitch randomized controlled trial. BMC Public Health **14**(1), 950 (2014). https://doi.org/10.1186/1471-2458-14-950

44. J.M. Bernhardt, J.D. Chaney, B.H. Chaney, A.K. Hall, New Media for Health Education. Health Educ. Behav. **40**(2), 129–132 (2013). https://doi.org/10.1177/1090198113483140

45. N.E. Stanczyk, C. Bolman, J.W. Muris, H. de Vries, Study protocol of a dutch smoking cessation e-health program. BMC Public Health **11**, 847–847 (2011). https://doi.org/10.1186/1471-2458-11-847
46. A. Zubala, S. MacGillivray, H. Frost, T. Kroll, D. Skelton, A. Gavine, N.M. Gray, M. Toma, J. Morris, Promotion of physical activity interventions for community dwelling older adults: A systematic review of reviews. PLoS One **12**(7), e0180902 (2017)
47. R.E. Ostrander, H.J. Thompson, G. Demiris, Using targeted messaging to increase physical activity in older adults: A review. J. Gerontol. Nurs. **40**(9), 36–48 (2014). https://doi.org/10.3928/00989134-20140324-03
48. Liu, J., Modrek, S., Anyanti, J., Nwokolo, E., Cruz, A. D., Schatzkin, E, Isiguzo C, Ujuju C, . Montagu, D. (2014). How do risk preferences relate to malaria care-seeking behavior and the acceptability of a new health technology in Nigeria? BMC Health Serv. Res., 14(1). 374. doi:https://doi.org/10.1186/1472-6963-14-374
49. A.C. King, J.M. Guralnik, Maximizing the potential of an aging population. JAMA **304**(17), 1944 (2010). https://doi.org/10.1001/jama.2010.1577
50. R. Campbell, D. Nolfi, D. Bowen, Teaching elderly adults to use the internet to access health care information: Before-after study. J. Med. Internet Res. **7**, 2 (2015)

Technologies for Motion Measurements in Connected Health Scenario

Pasquale Daponte, Luca De Vito, Gianluca Mazzilli, Sergio Rapuano, and Ioan Tudosa

Abstract Connected Health, also known as Technology-Enabled Care (TEC), refers to a conceptual model for health management where devices, services, or interventions are designed around the patient's needs and health-related data is shared in such a way that the patient can receive care in the most proactive and efficient manner. In particular, TEC enables the remote exchange of information, mainly between a patient and a healthcare professional, to monitor health status, and to assist in diagnosis. To that aim recent advances in pervasive sensing, mobile, and communication technologies have led to the deployment of new smart sensors that can be worn without affecting a person's daily activities. This chapter encompasses a brief literature review on TEC challenges, with a focus on the key technologies enabling the development of wearable solutions for remote human motion tracking. A wireless sensor network-based remote monitoring system, together with the main challenges and limitations that are likely to be faced during its implementation is also discussed, with a glimpse at its application.

Keywords Motion measurements · Connected health · Body area sensor network · IMU · Healthcare

1 Introduction

Healthcare challenges get increasingly complex due to the growing and aging population, the rising cost of advanced medical treatments and the severely constrained health and social care budgets. In such scenario, TEC is capable of providing cost-effective solutions such as telehealth, telecare, and telemedicine with the aim of providing care for people in convenient, accessible, and cost-effective manner.

P. Daponte · L. De Vito · G. Mazzilli · S. Rapuano (✉) · I. Tudosa
Department of Engineering, University of Sannio, Benevento, Italy
e-mail: daponte@unisannio.it; devito@unisannio.it; gmazzill@unisannio.iti;
rapuano@unisannio.it; itudosa@unisannio.it

© Springer Nature Switzerland AG 2020   191
A. El Saddik et al. (eds.), *Connected Health in Smart Cities*,
https://doi.org/10.1007/978-3-030-27844-1_10

One of the most challenging features of Connected Health is related to human motion measurements. Over the last few years, several motion tracking systems and techniques have been developed in order to allow clinicians to evaluate human motion across several biometric factors or obtaining accurate postural information about sport athletes. Recent developments in human motion tracking systems, mainly due to the modern communication capabilities, led to a number of exciting applications in Connected Health scenarios, in particular in the fields of medical rehabilitation and sport biomechanics.

In recent years, medical motor rehabilitation relevance grew fast as the average population age increased, along with a surge of chronicle diseases and accidents, as those related to sport activities. The ultimate goal of rehabilitation process, which includes several stages, should be to fully recover from temporary motor impairments, or to enhance the life quality of patients with permanent motor disorder by aiming at the highest possible level of independence [1].

In the rehabilitation of motor dysfunctions, a key role is played by the Range Of Motion (ROM) measurements whose evaluation constitutes the basis of the therapist's work. ROM is defined as the amount of movement through a particular plane, expressed in degrees, that can occur in a joint. Figure 1 depicts a flexion exercise apt to determine the ROM for elbow. Most times ROM measurements are carried out under subjective scrutiny of therapists who rely on their own sensitivity and expertise about visual analysis of human body and palpation of the concerned regions. The adoption of electronic measurement methods in rehabilitation offers the outstanding advantage of automatic measurements that allow to assist qualitative analysis of therapists with objectively measured quantities. Moreover, combining measurements via electronic instrumentation with the wide area networks set rehabilitation activities free of space and time constraints.

One of the fields where the automatic measurement of ROM could provide significant improvements in the treatment process and in the cost reduction of such

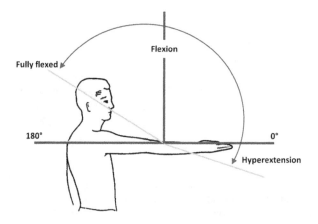

Fig. 1 Range of motion for elbow joint

treatment is home rehabilitation. Basically, home rehabilitation allows a patient to undergo treatment without the need to reach a specialized center. Apart from minimizing inconvenience and cost of commuting, a patient that has been given the opportunity of carrying out rehabilitation activities while staying at home is likely to show motivation and make progress thanks to the more comfortable conditions he/she enjoys. Moreover, avoiding for patient to share space, equipment, and therapists' attention with other people in a crowded center implies longer, and thus more effective, sessions. Ultimately, helping to improve the quality of treatment mainly means helping make recovery faster, which has a direct impact on the costs for healthcare systems [2].

Another emerging field that involves automatic human motion measurement techniques, often simply called motion tracking techniques, for studying biomechanical parameters of the human movement is sport biomechanics. In this context, the development of accurate activity monitoring techniques is performed to gain a greater understanding of the athletic performance. As an example, real-time monitoring of load and tiredness of athletes during their training sessions is important in order to maximize performance during competitions, as well as being important for the health of the athletes. Activity monitoring also plays an important role in injury prevention and rehabilitation. Due to the nature of sport activities, any monitoring device should be small and unobtrusive as possible.

Recent advancements in communication and network technologies have made possible the remote monitoring of motion tracking systems, both for home rehabilitation and sport applications. Authors in [3] describe a remote environment for athletes' training and support. By means of wireless sensors, the system provides the visualization to a remote advisor about runners' conditions, providing feedback functions to them by using kinematic feature of arm swing. A conceptual representation of a remote monitoring system for home healthcare in a Connected Health scenario is shown in Fig. 2. Small sensors, unobtrusively worn on designed clothing or accessories, are used to gather physiological and movement data. Sensors are placed according to the clinical application of interest. For instance,

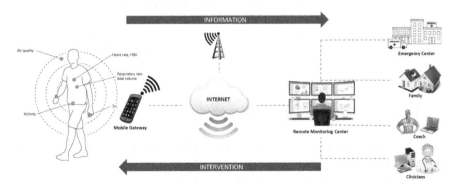

Fig. 2 Conceptual representation of a remote monitoring system for home healthcare in a Connected Health scenario

sensors for human motion measurements could be deployed on the body parts involved in a rehabilitation treatment. Wireless communication is enabled to stream health-related information to a mobile phone or an access point, forwarding them to a Remote Monitoring Center (RMC) via Internet. Warning situations are detected via dynamic data processing algorithms and an alert message is sent to an emergency center to provide immediate assistance. Caregivers and family members are alerted in case of an emergency but could also be notified in several situations when the patient requires assistance.

Despite the proven benefits of the remote monitoring systems relying on body-worn sensors like those described above, there are considerable open challenges that need to be addressed before such systems can be adopted on a large scale. These challenges include not only technological barriers, such as interoperability across different platforms and security issues but also serious cultural barriers such as the dislike of the use of medical devices for home-based clinical monitoring [4].

Some of the aforementioned technical challenges have already been dealt with satisfactorily, some others are being faced and some others are still under study. This chapter presents some solutions to those challenges focusing on a remote measurement system designed for motion tracking in home rehabilitation field that can be adopted for sport biomechanics and can easily be extended to other remote health applications. The main challenges will be presented first, than the available technologies, their lacks, and some possible solutions will be discussed in the next sections. In particular, Sect. 2 provides an overview of key sensing technologies enabling the development of wearable solutions for human motion tracking and remote monitoring systems. Although the most common enabling technologies can be classified as sensing and communication hardware, the influence of signal processing and software technologies can be significant when designing a remote monitoring system for home healthcare. Of course, the role of such technologies depends on the specific application case. Therefore, the chapter presents a case study from the choice of the sensors to the architecture design and implementation to the communication and usage optimization. In Sect. 3, a remote monitoring system capable of bringing a real-time 3D reconstruction of human posture is described. Section 4 deals with the problems of realizing such system relying on a standard wireless network. Section 5 shows an example of the application of advanced software technologies to improve the scalability and the communication performance of the remote monitoring system. Finally, Sect. 6 draws conclusions.

2   Key Enabling Technologies

Systems for human motion tracking and remote monitoring consist of three main blocks: (1) the sensing hardware to collect motion data; (2) the communication interface (both hardware and software) to gather data coming from sensing devices and relay them to a RMC, and (3) dynamic data analysis algorithms to extract clinically relevant information from motion data.

The advancements of sensors based on MEMS (Micro Electro-Mechanical Systems) technology, and in particular of inertial sensors have enabled a huge development of instruments and systems for motion tracking, in particular for applications in the fields of healthcare, rehabilitation, and biomechanics. MEMS inertial sensors have been recently used to design personal and body area motion measurement systems to continuously monitor the patients during the rehabilitation treatment. Monitoring allows the doctors to be aware of the patient's progress, as well as to collect data for biofeedback systems, where the patient's motivation can be increased by looking at his/her results [5]. MEMS inertial sensors are usually composed of a 3-axial accelerometer, able to measure the static acceleration, and a 3-axial gyroscope, able to measure the angular rate, to form an Inertial Measurement Unit (IMU). Often such sensors are combined with a 3-axial magnetometer, able to measure the Earth magnetic field. In this case, the sensor unit takes the name of MARG (Magnetic, Angular Rate, and Gravity).

The values measured by the different sensors need to be combined to obtain an estimation of the orientation of the unit. Although, in order to obtain the orientation, just the 3-axial accelerometer and the 3-axial magnetometer would be needed, it is useful to merge the measurements from such sensors with those from the gyroscope, with the aims of reducing the noise on the accelerometer and magnetometer readings, and of compensating for the gyroscope offset, that causes a drift of the orientation estimation. Moreover, the magnetometer is often prone to disturbances coming from external magnetic fields and ferromagnetic materials in the environment.

A motion capture suit composed of inertial sensors has been presented in [6]. The suit has been specifically introduced for home and hospital rehabilitation, with the aim of providing real-time support to health assessment by supplying motion-related quantities. The embedded sensors communicate with a personal computer via CAN bus at 1 Mb/s. In their latest revision, authors replaced CAN interface with a Bluetooth module.

Sensor nodes must be noninvasive to be accepted by the patient, and they have to avoid restraining the movements that the patient does in normal conditions, otherwise the measurement results will be altered by the system itself. For this reason, wireless technologies have been recently adopted in many health applications because of the flexibility offered by reduced wiring, which gets costs lower and patient more friendly to instruments he/she has to interact with. Furthermore, wireless equipment is usually based on low-power consumption technologies enabling long-term monitoring. A review of wireless-based solutions for health applications is available in [7].

Authors of [8] experimented with a wireless system using an accelerometer to monitor vital signs of people staying at home. Post analysis unveiled that different types of human movements (i.e., walking, falling, jumping, and so forth) generate different patterns in acceleration data, and that information can be used to recognize abnormal activities and warn against them. Patients with Parkinson disease were monitored during everyday activities to evaluate their in-home mobility [9]. To capture the whole-body motor function and identify movement patterns in scripted and unscripted tasks, inertial units were attached to body parts and communicated with a laptop computer in the range of action. Results obtained with principal component analysis showed a wide variability across tasks for several subjects, and within subjects for each task. IMUs have also been integrated into consolidated equipment accompanying rehabilitation treatment, like those applied to forearm crutches being used in lower limb rehabilitation [10] to sense the force applied by patient, the crutch tilt and the handle grip position. These parameters have been proven to deeply affect the recovery rate, thus, monitoring them and giving biofeedback can help the patients to adjust their crutch walking to the proper way.

Several studies can be found in the literature addressing the use of wireless IMUs in sport applications. The speed and energy expenditure of athletes over ground running can be obtained through the use of wearable accelerometers [11]. Authors in [12] combined a suite of common, off-the-shelf, sensors with body sensing technology and developed a software system for recording, analyzing, and presenting sensed data sampled from a single player during a football match. Readings are gathered from heart rate, galvanic skin response, motion, respiration, and location using on-body sensors.

Although they are not the most accurate instrument to track human movements [13], wireless IMUs have long turned out comfortable for home rehabilitation applications, as they can work under the most common circumstances, without any particular constraint on lighting or space. Many approaches to motion tracking have been introduced over the years based on wearable motion sensors, whose measurements have mostly been validated against well-known camera-based systems with markers. A wearable wireless sensor network able to keep track of arm motion in sagittal plane was proposed in [14]. Two nodes, equipped with a biaxial accelerometer, were used as inclinometer and sensed the orientation of the upper and lower arm while extending and flexing the limb. The angle estimate error due to misalignment of nodes along the arm was modeled, and a calibration to determine accelerometer offsets was carried out by mounting the sensor on a high-precision rotary motor. Furthermore, system accuracy was evaluated by making the motor produce swinging motion with different oscillation speeds.

Motion tracking applications by means of wearable systems most often employ multiple sensors typically integrated into a Body Area Sensor Network (BASN). An example of this technology is the motion tracking system described in [15, 16]. The described home rehabilitation system produces, by means of a BASN, ROM measurements for patients performing rehabilitation exercises. A set of wireless nodes (or motes) constitutes a wearable device that keeps track of orientation produced by different body segments. Given a joint to monitor, both of the involved limb segments are equipped with a mote embedding an IMU, so that the ROM is determined from the absolute orientation of two motes. The primary functions of the sensor nodes in a BASN are (1) to unobtrusively sample motion signals and (2) to transfer relevant data to a personal gateway by means of a wireless connection. A personal gateway, implemented on a smartphone or a personal computer, sets up and controls the BASN, transferring health-related information to the RMC through the Internet.

The availability of mobile telecommunication networks (e.g., GRPS, 3G, 4G) allows pervasive user monitoring when he/she is outside the home environment. During the last few years, several communication standards for low-power wireless communication have been proposed in order to fulfill three main requirements: (1) low cost; (2) small size of transmitter and receiver devices; and (3) low-power consumption. The recent developments of IEEE 802.15.4 (ZigBee) and IEEE 802.15.1 (Bluetooth) have the major focus on increasing network throughput. Moreover, network lifetime has a greater importance in BASNs since devices are expected to perform over long periods of time [17].

The large amount of data gathered using wearable systems for user's status monitoring has to be managed and processed in order to derive clinically relevant information. Signal processing, data mining, and pattern recognition are examples of data analysis techniques that enable remote monitoring applications that would have been otherwise impossible. Although an exhaustive discussion of the various data processing algorithms used to process and analyze wearable sensor data is outside the scope of this chapter, one cannot emphasize enough the fact that data processing and analysis techniques are an integral part of the design and development of remote monitoring systems based on wearable technology.

3 A Remote Monitoring System for Home Rehabilitation

An example of joint adoption of the key technologies introduced in the previous section can be found in [18], proposing an integrated wireless system gearing toward the human motion tracking in home rehabilitation. The study described in [18] deals with the design and implementation, from scratch, of a remote monitoring system allowing the real-time 3D reconstruction of the patient's motion. The key contribution of the proposal, in addition, to help improving treatment conditions and to reduce healthcare costs, lies in producing outputs that can be evaluated both qualitatively and quantitatively by an operator. The system has been designed in order to reduce costs, as well as occupancy, of home-side instrumentation. In such a scenario, a subject in treatment may stay at home performing rehabilitation exercises while wearing small motion sensors, which are included in a BASN. Of course, nothing prevents the same system from being used also within the rehabilitation centers, where many patients could be contemporarily accommodated.

Being properly strapped to the body segments of interest, the sensor nodes provide information about their own respective motions. Through a network connection, sensed data are delivered to a dedicated server (Posture Reconstruction Server—PRS), housed at the RMC, that processes the raw measurements to determine the corresponding human posture. The evolution of human body part orientation and posture in time is afterwards stored in a database so that the motor behavior can be replayed for post analysis. The patient's motor behavior is projected at the RMC on a 3D digital representation.

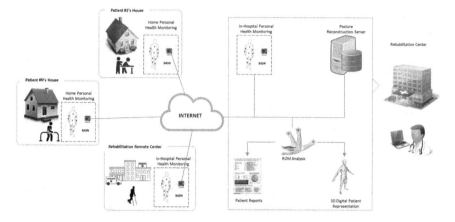

Fig. 3 System architecture of the human motion tracking system proposed in [18]

By interacting with a ROM analysis graphical user interface, the clinical staff can watch, without leaving the workplace, the movements of several subjects under analysis as they are executed at the same time. Augmenting the observation experience of physiotherapists with objective ROM measurements may stand for an unprecedented way to evaluate functional recovery, both between and within subjects.

The components of the remote monitoring system are detailed in the following subsections (Fig. 3).

3.1 Body Area Sensor Network

The proposed BASN (Fig. 4) includes as many sensor nodes as body segments to track, in addition to a gateway node. Each sensor node is responsible for providing the data needed to determine the absolute orientation in the space of the body segment. All the motes taking part in the BASN are Zolertia Z1 modules, having the size of $34.40 \times 57.00 \times 11.86$ mm^3, and transmitting data via IEEE 802.15.4 interfaces to the gateway node. Each of them is programmed with TinyOS, and equipped with a 9 degrees of freedom IMU. Such an IMU comprises three sensors connected by I2C bus to a Texas Instruments© MSP430 microcontroller: a 3-axis accelerometer measuring linear acceleration with 12-bit resolution, a 3-axis gyroscope measuring angular rates with 16-bit resolution, and a 3-axis magnetometer sensing the magnetic field with 16-bit resolution, all being sampled at 50 Hz along the same local reference system. Apart from size and weight of motes being limited, the fact that the whole communication relies exclusively on wireless technology goes a long way toward getting the usage as tidy and comfortable as possible. Consequently, the patients may enjoy more mobility than wearing a wired

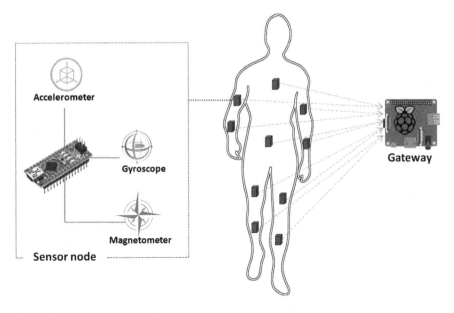

Fig. 4 Body area sensor network

measurement system, which may play an essential role in motivating patients. The gateway node consists of a mote, wirelessly receiving data from sensor nodes, that is attached via USB to a Raspberry Pi, a very cheap banknote-sized single-board computer, having TCP/IP capabilities and being connected to the power grid. The single-board computer, equipped with a 32-bit ARM 700 MHz processor and 512 MB RAM, gathers and handles raw sensed data from IMUs that are then streamed to the PRS via Real-time Transport Protocol (RTP).

3.2 Posture Reconstruction Server

The PRS, housed in the RMC, is a processing unit that is in charge of three different functions: (1) it handles raw sensed data from several BASNs to obtain absolute orientation of single body segments and, as a result, the whole body orientation and posture of multiple patients tracked at once; (2) it runs a Real Time Streaming Protocol (RTSP) server offering to the users the possibility of controlling the 3D representation playback; and (3) it operates a database storing the patient's posture as it evolves in time, thus making up a sort of personal motor history. The PRS represents a powerful resource that allows both for offline analysis of progresses made by a given subject over time and for comparison of quantities concerning the same rehabilitation stage in a given treatment from different patients. The RTSP server can be required by the user to stream either "live" playback, directly from a BASN, or some content stored in the database.

3.3   ROM Analysis Software

The software application for posture and ROM analysis runs at the physician's workstation and offers several analysis interfaces to the medical staff by interacting with the PRS. For example, patient reports including data and statistics on current treatment can be composed and displayed by the software upon accessing the history database in the PRS. Intra-subject analyses can be conducted by aggregating data from that source as well. The digital reconstruction of human posture is realized by means of a free 3D engine. The application can be set to feed the animation either with the data from one of the operating BASNs (real-time playback), or with stored posture information (delayed playback). It is worth adding that the operator is given the possibility of defining a set of joint angles he/she is interested to watch. The 3D animated model can be observed in Fig. 5 while set for measuring right upper limb motion. In this way, while the 3D animation is going on, objective quantities about those angles are displayed in virtual labels. The labels also show the maximum value reached since the therapy session has started, giving highly valuable support for immediate ROM assessment.

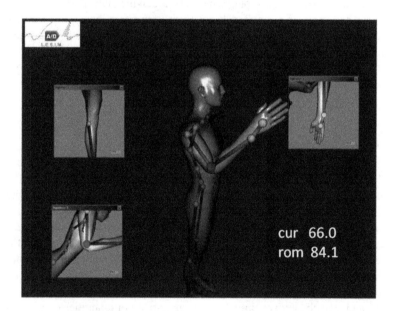

Fig. 5 A screenshot from the 3D animation of the right upper limb in action. The joint under analysis is the blue node in the screen

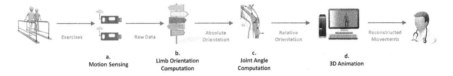

Fig. 6 Stages of real-time processing to animate the 3D reconstruction

3.4 Stages in Processing the Measurement Signals

Figure 6 outlines the stages that the real-time 3D reconstruction goes through, from home to the RMC. At the first stage (a), the movements produced by the patient are captured by the IMUs, whose raw data are collected and sent by the gateway to PRS. Subsequently (b), the PRS filters the compensated sensor outputs to determine, in real time, the orientation of the several body segments in the Earth's coordinate frame. The segment orientations are then combined to compute relative orientations and joint angles for reconstructing the posture of the subject (c). In the final stage (d), limb orientation and posture feed the ROM analysis application running on clients that show a 3D real-time animated model representing the patient. A therapist working at the rehabilitation center can finally observe from his/her workstation the movements as they are executed, maximizing productivity by observing multiple subjects at once.

3.5 Quaternion-Based Processing

Avoiding to engage them in any orientation computation lets the nodes of the BASN spend most of their working time in low power consumption mode, thus preserving battery life. Therefore, the PRS turns raw sensor data into body segment orientation and posture.

The orientations are expressed with quaternions $\mathbf{q} \in \mathbb{R}^4$ as representations based on Euler angles (i.e., pitch, roll, and yaw) suffer well-known singularity problems [19]. Although angular rates produced by a 3-axis gyroscope suffice to sense movements in the three planes, bias drift affecting the measurement prevents the accuracy necessary in human motion tracking applications. This is why the adopted algorithm uses data from accelerometer and magnetometer to estimate and compensate the gyro drift. On the other hand, external acceleration and magnetic disturbance usually make outputs from those two sensors noisy. To tackle these problems, step b of Fig. 6 is carried out by a quaternion-based implementation of extended Kalman filter [20]. Before an orientation estimation might be produced by a filter, a quaternion corresponding to each set of accelerometer (a) and magnetometer measurements (m) $y_m = [a\ m]^T$ should be computed. This is done by the Factored Quaternion Algorithm (FQA) [21], which offers good performance by avoiding to compute trigonometric functions. Moreover, since magnetic disturbance might be remarkable in indoor environments such as home and medical settings, the adoption of FQA is significant for the application as it limits the influence of magnetometer and, consequently, of disturbance to one plane of motion. The computed quaternion, along with angular rate from gyroscope, represents the input of the Kalman filter. Relative orientation quaternions necessary to the 3D representation are obtained at step c of Fig. 6 from global coordinate orientations through a reference system conversion. For example, let $\mathbf{q}_u$ and $\mathbf{q}_f$ be, respectively, the quaternions providing the absolute orientations of the upper arm and forearm segments, then $\mathbf{q}_f^u$ is the forearm orientation expressed in the upper arm's local reference system and is given by:

$$\mathbf{q}_f^u = \mathbf{q}_u^* \bigotimes \mathbf{q}_f \tag{1}$$

where $\bigotimes$ is the quaternion multiplication and $\mathbf{q}_u^*$ represents the conjugate of $\mathbf{q}_u$. Relative quaternions are also used to determine the joint angles that the operator requires to measure. For example, elbow joint angle θ can be expressed as pitch angle of the forearm segment in the upper arm's reference frame, that is:

$$\theta = \arcsin\left(2wy - 2xz\right) \tag{2}$$

with $\mathbf{q}_f^u = [\,w\ \ x\ \ y\ \ z\,]^T$.

4   Orientation Estimation in BASN Affected by Packet Loss

In order to achieve battery life extension, leading commitment in designing a BASN, a node is generally equipped with a low-power radio transceiver implementing IEEE 802.15.4 communication [22]. After all, extended battery life comes at a price: the less power is used, the lower is the communication reliability, meaning that the probability of packet loss may be significant. In most of wireless sensor network applications, communication occurs once in a while and retransmission is a viable way to overcome losses. Unfortunately, the strict time constraints on sampling, processing, and sending in real-time systems do not allow to broadcast once again a packet supposed to be not delivered. This happens any time a processing task cannot be postponed due to the needs for immediate feedback to provide. For instance, augmented reality applications have to adapt their outputs according to the change of spatial position and orientation as it happens [23].

In those cases, the only action one can take to face loss is to deal with it: loss tolerance countermeasures must aim at the reduction of the relative effects on the system outputs. Packet loss in real-time motion tracking applications basically results in a temporary decrease of the sampling rate, whose value is essential to capture a subject's movement adequately. In particular, for remote monitoring systems like the one described in the previous section, it can seriously harm the capability of the system to provide the user with accurate real-time measurements (e.g., a 3D model in motion tracking may happen to pose incorrectly). The problem is even bigger in applications with tens of nodes jointly working to trace the whole-body motion.

The problem of tracking and reconstructing the subject's movements can be modeled as the problem of finding out the spatial orientations, at any given time, of each of the segments the body is composed of. Theoretically, two main approaches are possible in order to estimate an orientation: either integrating the angular rates or referring to the projections of the Earth's gravity and magnetic field onto the sensor frame. In the former case, estimation relies exclusively on gyroscope data, in the latter accelerometer and magnetometer measurements are used as the inputs. Integrating angular rates means keeping an internal state (*stateful*) relying on the history of gyroscope data, while one sample of acceleration and magnetic field suffices to find orientation (*stateless*). In practice, both approaches, when working separately, fail to come up with a result being fit to represent human motion accurately. Gyroscope data are affected by bias that changes unpredictably in time, leading to an integration error that drifts remarkably in a few seconds. On the other hand, accelerometer and magnetometer data are basically noisy, and so are the resulting orientations, in addition, to suffering from interference caused by external acceleration and magnetic perturbations.

Every time a packet gets lost, a gap in the history of angular rates some of the body segments of the 3D model fall behind the actual movement, and in some cases awkward postures may show up. Figure 7 shows the ideal humerus pitch angle obtained when a loss occurs after 40 s, against the humerus pitch angles produced by single-frame algorithm (red line) and data-fusion algorithm (blue line). As can be seen, the ideal pitch angle grows linearly with time, while single-frame trajectory gets back on its track reacting to the same loss faster than what happens for data-fusion trajectory. A trade-off has to be found between choosing single-frame or data-fusion algorithms that could cause lower orientation accuracy and/or better loss resilience. In order to deal with that problem, a method based on the interpolation of quaternions computed by two algorithms, as depicted in Fig. 8, has been proposed in [24].

Having two unit quaternions representing rotations, an intermediate rotation can be found by interpolating them. Linear interpolation is not the best solution since a rotating joint is expected to move along a smooth curve. *Spherical Linear IntERPolation (SLERP)* is defined as a linear interpolation performed on the surface of a unit sphere, used in the field of computer graphics to obtain smooth motion. Analytically, let $\mathbf{q}_A$ and $\mathbf{q}_B$ be two unit quaternions, θ be the rotation angle, and $\mu \in [0, 1]$ be a real scalar value, the *SLERP* resulting from

$$\mathbf{q}_C = SLERP\,(\mathbf{q}_A, \mathbf{q}_B, \mu) = \frac{\sin\,(1 - \mu)\,\theta}{\sin\theta}\mathbf{q}_A + \frac{\sin\mu\theta}{\sin\theta}\mathbf{q}_B \tag{3}$$

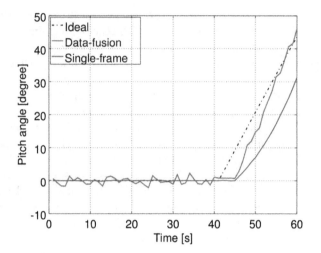

Fig. 7 Humerus pitch angle trajectories

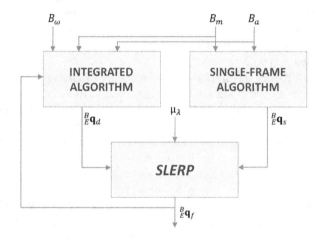

Fig. 8 Interpolation between data-fusion and single-frame quaternion

carries out a spherical interpolation between $\mathbf{q}_A$ and $\mathbf{q}_B$ by an amount μ, with $\mathbf{q}_C$ determined as a point along the circle arc on the surface of the unit sphere.

Early experiments have been carried out and their results have been presented in [24]. The sensor platform used in experiments consists of the same Zolerzia Z1 described above. The raw data have been organized in 6-sample packets, collected by a personal computer from a sensor via wired serial communication in order to get continuous lossless sequences of samples. These sequences then have been artificially injected with several profiles of loss, so as to create artificial lossy sample sequences and analyze the algorithm performance under different conditions of network reliability. In order to assess effects not only on the single node orientation, but also on joint angle measurement, sequences from two adjacent nodes have been acquired. In particular, raw data related to a 90° arm extension have been acquired and the pitch angles of humerus and forearm have been analyzed. The raw data sequence of the humerus trajectory has been injected with a loss of four packets right after 80 samples.

Figure 9a reports the performance of the data-fusion algorithm proposed in [24]. It can be seen that the occurrence of packets loss results in humerus pitch angle (red line) different from forearm one (blue line). As reported previously, this results in a growing elbow joint angle (black line). Moreover, the slow convergence rate causes a considerable deviation of the elbow joint angle for more than 2 s (about 100 samples), which is not desirable in human motion capture. The noisy single-frame orientations are shown in Fig. 9b to reduce the upper bound of elbow joint error below 20°, even though they return trajectories being unacceptably jerky. The performance of the interpolation method is shown in Fig. 9c, where the error of elbow joint angle reaches 10° for about 1 s only. It is worth remarking that these

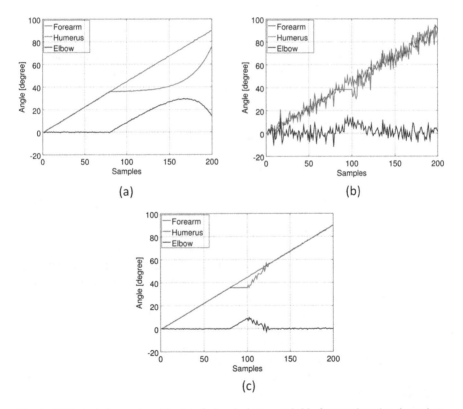

Fig. 9 (**a**) Trajectories produced by data fusion deviate remarkably from real motion due to loss. (**b**) Single-frame algorithm produces jerky trajectories. (**c**) Interpolation algorithm preserves the smoothness and limits the maximum deviation

early results seem to confirm that quaternion interpolation is a viable way to reduce the packet loss effects.

5 Remote Health Monitoring Systems and IoT

The example shown above follows a general paradigm based on a three-layer architecture. The first layer of the architecture is composed of the sensing nodes of the BASN. Each mote receives initialization command and responds to queries from its coordinator, also called gateway. The network nodes continuously sample and process raw information, sending data to the gateway. The operative frequencies for sampling, processing, and communicating are established according to the nature of the application. The second layer is the gateway that interfaces the BASN sensor nodes and communicates with services at top level. Typically, the gateway is responsible for the following tasks: (1) sensor node registration (number and type of sensors), (2) initialization (e.g., specify sampling frequency and operational mode), and (3) setup of secure communication. Once the network is configured, the gateway manages the BASN, taking care of channel sharing, time synchronization, data retrieval, and processing. At top level, a wide area network of several computers receives user' electronic health data and provides several services, such as data storage, user authentication, data pattern analysis, and recognition of serial health anomalies.

In addition to technology for data collecting, storage and access, healthcare-related information analysis and visualization are critical components of remote health monitoring systems [25]. Dealing with huge amount of data often makes their analysis quite frustrating and error prone from the clinician point of view. A solution for the aforementioned challenges can be found in data mining and visualization techniques [26]. The integration of Internet of Things (IoT) paradigm into remote monitoring systems can further increase intelligence, flexibility, and interoperability [27]. A device adopting the IoT scheme is uniquely addressed and identifiable anytime and anywhere through the Internet. IoT-based devices in remote health monitoring systems are not only capable of sensing tasks but can also exchange health information with each other. As exemplified in [28], IoT-enabled remote monitoring systems are able to provide services such as automatic alarm to the nearest emergency center in the event of a critical accident for a supervised patient.

A paradigm that breaks the rigid layered architecture shown above can be helpful when human motion of multiple users is simultaneously monitored by multiple observers. In such cases, a solution that takes advantages from the IoT and the Publish-Subscribe communication paradigm has been proposed in [29]. According to this last paradigm, the information produced by users, also known as *publishers*, is delivered to one or multiple observers, as a function of their interests. To this aim, the user labels the information with a topic before publishing it. The subscription

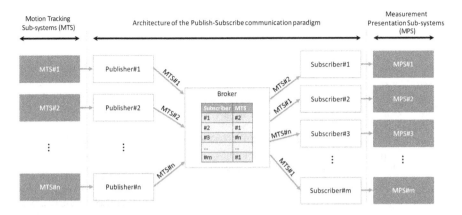

Fig. 10 Architecture of the remote health monitoring system based on IoT and Publish/Subscribe communication paradigm

of the interest to a certain topic enables the observers, also called *subscribers*, to receive notification when publications on such topic occur.

In Fig. 10, a different architecture of the remote health monitoring system based on IoT and Publish/Subscribe paradigms is shown. It is made of several Motion Tracking Sub-systems, devoted to acquire measurement information about the body segments of a single user (i.e., the BASNs described previously) and several Measurement Presentation Sub-systems, devoted to display the results to the clinicians. Among them the communication is ensured by software modules called publishers, subscribers, and broker. Differently from traditional human motion tracking systems, in the proposed one: (1) many Motion Tracking Sub-systems operate simultaneously and (2) each Motion Tracking Sub-system does not send the measurement information directly to the Measurement Presentation Sub-system but to the publisher. The publisher, once received the measurement information, labels it with a topic, e.g., the identification number of the subject being monitored and sends it to the broker by means of Internet. The broker reads the label of the received measurement information and sends it, using Internet, to further the subscribers that have previously declared their interest in that topic. Each subscriber operates in two successive phases: (1) it declares its interest by sending a message with the topic in which it is interested to the broker, and (2) it receives the measurement information in which it is interested from the broker and sends them to the Measurement Presentation Sub-system.

In the proposed solution, the human motion measurements coming from several Motion Tracking Sub-systems are published onto topic-based channels. A topic can refer to measurement information concerning a single user, multiple users, a body part of one or more users. Subscribers express their interest in one or more topics and then receive all information published to such topic.

In order to manage the information delivery, the Message Queue Telemetry Transport standard (MQTT) protocol has been selected. It was designed for networks with low bandwidth and high-latency, as in the case of Internet. The reduced size of header and payload in MQTT messages makes it useful for the transmission of data in a real-time mode. Further advantages of using MQTT relate to hiding the implementation details about networking aspects and to confine the difficulties in the data recruitment only to a topic identification. In this way, different subscribers can easily access data from different publishers. To this aim, MQTT makes use of different components, as described in the following:

- The publisher software module: (1) Creates a message, (2) labels the message with a topic, and (3) sends the message to the broker.
- The subscriber software module: (1) Subscribes to receive messages that it is interested in, (2) unsubscribes to remove a request for messages, and (3) receives from the broker the messages labeled with the topic in which it is interested in.
- The broker software module routes the messages from publishers to subscribers according to each message label and the topic in which each subscriber is interested in.

The novelty of such a paradigm lies in the fact that a client will no longer need to contact the server periodically to check new data availability. Instead, the server sends the specific data requested by the client, as soon as it has them available.

The performance of the previously described remote health monitoring system has been evaluated by considering the one-way delay from publisher to subscriber. In order to characterize such packet delays in the IoT scenario, multiple instances of MQTT publishers and subscribers have been executed providing multiple message flows from publisher to broker and from broker to subscriber. Figure 11 depicts the architecture of the test bench. Several instances of MQTT publishers have been executed on a dedicated computer (PC#1 in Fig. 11). One instance of the MQTT broker has been running on a further computer (PC#2 in Fig. 11). Several instances of MQTT subscribers have been executed on another computer (PC#3 in Fig. 11). Finally, a delay measurement system has been installed on a further computer (PC#4 in Fig. 11), in order to analyze the network traffic. It consists of an open-source network analyzer tool, *Wireshark*, able to capture network packets in real time, filtering them, and displaying the acquired information in human-readable format. It is worth noting that the packets are time stamped by *Wireshark* having as reference the same clock, i.e., the one of PC#4. This solution avoids the use of protocols to synchronize the clock of the PC sender and the clock of the PC receiver in order to evaluate the packet delay [30]. All computers in the test bench are connected together to a network hub. This choice allows to capture each packet as soon as it is sent by PC#1 and PC#2 and then to consider the behavior of the broker as function of the message flows, only. In the test scenario of this preliminary experimental analysis, a computer has been used for all the publishers and a further computer for all the subscribers. This does not happen in actual applicative scenario, where a dedicated machine is typically used for each publisher and subscriber. The usage of a single computer, however, represents a worst case, for two main reasons: (1) all the publishers/subscribers, share the same computational resources, and (2) the messages sent by all the publishers are queued to the same network interface.

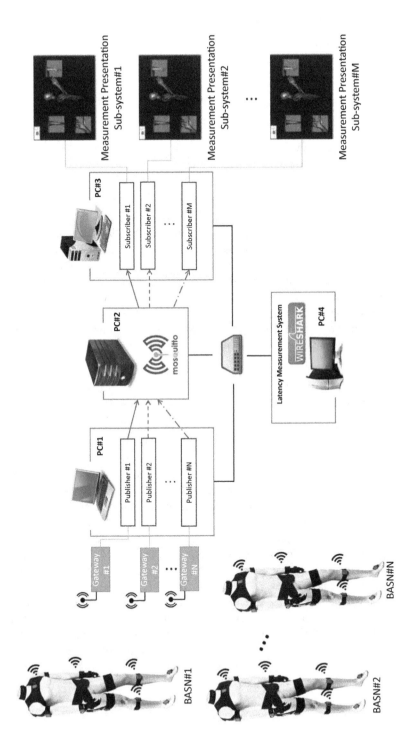

Fig. 11 The architecture of the experimental test bench

Table 1 Packet delays with respect to multiple publishers and subscribers [29]

# Publisher	# Subscriber	Max. (ms)	Min. (ms)	μ (ms)	σ (ms)
1	1	14.54	0.01	0.08	0.96
1	3	13.45	0.01	0.05	0.63
3	3	13.29	0.01	0.41	2.05
5	5	55.33	0.01	9.98	7.47
5	10	24.53	0.01	3.61	4.48
10	5	21.16	0.01	5.29	4.40
10	10	20.49	0.01	7.38	6.28

Table 1 shows the results of the experimental test bench considering different numbers of message flows produced by the publishers and received by the subscribers. As expected, the values of mean and standard deviation increase by increasing the number of message flows. No strict requirements are needed about the end-to-end delay, as the streaming is one way from the Motion Tracking Subsystems to the Measurement Presentation Sub-system. About the delay variation, requirements are related to the capability of a jitter buffer of removing such variation. This can be easily done until values of the variation in the order of 50 ms, therefore, the obtained results, reporting a maximum standard deviation of less than 8 ms, are fully acceptable for the 3D movement reconstruction application.

6 Conclusions

Driven by the widespread adoption of information and mobile communication technologies for health-related applications, the healthcare system could see a radical changing from current professional centric healthcare system to a distributed networked and mobile healthcare system. In such a context, the pervasive access to health-related data will be essential for diagnosis and treatment procedure in healthcare system. Wearable sensors, particularly those equipped with IoT capabilities, are the key players of such challenge. In this chapter, an unobtrusive sensing solution based on MEMS technologies with the aim of providing human motion measurement has been presented, together with motion measurement related research field and open issues. In particular, technological solutions related to packet loss in wireless networks, network scalability, and remote control in existing network infrastructures have also been discussed. It is easy to imagine extending the type and number of measurements by embedding other kinds of sensors in the wireless motes, like EMG electrodes and force sensors, in order to monitor and process vital signs related to motor activity.

References

1. P. Daponte, J. De Marco, L. De Vito, B. Pavic, S. Zolli, Electronic measurements in rehabilitation, in: *Proceedings of 2011 IEEE International Symposium on Medical Measurement and Applications (MeMeA)*, Bari, Italy, May 2011, pp. 274–279
2. S.F. Jencks, M.V. Williams, E.A. Coleman, Rehospitalizations among patients in the medicare fee-for-service program. New Engl. J. Med. **360**(14), 1418–1428 (2009)
3. N. Gotoda, K. Matsuura, S. Otsuka, T. Tanaka, Y. Yano, Remote training-support of running form for runners with wireless sensor, in: *2010 Proceedings of International Conference on Computers in Education*, Putrajaya, Malaysia, pp. 417–421
4. S. Patel, H. Park, P. Bonato, L. Chan, M. Rodgers, A review of wearable sensors and systems with application in rehabilitation. J. Neuroeng. Rehabil. **9**(12), 1–17 (2012)
5. L. De Vito, O. Postolache, S. Rapuano, Measurements and sensors for motion tracking in motor rehabilitation. IEEE Instrum. Meas. Mag. **17**, 30–38 (2014)
6. S. Sessa, M. Zecca, Z. Lin, T. Sasaki, K. Itoh, A. Takanishi, Waseda bioinstrumentation system #3 as a tool for objective rehabilitation measurement and assessment—development of the inertial measurement unit, in *Proceedings of 2009 IEEE International Conference on Rehabilitation Robotics*, Kyoto, Japan, June 2009, pp. 115–120
7. E. Zubiete, L. Luque, A. Rodriguez, I. Gonzalez, Review of wireless sensors networks in health applications, in: *Proceedings of 2011 Annual International Conference on in Engineering in Medicine and Biology Society*, Boston, MA, USA, September 2011, pp. 1789–1793
8. C. Chen, C. Pomalaza-Raez, Design and evaluation of a wireless body sensor system for smart home health monitoring, in *Proceedings of IEEE Global Telecommunications Conference*, Honolulu, HI, USA, December 2009, pp. 1–6
9. F. Rahimi, C. Duval, M. Jog, C. Bee, A. South, M. Jog, R. Edwards, P. Boissy, Capturing whole-body mobility of patients with Parkinson disease using inertial motion sensors: Expected challenges and rewards, in *Proceedings of 2011 Annual International Conference in Engineering in Medicine and Biology Society (EMBC)*, Boston, MA, USA, 2011, pp. 5833–5838
10. G.V. Merrett, M. Ettabib, C. Peters, G. Hallett, N. White, Augmenting forearm crutches with wireless sensors for lower limb rehabilitation. Meas. Sci. Technol. **21**(12)
11. J. Neville, A. Wixted, D. Rowlands, D. James, Accelerometers: An underutilized resource in sports monitoring, in *Proceedings of 2010 International Conference on Intelligent Sensors, Sensor Networks and Information Processing (ISSNIP)*, Brisbane, Australia, December 2011, pp. 287–290
12. A.F. Smeaton, D. Diamond, P. Kelly, K. Moran, K.T. Lau, D. Morris, N. Moyna, N.E. O'Connor, K. Zhang, Aggregating multiple body sensors for analysis in sports, in *Proceedings of 5th International Workshop on Wearable Micro and Nanosystems for Personalised Health*, Valencia, Spain, May 2008, pp. 1–5
13. M.A. Brodie, A. Walmsley, W. Page, The static accuracy and calibration of inertial measurement units for 3d orientation. Comput. Methods Biomech. Biomed. Engin. **11**(6), 641–648 (2008)
14. G.X. Lee, K.S. Low, T. Taher, Unrestrained measurement of arm motion based on a wearable wireless sensor network. IEEE Trans. Instrum. Meas. **59**(5), 1309–1317 (2010)
15. P. Daponte, L. De Vito, C. Sementa, A wireless-based home rehabilitation system for monitoring 3D movements, in *Proceedings of 2013 IEEE International Symposium on Medical Measurements and Applications (MeMeA)*, Gatineau, Canada, 4–5 May 2013, pp. 282–287
16. P. Daponte, L. De Vito, C. Sementa, Validation of a home rehabilitation system for range of motion measurements of limb functions, in *Proceedings of 2013 IEEE International Symposium on Medical Measurement and Applications*, Gatineau, Canada, 2013, pp. 288–293
17. S. Movassaghi, M. Abolhasan, J. Lipman, D. Smith, A. Jamalipour, Wireless body area networks: A survey. IEEE Commun. Surv. Tutor. **16**(3), 1658–1686 (2014)

18. P. Daponte, L. De Vito, M. Riccio, C. Sementa, Design and validation of a motion-tracking system for rom measurements in home rehabilitation. Measurement **55**, 82–96 (2014)
19. J.B. Kuipers, *Quaternions and Rotation Sequences : A Primer with Applications to Orbits, Aerospace, and Virtual Reality* (Princeton Univ. Press, Princeton, NJ, 1999)
20. J.L. Marins, X. Yun, E.R. Bachmann, R. McGhee, M.J. Zyda, An extended kalman filter for quaternion-based orientation estimation using Marg sensors, in *Proceedings of 2001 IEEE/RSJ International Conference on Intelligent Robots and Systems*, Maui, HI, USA, 2001, pp. 2003–2011
21. X. Yun, E.R. Bachmann, R.B. McGhee, A simplified quaternion-based algorithm for orientation estimation from earth gravity and magnetic field measurements. IEEE Trans. Instrum. Meas. **57**(3), 638–650 (2008)
22. P. Daponte, L. De Vito, G. Mazzilli, S. Rapuano, C. Sementa, Investigating the on-board data processing for IMU-based sensors in motion tracking for rehabilitation, in *Proceedings of IEEE International Symposium on Medical Measurement and Applications*, Torino, Italy, May 2015, pp. 645–650
23. J. Grubert, T. Langlotz, S. Zollmann, H. Regenbrecht, Towards pervasive augmented reality: Context- awareness in augmented reality. IEEE Trans. Vis. Comput. Graph. **23**(6), 1706–1724 (2017)
24. L. De Vito, G. Mazzilli, M. Riccio, C. Sementa, Improving the orientation estimation in a packet loss-affected wireless sensor network for tracking human motion, *in Proceedings of 21st IMEKO TC4 International Symposium on Understanding the World through Electrical and Electronic Measurement*, Budapest, Hungary, September 2016, pp. 184–189
25. M. Hassanalieragh, A. Page, T. Soyata, G. Sharma, M. Aktas, G. Mateos, B. Kantarci, S. Andreescu, Health monitoring and management using Internet-of-Things (IoT) sensing with cloud-based processing: Opportunities and challenges, in *2015 Proceedings of IEEE International Conference on Services Computing*, pp. 285–292
26. L. Wei, N. Kumar, V. Lolla, E. Keogh, S. Lonardi, C. Ratanamahatana, H. Van Herle, A practical tool for visualizing and data mining medical time series, in *Proceedings of 18th IEEE Symposium on Computer-Based Med. Sys.*, June 2005, pp. 341–346
27. M. Bazzani, D. Conzon, A. Scalera, M. Spirito, C. Trainito, Enabling the IoT paradigm in e-health solutions through the VIRTUS middleware, in *Proceedings of IEEE 11th International Conference on Trust, Security and Privacy in Computing and Com. (TrustCom)*, June 2012, pp. 1954–1959
28. N. Bui, M. Zorzi, Health care applications: A solution based on the internet of things, in *Proceedings. of 4th International Symposium on Applied Sciences in Biomed. and Com. Tech.*, New York, USA, 2011, pp. 1–5
29. L. De Vito, F. Lamonaca, G. Mazzilli, M. Riccio, D.L. Carnì, P.F. Sciammarella, An IoT-enabled multi-sensor multi-user system for human motion measurements, in *2017 IEEE International Symposium on Medical Measurements and Applications (MeMeA)*, Rochester, USA, May 2017, pp. 210–215
30. L. De Vito, S. Rapuano, L. Tomaciello, One-way delay measurement: State of the art. IEEE Trans. Instrum. Meas. **57**(12), 2742–2750 (2008)

Healthcare Systems: An Overview of the Most Important Aspects of Current and Future m-Health Applications

Giovanna Sannino, Giuseppe De Pietro, and Laura Verde

Abstract This chapter explores the most relevant aspects in relation to the outcomes and performance of the different components of a healthcare system with a particular focus on mobile healthcare applications. In detail, we discuss the six quality principles to be satisfied by a generic healthcare system and the main international and European projects, which have supported the dissemination of these systems. This diffusion has been encouraged by the application of wireless and mobile technologies, through the so-called m-Health systems. One of the main fields of application of an m-Health system is telemedicine, for which reason we will address an important challenge encountered during the realization of an m-Health application: the analysis of the functionalities that an m-Health app has to provide. To achieve this latter aim, we will present an overview of a generic m-Health application with its main functionalities and components. Among these, the use of a standardized method for the treatment of a massive amount of patient data is necessary in order to integrate all the collected information resulting from the development of a great number of new m-Health devices and applications. Electronic Health Records (EHR), and international standards, like Health Level 7 (HL7) and Fast Healthcare Interoperability Resources (FHIR), aims at addressing this important issue, in addition to guaranteeing the privacy and security of these health data. Moreover, the insights that can be discerned from an examination of this vast repository of data can open up unparalleled opportunities for public and private sector organizations. Indeed, the development of new tools for the analysis of data, which on occasions may be unstructured, noisy, and unreliable, is now considered a vital requirement for all specialists who are involved in the handling and using of information. These new tools may be based on rule, machine or deep learning, or include question answering, with cognitive computing certainly having a key role to play in the development of future m-Health applications.

G. Sannino (✉) · G. De Pietro · L. Verde
Institute of High Performance Computing and Networking (ICAR) of the National Research Council (CNR), Naples, Italy
e-mail: giovanna.sannino@icar.cnr.it; giuseppe.depietro@icar.cnr.it; laura.verde@icar.cnr.it

© Springer Nature Switzerland AG 2020
A. El Saddik et al. (eds.), *Connected Health in Smart Cities*,
https://doi.org/10.1007/978-3-030-27844-1_11

Keywords Electronic health records · Mobile apps · Security privacy ·
Physiological signals

1 e-Health and the Requirements of a Healthcare System

The term e-Health [1] indicates the use of Information and Communication
Technology (ICT) to provide a healthcare service. During recent decades, a series
of e-Health applications have been designed and developed, ranging from Health
Information Systems (HIS) and EHRs to wearable and portable monitoring systems
and telemedicine services.

Governments, non-governmental organizations (NGOs), and international development organizations are working to improve health outcomes through better
national health systems. One of the six building blocks for a strong national health
system, according to the World Health Organization (WHO), is the use of an
HIS. A well-functioning HIS will provide timely and relevant information about
health outcomes and the performance of the components of the health system
[2]. Therefore, it is necessary to search for solutions to improve data availability
and accessibility [3]. Additionally, the development of tools and systems that can
help healthcare workers become more efficient and effective is crucial in order to
compensate for health personnel shortages [4].

According to [5], a healthcare system must satisfy six quality principles,
schematized in Fig. 1, to provide high-quality healthcare, namely:

- Safety: The healthcare delivered should be as safe for the patient in the health
care facility as it would be in her/his own home.

Fig. 1 The six quality
principles that a healthcare
system must satisfy

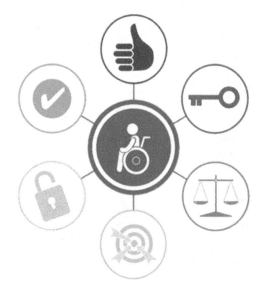

- Effectiveness: The current state of scientific knowledge in relation to healthcare should be applied and should set the standard for the delivery of care.
- Efficiency: The healthcare service should, as far as possible, be cost effective, and any excessive waste should be eliminated from the system.
- Timeliness: Patients should experience the fewest possible delays and the shortest possible waiting times in relation to their access to the healthcare service.
- Patient-centeredness: The system of care should, as far as possible, be focused on the patient, putting her/him in control and respecting her/his preferences.
- Equitableness: All unequal treatment and any disparities in healthcare provision should be eliminated.

1.1 International and European Healthcare Projects: A Review

The design and development of e-health applications have been supported by appropriate International and European healthcare projects. Numerous international and national projects are, in fact, investigating and promoting new ICT solutions to affect a paradigm shift in healthcare services, whereby patients are increasingly empowered to take control of the healthcare service they receive. In relation to the European Community's Seventh Framework Programme (FP7), the funded projects include 339 focusing on Hypertension (HT) (mostly related to medical issues and practices) and 1413 on applications for disease management.

In the following section, we will provide a brief summary of some of the most representative projects of each category:

- HEARTCYCLE (www.heartcycle.eu) aims to provide a closed-loop disease management service for both Heart Failure (HF) and Coronary Heart Disease (CHD) patients, possibly also afflicted by comorbidities such as HT, diabetes, and arrhythmias. This objective will be achieved through the multi-parametric monitoring and analysis of vital signs and other measurements.
- HATICE (www.hatice.eu) aims to develop an innovative, interactive Internet intervention platform targeted at enhancing the treatment of cardiovascular diseases in the elderly. The application will be evaluated by means of a randomized controlled trial with the objective of investigating whether the onset of new cardiovascular disorders and cognitive decline can be delayed or prevented.
- PRIMA-EDS (www.prima-eds.eu) aims to optimize the treatment of elderly patients with a combination of chronic diseases and the concurrent use of multiple medications. PRIMA-EDS provides an electronic tool to assist physicians to take advantage of the best evidence available.
- NAAN (www.hu.edu.eg/node/180) aims to define the most active elements of two specific plant extracts and to determine whether, in terms of their mechanism of action, they have potential applications either as antihypertensive or as antidiabetic drugs.

- ICT4DEPRESSION (www.ict4depression.eu) provides an innovative mobile solution for the treatment of depression by using mobile phones and web-based technologies.
- MOVINGLIFE (www.moving-life.eu) aims to consolidate and disseminate the use of mobile e-Health solutions targeted at supporting lifestyle changes. To contribute to the achievement of this objective, MOVINGLIFE has delivered roadmaps to guide technological research, implementation practice, and policy support.
- EU-MASCARA (www.eu-mascara.eu) aims at enhancing, by means of the analysis of a panel of biomarkers, the accurate prediction of cardiovascular risk, and the diagnosis of cardiovascular diseases.
- SmartHealth 2.0 aims at realizing a technological system that implements an innovative model of healthcare based on a digital, open, modular, and scalable architecture.
- CHRONIOUS aims at providing a smart wearable platform, based on multiparametric sensor data processing, for the monitoring of patients afflicted by a chronic disease and based in a long-stay residential setting.
- eHealthNet (www.ehealthnet.it) aims at enhancing the interoperability necessary for communication and interconnection with any existing health systems, focusing on technologies for remote monitoring and telemedicine, knowledge technologies, and technologies for predictive medicine.
- SHARE is focused on the development of a Decision Support System (DSS) for the early detection of cardiovascular events that, if not recognized at an early stage, may lead to the onset of more severe cardiovascular conditions in hypertensive patients.
- Standing Hypotension is focused on modeling physiological signals to prevent secondary adverse events (e.g., falls) in patients suffering from HT and other metabolic diseases.
- EMBALANCE is focused on the realization of a DSS and related supporting tools such as Virtual Physiological Human (VPH) models, monitoring solutions, and Human–Computer Interaction (HCI) methods for data management in relation to balance disorders.
- Monica Healthcare (www.monicahealthcare.com) is a university spin out company devoted to developing innovative wearable devices for fetal heart rate monitoring using Electrocardiography (ECG) with the goal of facilitating globally accessible obstetric services at home and in the hospital.
- MATCH is a research project aimed at developing methods and tools for the early stage Health Technology Assessment (HTA) of healthcare technology and particularly for personalized interventions and home monitoring. One of the main activities of the MATCH project has been the development of methods and tools for user need elicitation in relation to early stage HTA and for the design of healthcare technologies.
- HYPERGENES (http://www.hypergenes.eu) is a research project aimed at identifying genes responsible for essential HT and target organ damage, through the use of a whole genome association/entropy-based approach. The plan is,

first, to develop an integrated disease model, taking the environment into account, by means of an advanced bioinformatics approach, and, secondly, to test the predictive ability of the model in terms of the accurate identification of individuals at risk. Two of the partners in this project are also partners in our present proposal.

- EuResist (http://www.euresist.org/) is a research project funded within the European Community's Sixth Framework Programme (FP6), aimed at building a DSS for the treatment management and prediction of the human immunodeficiency virus (HIV). The EuResist network GEIE manages the EuResist Integrated Data Base (EIDB) and the EuResist treatment response prediction engine, a data-driven system that has the function of predicting the response to any combination drug therapy prescribed for a patient with a given viral genotype.

2 m-Health: Emerging Healthcare Solutions

The development of new and advanced e-health solutions has been stimulated and facilitated by the application of wireless and mobile technologies. Nowadays, we are experiencing an unprecedented increase in the number of users of smartphones and Internet technologies, while the price of devices and services is in constant reduction. This provides new opportunities to support healthcare delivery by means of mobile technology, a phenomenon referred to as m-Health.

m-Health solutions have been defined by the WHO as "the use of mobile devices, such as mobile phones, patient monitoring devices, personal digital assistants (PDA) and wireless devices, for medical and public health practice" [6]. As such, they can contribute to the achievement of universal health coverage, facilitating the access to care, improving care delivery, empowering patients through targeted messaging, and collecting real-time data to optimize resources and decision-making [7]. As a result, health programs are exploring ways of harnessing mobile technology to achieve these objectives, while reducing healthcare costs.

For m-Health to assume a fully integrated role in healthcare, it must be provided in a way that gives patients and providers' confidence that patient privacy will be protected and the confidentiality and security of patient information will be assured. The data need to be credible and consistent, and collected and stored securely in a trusted electronic health record with managed access for patients, caregivers, and healthcare professionals [8]. Smartphones, tablets, and other mobile devices are already being used to collect and transmit individual and aggregate data from points of collection to centralized HISs. Indeed, m-Health is becoming an important strategy for the delivery of health services and for the collection, reporting, analysis, and use of data in near real time.

However, the mobile devices used effectively in healthcare may also be used for personal activities such as calling, texting, playing games, taking photos, browsing the web, sending e-mails, and accessing social media. Such activities may take place through personal telephone services and Internet transmission systems that are vulnerable to viral attacks and other security risks that could lead to data breaches.

While some smartphones and tablets have as much power as computers, they may not be as well maintained and secure. Without proper security safeguards, the personal use of mobile devices and the sharing of devices with other people (such as family and friends) could jeopardize the quality, security, and confidentiality of any health data.

Nonetheless, the use of m-Health solutions has spread rapidly. In fact, while in 2000 there were fewer than [1] one billion subscriptions, by 2011 WHO officials were proclaiming that mobile technology for health has the potential to transform the face of service delivery across the globe [8, 9]. Indeed, the functions of m-Health span many of the components of a healthcare system:

- Client education and behavior change communication
- Sensors and point-of-care diagnostics
- Registries/vital events tracking
- Data collection and reporting
- Electronic health records
- Electronic decision support
- Provider-to-provider communication
- Provider work planning and scheduling
- Provider training and education
- Human resource management
- Supply chain management
- Financial transactions and incentives.

Data generated from these functions could contribute to a country's national HIS. Four types of mobile phone solution are already in use for the effective operation of an HIS: Interactive Voice Response (IVR), plain text SMS (Short Message Service), locally installed applications on handsets and SIM cards (data storage cards), and browser-based applications [10]. Many countries and organizations are testing ways in which m-Health can extend the reach of Internet-based HISs to mobile devices. Health systems are transitioning from paper-based systems to the real-time reporting of routine health data by health workers [11]. This involves the use of mobile devices such as phones or PDAs to collect data, which are then transmitted to a server that aggregates them across many sites and levels. Such aggregated data can be accessed on a computer program or web-based application that enhances data analysis across many variables. For example, DHIS [12], an open-source health management information system used in more than 40 countries, has options to adopt mobile extensions so that local health workers can report data into the system.

3   m-Health for Telemedicine

m-Health solutions are widely used in the telemedicine service, thereby considerably improving the quality of the care process. Telemedicine can be defined as the provision of healthcare remotely by means of a variety of telecommunication tools, including telephones, smartphones, and mobile wireless devices, with or without a video connection. The use of telemedicine is expanding rapidly, with the potential to affect a complete transformation in the means and quality of the delivery of healthcare for millions of people. The advances and achievements of telemedicine, to date, have been considered in a number of recent reviews [13–16].

Currently, three interconnected trends are influencing the development of telemedicine, each representing a significant shift in emphasis. First, there seems to a change of interception from merely increasing access to healthcare to enhancing convenience and, ideally, reducing cost. Secondly, the expansion of telemedicine is being accompanied by the aim of addressing not only acute diseases but now also episodic and chronic conditions. Thirdly, telemedicine is enabling a transformation in location, moving care from hospitals and clinics to the home, obviously with the support of mobile devices.

The principle objective of telemedicine, from the viewpoint of the patients, is to increase levels of access to care [17]. In such terms, it has already achieved considerable success, extending healthcare to population groups, and in respect of particular conditions, where previously no treatment was available. Examples include the provision of tele-healthcare programs to people in the military, prisons, and rural locations [18].

However, the objective is not only to increase healthcare access, but also to transform the character and effectiveness of the delivery. In such terms, the Internet is revolutionizing the provision of healthcare [19] in much the same way as has been the case with respect to service delivery in the travel, retail, and financial services sectors. Many healthcare organizations, from prestigious public institutions to recently established small businesses, are now offering low-cost virtual examinations available throughout the day and night, often at a cost of less than $50 for each appointment, for the most common and troublesome conditions. By way of comparison, it should be considered that patients often have to wait, sometimes for a considerable time, to secure even a short appointment with a general or specialist doctor (the average delay has been estimated at 20 days [20]), and the average duration of the appointment experience, including travelling and waiting times, 2 hours [21]. Bearing in mind, also, that there is always a significant emphasis on reducing costs, telemedicine must be regarded as an essential development, considering that it is expected, in the near future, to have the capacity to deliver intensive services to the 20% of the population who account for 80% of healthcare expenditure [22].

A second significant trend in current telehealth development relates to the adoption of telemedicine in the management and treatment of chronic and acute conditions. In fact, advanced wireless and mobile technologies, comprising the ability to store a vast repository of information on a mobile device, can be exploited, in combination with radio-enabled watches and a grid of body sensors, in the areas of health promotion and maintenance, and illness detection and prevention, as suggested in [23–27]. Such solutions envisage the storage, and updating as necessary, of all a patient's relevant medical information on her/his mobile device, including critical information such as blood group, allergies, heart rate, and existing

Fig. 2 A generic
telemedicine m-Health
application

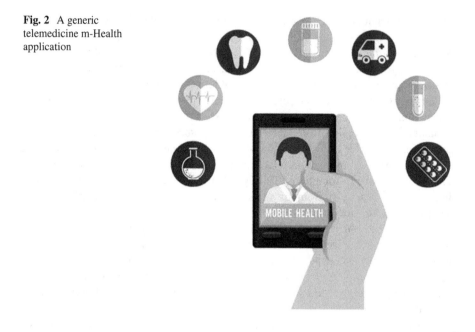

medical conditions, as shown in Fig. 2, thereby facilitating the provision of personalized healthcare monitoring and management, and providing vital data, which can be easily accessed to ensure that the correct medical care is administered in any medical emergency.

In reality, telehealth applications were first introduced in relation to the treatment of acute conditions, such as trauma and stroke [28]. The first significant example, Telestroke, was established in 1999, involving the provision of acute stroke care to a patient in an emergency department, by means of fibrinolytic therapy (a tissue plasminogen activator), with the assistance of a remote neurologist. In just 15 years, Telestroke has become an established telemedicine company, a major care provider for patients with stroke. More recently, telehealth has expanded, through the application of different care models, including school visits by medical assistants [29], video calls [30], telephone calls [17], and online algorithms [31], to encompass the treatment of episodic conditions, such as sinusitis. Interest in telehealth has been increasing rapidly for many chronic conditions, the treatment of which accounts for 80% of healthcare expenditure [32]. It is envisaged that in the future there will be a shift in development, a transition from the predominantly conversational features of current models to advanced versions that include rich data transfer from remote monitoring, delivered through the use of wearable sensors and mobile diagnostic systems, such as electrocardiograms. Such models will comprise the education and monitoring of patients, supported by frequent virtual and in-person visits from physicians, nurses, therapists, and social workers.

Finally, an important third telehealth trend will involve the shift in the location of care provision away from the hospital or other medical institution. The first telemedicine applications delivered care to patients in establishments such as hospitals and day surgery clinics, which frequently required expensive technological systems and on-site clinical or technical support. The increased availability of broadband and portable diagnostic technologies means that telemedicine is now moving into the home. For people with chronic conditions, including elderly patients, who are essentially homebound, the patient's home is fast becoming a patient-centered medical environment, with the provision of treatment, even for acute conditions such as stroke and pneumonia, provided by means of video examinations either in the house or in the ambulance. Providing healthcare to patients in clinics or at home, or simply over the telephone, mirrors the trend in a sector such as banking, where the Internet and automatic cash machines have moved financial services away from the bank lobby onto the customer's mobile device.

3.1 Requirement Analysis for m-Health Applications

A crucial aspect in the realization of an m-Health application is the analysis of its requirements. To achieve this aim, we have investigated the functionalities that an m-Health app has to provide, by means of an overview of a generic m-Health application, depicted in Fig. 3. In particular, an m-Health application is composed of a series of sensors that are worn by a patient with the objective of monitoring her/his vital signs, including the electrical activity of the heart (by ECG), blood pressure (BP), respiration rate (RR), and temperature. Each device may be designed for the measurement of only one particular vital sign, such as temperature, or for several. Such devices can have two different kinds of transmission: push or pull. In the first case, the vital sign is continuously monitored and the monitoring data are transmitted by the device on the expiry of a given sampling period. On the contrary, in the second case, the vital sign is measured by the device only after an explicit command received by the patient of the monitoring application; therefore,

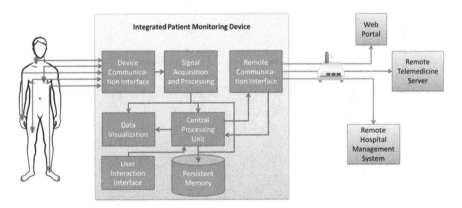

Fig. 3 Overview of a generic m-Health application

the monitoring data are sent only after an explicit request. Besides the monitoring sensors, we can find a monitoring application, which can run on a desktop machine, and also nowadays on a mobile device such as a tablet or smartphone.

In Fig. 3, we can see all the components that constitute a generic m-Health application:

- The Device Communication Interface (DCI): This has the duty of collecting the monitoring data coming from a certain monitoring sensor. Since monitoring sensors differ from each other in terms of the communication protocol and data format adopted, we can have as many DCIs as there are sensors deployed on the patient. Alternatively, there may be a more sophisticated design that uses the adapter design pattern, shown in Fig. 4. The communication details for interacting with a given sensor are wrapped within an adapter, which is masked from the rest of the application by a proper interface. In this way, the communications with the sensors are transparently managed by the application and new sensors can be inserted without changing the application code but only by adding new adapters.

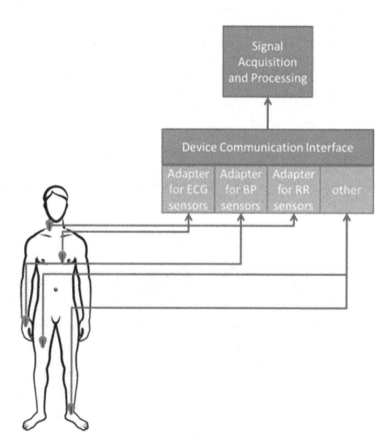

Fig. 4 Adapter Pattern applied for the acquisition of the monitoring data

- The Signal Acquisition and Processing (SAP) unit: This is the component that can apply additional processing operations to the data received from the DCI component, such as normalization or spike removal.
- The Remote Communication Interface (RCI): This is useful to provide a remote communication. An m-Health application, in fact, can be a stand-alone, but in most cases it is positioned on the Internet for a series of different reasons. For example, the monitoring data may have to be sent to a remote doctor for telemedicine or a remote Hospital Management System for the remote assistance of patients. Alternatively, the m-Health application can be controlled remotely by means of a web portal. In all these cases, the m-Health application has to provide remote communication.

Such processed data can be given to:

- A Data Visualization (DV) component: This contributes to the accurate presentation of the data to the user. A concrete example is a chart of the ECG signal.
- A Persistent Memory (PM): This stores and reuses processed data for future operations. To integrate data coming from several patients, it is necessary to store these data according to the guidelines of an opportune format standard. An HER is an organized collection of health data that facilitates this integration by using appropriate standards, as discussed in the following subsection.
- A Central Processing Unit (CPU): This is useful for the further processing of the data to achieve the function of the m-Health application. During its operational phase, the CPU can retrieve the data stored in the PM, and use DV to present to the user the outcome of its elaborations. As a concrete example, let us consider a monitoring application for a cardiac patient. The CPU continuously receives the ECG signal, from which it can detect any possible abnormal heart behavior by verifying if the current heart rate is below a given threshold or by comparing the current ECG with previous ones to check for possible degradations.
- A User Interaction Interface (UII): An m-Health application has to include the possibility for the user to derive its logic; therefore, we can find a UII, which may, or may not, be a Graphical User Interface (GUI), for the collection of inputs and choices from the user, and the passing of these to the CPU that will adapt its behavior as a result.

3.2   m-Health and Electronic Health Records

m-Health solutions offer healthcare professionals the opportunity to have instant access to a wide range of sources of clinical information such as the patient's medication history or test results. An EHR is the keystone of a medical information system, constituting an organized and systematic collection of the patient's health information electronically. The connection between an EHR and an m-Health solution is an important development in the advance of mobile healthcare.

On the one hand, mobile healthcare apps have a greater number of abilities and resources to draw from, thereby improving the efficiency of the system. On the other, with the vast array of new devices and applications to gather data on patient health, physicians and medical professionals have been confronted with massive amounts of data and little time to analyze and incorporate them into treatment plans. Physicians generally see time spent on administrative tasks as time taken away from the contact time available to be spent with patients. The technological infrastructures within hospitals and other medical facilities have not been standardized, and, therefore, the staffs have found it difficult to integrate the data coming from different departments on individual patients, let alone incorporate the new data coming from health devices external to their specific healthcare organization. EHRs are aimed at addressing the former demand, whereas start-ups have begun to emerge to satisfy the latter requirement.

Improvements to the service could be achieved by linking it to an EHR at the Information Management Center (IMC) in order to facilitate the delivery of a higher level of integrated care for the patient. For example, the EHR could, with the patient's informed consent, store and share her/his contact records. Medical staff would also be able, again with the patient's informed consent, to access her/his historical records in accordance with the Health Level 7 (HL7) v3.0 standard, or the emerging Fast Healthcare Interoperability Resources (FIHR) standard [33]. Such a facility would undoubtedly enhance the ongoing care management for the patients and would provide, in addition to traditional face-to-face contact, an alternative communication route between the patients and the medical staff. Additional services could also be integrated, such as the Remote Monitoring already described. This development mirrors the evolution seen in the general mobile industry, where further services have progressively been added on the foundation of the initial service baseline. Mobile technology commenced with voice and SMS services, but then progressed to encompass other facilities, such as email delivery, cameras, and the vast array of application-based services. A possible connection between mobile apps and an EHR is presented in Fig. 5.

If a patient has a personal health record (PHR), this can be shared with her/his clinical specialists. It will contain an aggregated summary of the EHR information deriving from different hospital and other clinical appointments and, where relevant, statistical information deriving from personal systems, such as health, wellness, or fitness apps. Even in its present configuration, this is an indispensable service since it can provide access to medical information in an unified format, expedient when the user may not be able to attend a face-to-face appointment or maybe seeking medical advice in a nonemergency context. Such an availability of data, at any time and in any place, will obviously be especially significant in areas where large sections of the community only have limited access to healthcare provision.

The interaction between the hospital information and EHR systems will certainly facilitate the realization of many of the benefits envisaged for a digital health solution. However, the design and implementation of such a hospital information service–EHR connectivity, which is fully interoperable and integrated, including semantic exchanges of information with locations internal and external to a single

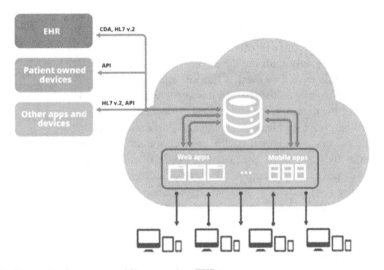

Fig. 5 Connection between a mobile app and an EHR

hospital, is a complex and arduous task. The realization of such a service requires the evaluation and, in some cases, redesign of clinical workflows, with the replacement of any existing paper-based or electronically siloed workflows, to enable an appropriate definition of the features of the different system interfaces, so allowing their effective integration.

The aim of such integration is to ensure that hospital clinicians are supported by the most advanced information systems, rather than hindered in the delivery of their main responsibility, the provision of care. On the assumption that this is permitted by local regulations, the application of standards in the development of this system presents the possibility of linking the data contained within both the regional and national HISs to enhance and extend the service, so providing a wider coverage. This development could also allow patients to access their own health information through a web portal, without having to rely on the more traditional means of access, i.e., telephone contact with a trained call center operator or member of staff at a local health service center. The FHIR standard, which is currently becoming more widely used, maybe more expedient in relation to the provision of access via a web portal since this standard has been designed to be more suitable for web-based applications.

3.3 Security and Privacy

The development of wireless communication and biosensor technologies has resulted in numerous benefits for mobile healthcare. However, as has already been indicated in the previous paragraphs, there are many anxieties in relation to security and privacy that have to be resolved in order to protect the user's information in any m-Health system. Smartphone and m-Health applications may be vulnerable to a vast array of security threats. Certainly, information security has not emerged as a new concept only with the development of m-Health systems. The particular drawback in this case, however, is that the most attractive characteristic of these devices, their mobility, also constitutes the greatest challenge in relation to the protection of the data stored on such devices or accessed with them.

According to the Health Insurance Portability and Accountability Act (HIPAA),"privacy" is defined as the respect for an individual's personal health information by limiting its use and disclosure to third parties, while "security" entails the physical protection of health information stored or transmitted electronically [34]. Keeping in mind the constant development of technology in relation to the capture and transmission of data, security plans, and procedures must be incorporated within m-Health solutions in order to provide protection for the patient's privacy and guarantee the security of the healthcare data. Breaches of protected data can only be minimized by the adoption of robust security protocols, involving encryption at all data points and multifactor authentication programs.

One promising technique that has achieved positive results in terms of improving a system's security is moving target defense (MTD) [35]. MTD's mode of operation is centered on the continuous randomization of a system's configuration in order to render any attack more expensive and reduce the prospects of successful strike. Eldosouky and Saad [36] used an MTD security framework in relation to an m-Health system, in which secret keys were used to encrypt data sent from the device to the gateway while a public key was used to encrypt data sent from the gateway over the Internet. Ferebee et al. [37], instead, proposed a security framework that exploits biometric parameters and the system history and context to identify any anomalies. Additionally, they made use of correlation networks to contextualize the sensed biometric values with the values of other related parameters.

In summary, it is clear that a variety of techniques have been used with the aim of protecting the collection and transmission of a patient's data. It is necessary to consider such techniques during the development and design of an m-Health application in order to minimize any possible damage that might be inflicted on the patients' data and any intrusions that might be made.

4   Toward the Next Generation of m-Health Cognitive Apps

Big Data is fast becoming one of the hottest topics at the cutting edge of research in several different fields including information management, data analytics and, indeed, healthcare. During the last decade, various different types of data have been coming to prominence, including unstructured data deriving from social networks, streaming data, and online publications, and massive data generated by sensors from the physical world. All such data are starting to outpace traditional forms of structured data, and certainly, this trend will continue with even faster growth in the future. Moreover, the insights that can be discerned from an examination of this vast repository of data can open up unparalleled opportunities for public and private organizations. Data, indeed, is now considered one of the most valuable resources in the contemporary environment, and, as data collection and delivery is expected to continue to develop at an even faster rate, the increasing prominence of data management will certainly maintain a significant influence in the determination of trends in business and society.

In the area of macroeconomics, the last century has seen a rapid expansion of the service sector, which now contributes more than 80 percent of the gross domestic product of many modern economies. Knowledge-based services are one of the major elements of this business sector. Knowledge work, which is the foundation of knowledge-based service growth, will be completely transformed with the emergence of big data. The value of businesses in the future will be increasingly determined by the extent to which such organizations empower their knowledge workers to exploit the advantages deriving from big data. Knowledge workers who possess such skills will have the potential to be considerably more effective in the management of data than they have ever been previously.

However, new tools will be necessary to extract the insights deriving from modern big data, which is generally unstructured, noisy, and unreliable. These new tools cannot be constructed from the same manually specified rule-based symbolic computing techniques that have allowed us to manage the clean, structured data, which have been predominant to date. Such new tools will employ machine learning and will interact with the user in a more natural way, furnishing evidence-based explanations of candidate insights. Knowledge represented explicitly will itself become big data, and its exploitation will bring to light both conventional and innovative insights. These new knowledge systems, which learn and interact naturally with the user, are referred to as knowledge work cognitive systems. As a representative case, IBM's Watson Business Unit is currently engaged with its clients in the development of a family of systems that are capable of learning and interacting naturally in a variety of different domains.

In the future, cognitive systems will advance beyond simple question answering to provide support for the discovery of insights concealed in big data, e.g., in the vast repositories of scientific literature, reasoning with the evidence to confirm or refute the topics of discussion, advancing beyond textual data to encompass images and videos. In the near future, cognitive systems are expected to be able to assist us in the completion of complex tasks in almost every work environment, from business to education, and including, significantly in this context, healthcare. Knowledge workers in almost every field of application will have the tools, the cognitive assistants, to enable them to penetrate and interpret huge amounts of data, thereby solving complex problems and creating new ideas. For example, a physician will be able, with the help of a cognitive system, to connect information about a patient's genome and clinical history with the repository of experimental literature, in order to obtain an improved diagnosis of a medical problem or alternative treatment options. Likewise, an educator will be able to enhance the learning experience by linking educational content to an individual's needs and goals or, as another example, a business leader will be able to extract insights like demand patterns, product acceptance, and competitive differentiators within markets to inform tactical and strategic business decisions. Indeed, almost all knowledge-based professions will be able to benefit from this development in a similar fashion.

However, as we advance into this new era, anxieties will be expressed in relation to cybersecurity, privacy, and other important social considerations. Since malicious attacks can strike very rapidly, understanding how to react immediately in order to prevent severe damage to the system is a major challenge. Additionally, there is a constantly increasing divergence between the capability enabled by technology and the social and economic value that can be derived from it. Expressed in basic terms, it remains the case that educational and training institutions cannot provide appropriately trained knowledge workers in sufficient number and at sufficient speed in order to enable businesses and other organizations to exploit these new technologies immediately and effectively. To a great extent, this is a consequence of the fact that the development cycle of a technological innovation, and its subsequent diffusion throughout the economy, is now realized in a number of months rather than years. Moreover, the transformation is not only rapid but dramatic. As in every other new era of technological innovation, like, e.g., the industrial revolution, the advances introduced in the current age of the Internet are having a massive impact on the world, leading to, in addition to increases in productivity, a redefinition of occupations, with new professions being created and others becoming obsolete.

Cognitive computing will certainly have a significant influence on all the knowledge-based professions, including the healthcare environment. In this specific field, such advances will enable and enhance the coordination and organization of complex information useful for medical diagnosis and treatment [38]. As a concrete example, machine learning techniques and artificial neural networks will be able to provide invaluable support for the early detection of specific diseases through the identification of possible risk factors and determinist symptoms by means of an easy, fast, and portable m-Health application [39], as shown in Fig. 6.

5   Conclusions

Nowadays, the application of mobile tools and technologies is, more than ever, a key driver for innovation and development of a new way to provide a healthcare service. By promoting patient centricity and a redefinition of the patient role in clinical studies, as well as enhancing data collection or real-time remote monitoring, m-Health strategies are opening doors for huge advancements in the healthcare sector.

In this chapter, we presented the main functionalities and components of an m-Health solution, able to monitor or support the correct diagnosis of specific pathologies. Among these, the connection between m-Health systems and the great amount of patient data is fundamental for the development of mobile healthcare. This connection is realized by using appropriate international standards, such as Health Level 7 or Fast Healthcare Interoperability Resources. As well as, it is

Fig. 6 An example of a cognitive app

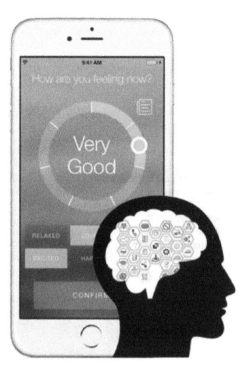

necessary to consider such techniques during the development and design of an m-Health application in order to minimize any possible damage to the privacy and security of patient.

In the next future, Artificial Intelligence and advanced algorithms will represent valid support to early detection of specific diseases. Their integration in m-Health systems provides a safer, faster, and more reliable support for monitoring and diagnosis of pathologies.

References

1. G. Eysenbach, What is e-health? J. Med. Internet Res. **3**, e20 (2001)
2. World Health Organization, *Everybody's Business—Strengthening Health Systems to Improve Health Outcomes: WHO's Framework for Action* (World Health Organization, Geneva, 2007)
3. T.A. Sanner, L.K. Roland, K. Braa, From pilot to scale: Towards an mHealth typology for low-resource contexts. Health Policy Technol. **1**, 155–164 (2012)
4. S. Agarwal, L. Rosenblum, T. Goldschmidt, M. Carras, A. Labrique, *Mobile Technology in Support of Frontline Health Workers. A Comprehensive Overview of the Landscape Knowledge Gaps and Future Directions* (Johns Hopkins University Global mHealth Initiative, Baltimore, MA, 2016)
5. L.T. Kohn, J. Corrigan, M.S. Donaldson, *To Err Is Human: Building a Safer Health System*, vol 6 (National Academy Press, Washington, DC, 2000)

6. World Health Organization, *Global Diffusion of eHealth: Making Universal Health Coverage Achievable: Report of the Third Global Survey on eHealth* (World Health Organization, Geneva, 2016)
7. World Bank, *Mobile Phone Access Reaches Three Quarters of planet's Population* (The World Bank, Washington, DC, 2012)
8. M. Kumar, S. Wambugu, *A Primer on the Security, Privacy, and Confidentiality of Electronic Health Records* (MEASURE Evaluation, University of North Carolina, Chapel Hill, NC, 2015)
9. M. Kay, J. Santos, M. Takane, *mHealth: New Horizons for Health through Mobile Technologies*, vol 64 (World Health Organization, Geneva, 2011), pp. 66–71
10. R.S. Istepanian, E. Jovanov, Y. Zhang, Guest editorial introduction to the special section on m-health: Beyond seamless mobility and global wireless health-care connectivity. IEEE Trans. Inf. Technol. Biomed. **8**, 405–414 (2004)
11. A.B. Labrique, L. Vasudevan, E. Kochi, R. Fabricant, G. Mehl, mHealth innovations as health system strengthening tools: 12 common applications and a visual framework. Glob. Health Sci. Pract. **1**, 160–171 (2013)
12. WHO Toolkit (2019). http://www.dhis2.org/
13. R. Wootton, Twenty years of telemedicine in chronic disease management—An evidence synthesis. J. Telemed. Telecare **18**, 211–220 (2012)
14. S. McLean, A. Sheikh, K. Cresswell, U. Nurmatov, M. Mukherjee, A. Hemmi, et al., The impact of telehealthcare on the quality and safety of care: A systematic overview. PLoS One **8**, e71238 (2013)
15. A.G. Ekeland, A. Bowes, S. Flottorp, Effectiveness of telemedicine: A systematic review of reviews. Int. J. Med. Inform. **79**, 736–771 (2010)
16. E.A. Krupinski, History of telemedicine: Evolution, context, and transformation. Telemed. J E Health **15**, 804–805 (2009)
17. R. Rayman, Telemedicine: Military applications. Aviat. Space Environ. Med. **63**, 135–137 (1992)
18. E.M. Brown, The Ontario telemedicine network: A case report. Telemed. J E Health **19**, 373–376 (2013)
19. L. Uscher-Pines, A. Mehrotra, Analysis of Teladoc use seems to indicate expanded access to care for patients without prior connection to a provider. Health Aff. **33**, 258–264 (2014)
20. M. Hawkins, Physician appointment wait times and Medicaid and Medicare acceptance rates, in *Report of Merritt Hawkins* (2014)
21. K.N. Ray, A.V. Chari, J. Engberg, M. Bertolet, A. Mehrotra, Disparities in time spent seeking medical care in the United States. JAMA Intern. Med. **175**, 1983–1986 (2015)
22. NIHCM Foundation, in *Health Care Is Big Spenders: The Characteristics behind the Curve* (2016). http://www.nihcm.org/topics/cost-quality/health-cares-big-spenders-chart-story
23. S. Naddeo, L. Verde, M. Forastiere, G. De Pietro, G. Sannino, A real-time m-health monitoring system: An integrated solution combining the use of several wearable sensors and Mobile devices, in *HEALTHINF* (2017), pp. 545–552
24. M. Forastiere, G. De Pietro, G. Sannino, An mHealth application for a personalized monitoring of one's own wellness: Design and development, in *International Conference on Innovation in Medicine and Healthcare*, (Springer, Cham, 2016), pp. 269–278
25. L. Verde, G. De Pietro, P. Veltri, G. Sannino, An m-health system for the estimation of voice disorders, in *IEEE International Conference on Multimedia & Expo Workshops (ICMEW)*, (IEEE, 2015), pp. 1–6
26. M.S. Hossain, G. Muhammad, A. Alamri, Smart healthcare monitoring: A voice pathology detection paradigm for smart cities. Multimedia Systems **32**, 1–11 (2017)
27. M.S. Hossain, Cloud-supported cyber–physical localization framework for patients monitoring. IEEE Syst. J. **11**, 118–127 (2017)
28. S.R. Levine, M. Gorman, Telestroke. Stroke **30**(2), 464–469 (1999)
29. K.M. McConnochie, N.E. Wood, H.J. Kitzman, N.E. Herendeen, J. Roy, K.J. Roghmann, Telemedicine reduces absence resulting from illness in urban child care: Evaluation of an innovation. Pediatrics **115**, 1273–1282 (2005)

30. T. Daschle, E.R. Dorsey, The return of the house CallThe return of the house call. Ann. Intern. Med. **162**, 587–588 (2015)
31. P.T. Courneya, K.J. Palattao, J.M. Gallagher, HealthPartners' online clinic for simple conditions delivers savings of $88 per episode and high patient approval. Health Aff. (Millwood) **32**, 385–392 (2013)
32. G.F. Anderson, *Chronic Care: Making the Case for Ongoing Care* (Robert Wood Johnson Foundation, Princeton, NJ, 2010)
33. D. Bender, K. Sartipi, HL7 FHIR: An agile and RESTful approach to healthcare information exchange, in *Proceedings of the 26th IEEE International Symposium on Computer-Based Medical Systems* (2013), pp. 326–331
34. R.L. Garrie, P.E. Paustian, Mhealth regulation, legislation, and cybersecurity, in *mHealth*, ed. by R. S. H. Istepanian, S. Laxminarayan, C. S. Pattichis, (Springer, Boston, MA, 2014), pp. 45–63
35. H. Okhravi, T. Hobson, D. Bigelow, W. Streilein, Finding focus in the blur of moving-target techniques. IEEE Secur. Priv. **12**, 16–26 (2014)
36. A. Eldosouky, W. Saad, On the cybersecurity of m-health IoT systems with LED bitslice implementation. in *2018 IEEE International Conference on Consumer Electronics (ICCE)*, 1–6 (2018)
37. D. Ferebee, V. Shandilya, C. Wu, J. Ricks, D. Agular, K. Cole, et al., A secure framework for mHealth data analytics with visualization, in *2016 IEEE 35th International Performance Computing and Communications Conference (IPCCC)*, (2016), pp. 1–4
38. G. Pravettoni, R. Folgieri, C. Lucchiari, Cognitive science in telemedicine: From psychology to artificial intelligence, in *Tele-Oncology*, ed. by G. Gatti, G. Pravettoni, F. Capello, (Springer, Cham, 2015), pp. 5–22
39. S. Pouriyeh, S. Vahid, G. Sannino, G. D. Pietro, H. Arabnia, J. Gutierrez, A comprehensive investigation and comparison of Machine Learning Techniques in the domain of heart disease," in *2017 IEEE Symposium on Computers and Communications (ISCC)* (2017), pp. 204–207

Deep Learning for EEG Motor Imagery-Based Cognitive Healthcare

Syed Umar Amin, Mansour Alsulaiman, Ghulam Muhammad, M. Shamim Hossain, and Mohsen Guizani

Abstract Electroencephalography (EEG) motor imagery signals have recently gained significant attention due to its ability to encode a person's intent to perform an action. Researchers have used motor imagery signals to help disabled persons control devices, such as wheelchairs and even autonomous vehicles. Hence, the accurate decoding of these signals is important to brain–computer interface (BCI) systems. Such motor imagery-based BCI systems can become an integral part of cognitive modules that are increasingly being used in smart city frameworks. However, the classification and recognition of EEG have consistently been a challenge due to its dynamic time series data and low signal-to-noise ratio. Deep learning methods, such as the convolution neural network (CNN), have achieved remarkable success in computer vision tasks. Considering the limited applications of deep learning for motor imagery EEG classification, this work focuses on developing CNN-based deep learning methods for such purpose. We propose a multiple-CNN feature fusion architecture to extract and fuse features by using subject-specific frequency bands. CNN has been designed with variable filter sizes and split convolutions for the extraction of spatial and temporal information from raw EEG data. A feature fusion technique based on autoencoders is applied. Cross-encoding technique has been proposed and is successfully used to train autoencoders for a novel cross-subject information transfer and augmenting EEG data. This proposed method outperforms the state-of-the-art four-class motor imagery classification methods for subject-specific and cross-subject data. Autoencoder cross-encoding

S. U. Amin · M. Alsulaiman · G. Muhammad
Department of Computer Engineering, College of Computer and Information Sciences (CCIS), King Saud University, Riyadh, Saudi Arabia
e-mail: samin@ksu.edu.sa; msuliman@ksu.edu.sa; ghulam@ksu.edu.sa

M. S. Hossain (⊠)
Department of Software Engineering, College of Computer and Information Sciences (CCIS), King Saud University, Riyadh, Saudi Arabia
e-mail: mshossain@ksu.edu.sa

M. Guizani
Department of Electrical and Computer Engineering, University of Idaho, Moscow, ID, USA

© Springer Nature Switzerland AG 2020
A. El Saddik et al. (eds.), *Connected Health in Smart Cities*,
https://doi.org/10.1007/978-3-030-27844-1_12

helps to learn subject invariant and generic features for EEG data and achieves more than 10% increase on cross-subject classification results. The fusion approaches show the potential of applying multiple CNN feature fusion techniques for the advancement of EEG-related research.

Keywords Motor imagery EEG classification · Deep learning · Convolution neural network · Multi-CNNs feature fusion

1 Introduction

Brain–computer interfaces (BCIs) [1–3] provide a mode of communication between the human brain and external devices [4]. BCI systems do not need action or muscular activity for communication [5], instead, a subject uses brain activity to communicate with external devices [6, 7]. Such systems can help patients with various types of motor disabilities [6, 7]. Electroencephalography (EEG)-based cognitive systems are being used in smart city applications for imparting human intelligence and cognitive behavior to such frameworks [8, 9].

A BCI system functions by reading and identifying different brain activity patterns produced by users, then translates these patterns into the desired commands. Most BCI systems rely on classification techniques [4] to identify brain activity patterns. The classification process involves automatic extraction of underlying features and then estimating the corresponding class for brain activity [5]. The noninvasive scalp EEG [10] is an easy and inexpensive technique for recording brain activity. EEG signals are recorded by using multiple electrodes placed on specific scalp areas. The signals have high temporal resolution in the millisecond range and are thus still impossible to decode even with the latest imaging techniques, such as computed tomography (CT) or magnetic resonance imaging (MRI). These properties make EEG an important area for research and diagnosis related to brain functions and disorders. Motor imagery tasks produce brain oscillations in specific brain areas. These oscillations are observed, in particular, frequency bands, such as alpha, beta, and gamma, and are subject-dependent characteristics. During motor imagery, band power changes for frequency components from single frequency band or multiple bands and varies from subject to subject, and thus active frequency bands for MI tasks are subject specific [11].

Motor imagery (MI) signals [12, 13] have recently attracted considerable interest due to its flexibility and its usefulness in discriminating various brain activations. MI EEG signals are brain activities recorded when the subject imagines or intends to perform actions such as hand or leg movements. MI EEG signals are produced in the brain's sensorimotor cortex area as a response to imagining or thinking tasks [11] and have been utilized by researchers to discriminate between different oscillatory brain activations for different tasks.

MI EEG-based BCIs have used machine learning to build systems that help stroke patients [14], epilepsy patients [15], and people with paralysis [16] to communicate and control external devices, such as wheelchairs and robots [13]. However, as motor imagery has limited spatial resolution, low signal-to-noise ratio (SNR), and dynamic characteristics, the extraction of relevant features is a crucial step in developing a successful BCI system. These issues and the large amount of noise in EEG data lead to difficulties in analyzing brain dynamics and classifying such data. Although conventional machine learning methods have successfully classified MI EEG data to a certain extent, good decoding accuracy has not been attained with handcrafted features. The recent success of deep learning methods has driven researchers to apply them to EEG classification. Automated features can produce better performance than handcrafted features. Deep learning models have achieved state-of-the-art results in different areas such as image and speech classification [17, 18]. For example, convolution neural networks (CNN) have the ability to find robust spatial features from images [19]. Recurrent neural networks (RNN) can extract temporal features better than other networks in applications, such as video and speech classification [20]. Networks, such as autoencoders, are suitable for unsupervised feature learning [21].

Recent studies have employed different deep learning techniques for automated feature extraction from EEG data [22–25]. Few EEG public datasets are available, and most of these datasets have limited sizes. Deep learning models may have millions of parameters that typically require huge training data, and thus applying them to small datasets is difficult. For this reason, limited research has been conducted on deep networks in this area. However, techniques, such as transfer learning, have provided researchers a way to use deep networks by pretraining on large datasets and then fine-tuning for small datasets. These techniques increase performance and reduce training time for deep models [26]. Deep Belief Networks (DBN) and CNN with transfer learning have been used for EEG and functional MRI (fMRI) datasets with a comparatively limited number of training samples [27]. Hence, deep learning models pretrained on similar EEG datasets could help increase decoding performance. However, the increased accuracy achieved by using deep learning models in fields, such as image or speech processing, is not evident in the case of EEG. Therefore, further research is necessary in this area.

Many variations in CNN have been effectively used for image classification. One variation is fusing multiple CNN streams for feature aggregation and improving accuracy. Different CNNs can specialize in extracting various spatial and temporal features, and network architecture and depth affect the performance and accuracy of a CNN. During the course of training, different convolution layers can extract features at different levels of abstraction. Initial layers learn local features, and end layers learn global features. CNN with different depths and filter sizes can extract different features. CNN has been applied for MI EEG classification, but the obtained improvement in accuracy is limited. The EEG signal is time-series data with multiple channels and low SNR and is difficult to interpret because of its nonstationary nature.

Feature fusion and multiple CNN architectures have not been explored for EEG data. In this paper, the proposed method reports performance improvement for MI data, showing that convolution features depend on CNN depth and filter size.

These features can be combined for the development of a robust EEG classification system. Transfer learning and pretraining can help alleviate issues of limited data and overfitting for the improvement of EEG decoding accuracy.

When designing an EEG-based automated classification system, several challenges related to EEG characteristics and classification techniques should be considered.

- EEG signal is nonstationary and has low SNR due to the presence of artifacts, such as muscle movement or eye blinking.
- EEG is recorded with multiple electrodes and thus highly dimensional. Limited training data and high dimensionality can render classification techniques to overfit the data.
- Classification of motor imagery signals is not easy due to the uncertainty of the exact time at which a subject performs a brain activity. Motor imagery is a purely mental task, so only the subject is aware of the exact time he performs the activity.
- The availability of public EEG datasets is limited, and thus the application of deep learning-based methods, which need a large amount of training samples, to EEG classification is extremely challenging.
- The class discriminative band power features for motor imagery tasks are present in different frequency bands for each subject. Therefore, cross-subject classification becomes increasingly complex.

Machine learning algorithms highly depend on patterns and features extracted from EEG data. Hence, with robust features, a machine learning technique can achieve good accuracy. However, as previously pointed out, various conventional machine learning methods have not obtained good decoding accuracy with handcrafted features. Thus, handcrafted features are inadequate for decoding EEG data. Therefore, the main motivation of this thesis is to improve the classification accuracy for MI EEG-based BCI systems.

Current classification techniques have reported results achieved on subject-specific data, as the EEG signal varies highly from subject to subject and even from session to session. The extraction of robust and generic features that do not depend on individual subjects and sessions is another motivation for this thesis.

Temporal information present in the EEG signal is neglected by most machine learning algorithms [28]. These complexities and challenges in EEG feature extraction and classification led to the use of deep learning methods, more precisely CNN, in this study. CNN has the ability to learn robust feature representations by using convolutions and can be designed to adapt to the temporal information and subject-independent characteristics of the EEG signal. Limited availability of public EEG datasets and the risk of overfitting on such small datasets prompted the use of pretraining and transfer learning techniques for deep learning, which have achieved good results in other domains but have not been tested for MI EEG datasets.

Deep learning-based techniques have achieved state-of-the-art performance in many image and speech processing applications [17, 18]. These techniques have the unique capability to extract features from data in a hierarchical manner. However, research using deep learning for EEG classification and, especially, motor imagery signals remain limited. CNN has already achieved similar accuracy as compared with conventional machine learning techniques. As CNN has the ability to find robust features from signals, such as images [19], a properly designed CNN can extract temporal and spatial features from EEG signals.

CNN feature fusion models have led to improvements in performance accuracy for various domains but have not been applied to EEG classification. Another motivation for this study is the performance of CNN with different depths and filters for MI EEG classification. Shallow and deep CNN [28–32] can provide good performance when tested with different filter sizes and for different EEG frequency bands. Different CNNs can specialize in extracting various spatial and temporal features, and the network architecture and depth affect its performance and accuracy.

2   EEG Signal Processing

EEG is a typically noninvasive electrophysiological technique for recording electrical brain activity [10]. Such electrical activity occurs due to the firing of neurons in specific brain areas as a result of the processing taking place inside the brain. The noninvasive EEG, sometimes referred to as scalp EEG, is an easy and inexpensive method in which multiple electrodes are placed on the scalp. The spatial resolution of the EEG signal indicates the spatial adjacency of electrodes, whereas temporal resolution indicates sampling frequency or the frequency at which data are recorded. In general, 21–64 electrodes are used for clinical or research purposes, but more can be added (up to 256 electrodes) to increase spatial resolution. EEG is a multichannel time series characterized by high temporal resolution in the millisecond range and is still impossible to decode with the latest imaging techniques, such as CT or MRI. However, EEG has low spatial resolution. Despite this, EEG remains an important tool for research and diagnosis related to brain function and disorders. EEG is preferred for BCI systems over other noninvasive imaging techniques, such as fMRI and magnetoencephalography (MEG), because it does not require costly instruments or does not require the patient to be stationary. Other noninvasive imaging techniques, such as functional magnetic resonance imaging (fMRI) and magnetoencephalography (MEG), require patients to be stationary and are carried out using costly and large-scale equipment.

A sample EEG recording done using multiple electrodes is shown in Fig. 1. The electrodes are placed on the scalp according to fixed positions. EEG output is typically measured in microvolts and it is a nonstationary time series having low SNR. Figure 2 shows the standard 10–20 system for electrode placement which uses 21 electrodes on particular locations on the scalp. EEG signals that record brain response to external stimuli or events are called Event-related potentials (ERP). Motor imagery is EEG signals recorded while the subject imagines the movement of various body parts, which can help BCI systems to find the subject's intent.

Researchers are also interested in the spectral or frequency content of the EEG signal. EEG signal is composed of several frequency bands. These frequency bands

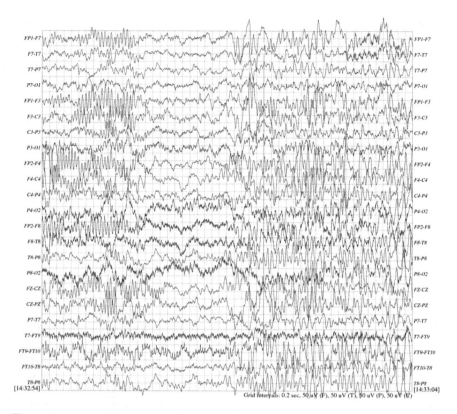

Fig. 1 Example of EEG recording

and spatial distribution of the electrodes are associated with different activities and states of the brain. The frequency bands exhibit distinct changes in amplitude during different tasks. The alpha band shows increase in amplitude when eyes are closed [5]. Table 1 shows different EEG frequency bands and their respective ranges.

Motor imagery and other similar activities which exhibit event-related phenomena show frequency-specific changes which consist of power decrease or increase in particular frequency bands during this EEG activity. This increase in power is called event-related desynchronization (ERD), and the decrease is called event-related synchronization (ERS) [11]. It is also observed that this energy decrease caused by MI task takes place in mu band (8–12 Hz) and energy increase can be observed in the beta band (13–31 Hz) [11]. MI tasks such as left- and right-hand movement show ERD and ERS in the right and left of the motor cortex area of the brain, respectively. Research has also shown that MI tasks also cause brain activity changes in the lower gamma band (32–40 Hz) [5]. ERD and ERS are observed in some frequency components from single frequency band or in multiple bands and which differ from subject to subject showing that the active frequency bands for MI tasks are subject specific [11].

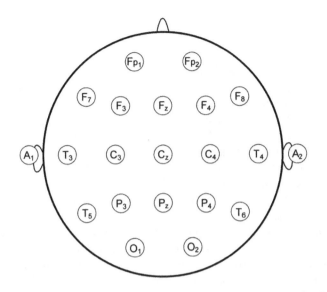

Fig. 2 International 10–20 system showing electrode positions on the scalp for 21 electrodes

Table 1 EEG Frequency bands

Band	Frequency (Hz)
Delta	<4
Theta	4–7
Alpha	8–15
Beta	16–31
Gamma	>32
Mu	8–12

Therefore Alpha, beta, and gamma frequency bands can be utilized to extract band power features, which could help in discriminating MI tasks. Unfortunately, the scalp EEG measurement method makes it susceptible to a number of noise artifacts such as electrocardiographic signals from the heart, electromyographic signals from muscle movement, or the eyes blinking, and tongue movement. These artifacts together with other noise from the environment or recording instruments make EEG analysis and its classification very difficult. However, recent research has demonstrated that machine learning and deep learning techniques can extract relevant EEG features and produce meaningful results.

3   MI EEG Classification

Motor imagery is defined as the mental process in which a subject simulates or rehearses a movement or an action without being executed [28]. Imagining hand, feet, or tongue movements without moving them is an example of MI. This process is widely used in MI-based BCI, neurological rehabilitation, and in research related to the investigation of brain activity, such as cognitive psychology and cognitive neuroscience [29]. The corresponding brain activity is most profound in the supplementary motor area and the primary motor cortex area of the brain. MI-based BCI systems have been developed to help disabled patients control devices, such as wheelchairs, or move the cursor on a screen [13–16].

In MI-based BCI systems, the subject is shown a cue on a screen and asked to perform the MI task shown. While the task is performed, the BCI system records the subject's brain activity, but the system cannot determine when exactly the subject starts imagining the task. Hence, the MI task is controlled only by the subject, which makes EEG interpretation quite difficult. Differences between the trials of the same subject may occur, and sometimes the subject may be unable to perform MI task. This occurrence is known as BCI illiteracy [29].

Most of the MI EEG classification systems based on machine learning techniques employ band-pass filters for time-domain filtering and spatial filters for spatial-domain filtering of the EEG signal. Then, feature extraction techniques are used to find and represent significant patterns in the filtered EEG signals. Feature selection techniques then determine the best feature subsets from the extracted features. Finally, the features are used for training a classifier.

In literature, different types of features have been proposed to represent EEG signals [30], and signals with band power and time point features are the most common. The power or energy of the EEG signal for a particular frequency band in a particular channel is represented by band power features, which are averaged over a time window (normally 1–2 s). These features exploit the oscillatory activity of the brain that is in the form of EEG amplitude changes. Band power features are extensively used for motor imagery BCI systems and for decoding mental tasks. Time point features are used for decoding Event-Related Potentials (ERP)-based BCI systems. ERP are time-domain amplitude changes in EEG signals that are time-locked to an event or stimulus [30]. Time point features are formed by the aggregation of all EEG samples for all channels. These features are extracted after the filtering and down-sampling of EEG signals.

Several studies have extracted band power and time point features after spatial filtering [31], which combines EEG signals from different electrodes and thereby increases the SNR as compared with that of the original EEG signal from each electrode. Using supervised learning to obtain spatial filters is the most common approach and has shown the best accuracy among all conventional feature extraction methods. Common spatial patterns (CSP) [31] are the most popular spatial filters obtained by using a supervised learning approach.

The CSP algorithm [31] uses amplitude changes observed when subjects perform MI tasks. In this algorithm, spatial filters are used to determine the linear transformations of electrodes with variances that can be used to discriminate left or right MI signals. The selected electrodes are spatially filtered, and the energy of selected electrodes is divided by the energy of all electrodes. This value acts as representations or features for the EEG data and can be used by support vector machine (SVM) to achieve good performance after dimension reduction [32]. The

CSP algorithm converts time-series EEG signals into a single value and ignores the temporal information in the signal. Another study extended the CSP algorithm, and the Filter Bank CSP algorithm (FBCSP) [10] was proposed using a linear combination of electrodes and frequency information present in the signal. The FBCSP algorithm is based on filter banks that are multiple band-pass frequency filters. The EEG signals pass through these band-pass filters and are converted into multiple frequency bands, from which CSP energy features are extracted. By using a feature selection algorithm, features are then selected with discriminative frequency bands and supplied to the SVM for classification. The temporal-spatial discriminative features help increase performance for MI classification. Among the machine learning-based MI classification algorithms, FBCSP has achieved the best performance. Other researchers have attempted to extend and improve the CSP algorithm.

Apart from the CSP-based algorithm, other popular algorithms for MI classification have achieved good performance. One such approach is the Riemannian geometry (RG), which uses data, apart from spatial CSP features, in the channel covariance space to classify EEG signals [28]. The RG algorithm employing subspace optimization has achieved good accuracy for MI EEG classification.

All the conventional machine learning algorithms for MI EEG classification and feature extraction discussed above have employed handcrafted features. Although these approaches and features are effective, the accuracy of motor imagery classification still requires improvements. Therefore, we investigated deep learning techniques to improve performance and find features that are more robust than handcrafted features.

4 Deep Learning for Motor Imagery Classification

EEG signals are recorded with multiple channels with a high sampling rate that accounts for its high dimensionality. A correlation exists between channels and low SNR due to the presence of artifacts and noise. Inspired by the success of deep learning models in numerous fields, many researchers have successfully applied deep learning models for EEG classification. Different methods for EEG data representation and dimensionality reduction have been proposed to prepare data at inputs to these models. Researchers have attempted to automatically extract temporal and spatial features from EEG signals. Multiple restricted Boltzmann machines that extract robust features from many EEG datasets have been proposed [32]. CNN has been a popular choice for analyzing spatial features and classifying EEG signals [23, 28] and has been used with RNN [32] to extract multidimensional features for capturing cognitive events from MI signals. CNN and autoencoders are used [22] in emotion recognition using EEG signals. Other researchers convert EEG signals into images and topological maps before they send the signals as inputs to deep learning models. A CNN and Long Short-Term Memory (LSTM)-based model was proposed and employed the Fourier transform of the EEG signal to represent them as scalp topological maps [33]. The resulting images act as inputs to the combined CNN and LSTM model. Novel image representations and the extraction of temporal features with the RNN model helped provide a good performance. A new set of features was proposed by combining spatial, spectral, and temporal information in EEG data. Another study [34] converted EEG signals into images by utilizing short-time Fourier transform (STFT), using a two-class public dataset with three EEG channels; the authors used mu and beta band features using CNN and stacked autoencoder (SAE) for MI classification. A CNN-based model was proposed for P300 EEG signal classification [35], which could extract temporal and spatial features by performing the first convolution spatially for all EEG channels and then the second convolution across time-samples for the entire EEG recording. This CNN structure is usually employed for the classification of steady-state visually evoked potentials (SSVEP). CNN is also used to extract features from raw EEG signals for music imagery classification [36]. In another paper, a convolutional autoencoder (CAE) was used for the same task, and a cross-trial and similarity constraint encoding method was proposed for subject-independent EEG music imagery classification [36]. These encoding techniques can be used for transfer learning and help train deep networks with limited EEG data. The CNN model is trained on log-energy features extracted from each frequency band. Raw EEG is used as input for deep and shallow CNN architectures for MI EEG decoding and visualization [37]. The study shows how to crop trials into small inputs to increase training data and accuracy. Similarly, recent CNN advancements are employed to achieve competitive accuracy for MI EEG classification.

The studies mentioned above have used various conventional machine learning and deep learning methods for motor imagery classification and decoding. Although deep learning methods have recently achieved state-of-the-art results for this task, a substantial improvement in accuracy similar to that achieved for image and speech processing has not been attained. Given that the maximum subject-specific accuracy is still less than 75%, and cross-subject accuracy is approximately 40% in public MI datasets [2], new inventions and architectures related to CNN are necessary for further improvement.

5   Multilayer CNN Feature Fusion for Motor Imagery Classification

This section describes the multilayer CNN feature extraction and fusion method proposed in this thesis. The CNN architecture, pretraining, extraction of convolution features, and weight-based feature fusion are discussed. Similarly, we present the experiments conducted, results obtained for MI EEG classification, and visual analysis of the features.

5.1 Input Representation

Most EEG datasets are recorded in many sessions for each subject, and each session consists of many trials. In subject-specific training and testing, each EEG data set supplied to the CNN model consists of labeled trials that belong to a given subject i. The data sets can be represented as $D_i = \{(X^1, y^1), \ldots, (X^{N_i}, y^{N_i})\}$ where N_i is the number of trials for each subject i. Each labeled trial j is a time segment of the EEG recording belonging to one of the K classes for motor imagery tasks. The EEG input for trial j is in the form of a matrix, $X^j \in \mathbb{R}^{E.T}$, where E and T denote the electrodes and time steps recorded for each trial, respectively. The output produced for each trial j is mapped onto one of the class labels y^j, which in our case corresponds to one of the imagined motor imagery tasks: left hand (class 1), right hand (class 2), both feet (class 3), and tongue (class 4).

Different input representations for EEG have been used to supply input to the CNN. One approach is to transform EEG recordings into topographic images in a time series. The scalp surface is flattened and voltage recordings are used to form a power spectrum, which then acts as inputs for the CNN [33]. The relevant EEG patterns are global and do not possess hierarchical composition in space [37]. EEG signals have been shown to correlate over multiple time scales. Hence, this study employs EEG representation, so that the CNN is able to automatically extract global spatial and temporal patterns from the EEG signal. The EEG signal is represented in the form of a 2D array with time steps across electrodes.

Electrode voltage has been used over the flattened scalp surface to convert EEG signals to topographical time-series images [38]. However, the conversion may result in the loss of important information and features. Evidence has shown that EEG signals are correlated to time scales that involve modulation in time [39]. Furthermore, CNN has recently achieved good accuracy for EEG data represented as 2D input with time-samples across channels [37].

5.2 CNN Architecture

The CNN architecture of the proposed method is inspired by popular CNN in computer vision, such as AlexNet [17]. A basic architecture is selected for the design of a CNN that can extract generic features from EEG data [28–30]. Our method has four blocks of convolutional- and max-pooling layers and a fully connected softmax classification layer at the end, as shown in Fig. 3. Compared with three-channel (RGB) image input, EEG signals have multiple channels; thus, the first convolution layer is split into two convolutions for the handling of a large number of channels. One-dimensional convolution and split convolution strategy have been successfully used for decoding many types of EEG [37, 40]. Without activation function in between, these two convolutions act like one logical convolution. Splitting the first convolution operation in this manner enables the division of the

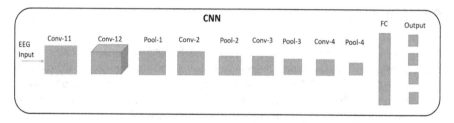

Fig. 3 Deep CNN architecture

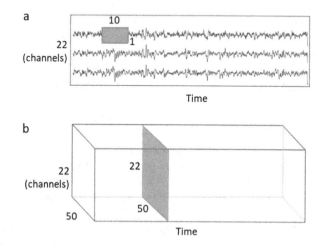

Fig. 4 (**a**) and (**b**) The first convolution operation split into two parts. (**a**) In the first part, convolution is performed across time steps. (**b**) In the second part, convolution is performed across all channels

linear transformation into temporal and spatial convolutions. The first part captures temporal features using filters for each channel, and the second part extracts spatial features for all channels similar to the CSP spatial filter. Split convolution shows better performance than normal convolution. The EEG input is in the form of 2D array with samples stored in time steps across channels (electrodes). Figure 4 shows the first convolution layer.

CNN has achieved good results on signals with a natural hierarchical structure, such as images. Initial convolution layers learn edges and boundaries for objects, and later convolution layers learn more complex object shapes. Pooling layers reduce the dimensions of the convolution features and thereby inducing translational invariance in the CNN. In this progressive manner, CNN can automatically learn hierarchical features layer by layer.

CNN consists of multiple convolutional layers composed of filters or kernels. These filters are convolved with the input signal. Stride is the parameter that determines the number of filter convolutions with the input. The output for convolution operation, which is a set of kernel or feature maps, can be expressed by Eq. (1) below.

$$y_{i'j'} = \sum_{i,j=0}^{n} w_{ij} x_{i+i', j+j'} \tag{1}$$

where $y_{i'j'}$ is the feature map produced at the position $i'j'$ of the input vector; w_{ij} is the kernel or filter matrix element; $x_{i+i', j+j'}$ is the input spatial region element; i, j denote the row and column index of the filter's current elements pair; and n denotes the number of filter elements. Exponential linear units are used as activation function, as shown in Eq. (2):

$$f(x) = x \text{ for } x > 0 \text{ and } f(x) = e^x - 1 \text{ for } x \leq 0 \tag{2}$$

Multilayer CNNs with different filter sizes and depths are designed and fused for the acquisition of robust features. CNN provides good results for particular frequency bands for each subject, indicating that the most active frequency bands for motor imagery tasks are subject specific. Thus, we used different frequency bands for different CNNs. The EEG signal is band-pass filtered into the frequency band with a range of 0–40 Hz.

The proposed methods comprise multilayer CNNs fused with an autoencoder, and collectively named as model CNN-A. In the first phase, each CNN is pretrained individually on the HGD [37]. In the second phase, these pretrained models are trained on the target BCID [41] dataset. After the training phases are complete, the CNN features are concatenated and passed as input to an autoencoder for fusion. The autoencoder-based fusion model is then trained separately with the combined CNN features. A softmax activation function layer is used as a classifier on top of the autoencoder fusion model, and the resulting networks are then fine-tuned for the acquisition of the output class labels for MI tasks. The architectural details for the different CNNs used are provided in Table 2.

Table 2 Structure of CNNs used for feature fusion

CNN-shallow	CNN-deep
Conv (30 × 1, 50 filters)	Conv (10 × 1, 50 filters)
Conv (1 × 22, 50 filters)	Conv (1 × 22, 50 filters)
Max Pool (3 × 1, stride 3)	Max Pool (3 × 1, stride 3)
Dense (1024)	Conv (10 × 1, 100 filters)
Softmax (4 classes)	Max Pool (3 × 1, stride 3)
	Conv (10 × 1, 100 filters)
	Max Pool (3 × 1, stride 3)
	Conv (10 × 1, 200 filters)
	Max Pool (3 × 1, stride 3)
	Dense (1024)
	Softmax (4 classes)

With the need to test different CNN design strategies, multiple CNNs are created and tested with a different number of layers and different filter size. The study started with a CNN with a single convolution, pooling block, and a dense classification layer at the end. The number of convolution and pooling blocks is increased until the performance of the models degrades. As shown in literature, most of the successful studies using CNN or other deep learning models for EEG classification have shallow architectures [28–32] and few models that have one or two layers [37, 40]. A deep CNN [37] was implemented to act as a baseline and to compare results with this model, because this study is so far the best deep learning technique available for MI EEG classification.

MI recordings have multiple channels that range from 3 to 128, thus this strategy is useful in the management of multisource inputs. As previously explained, in this strategy, the first convolution operation is performed on each channel or across some time-samples, and the second convolution is conducted for all the channels, one sample at a time. The resulting effect is a convolution across all input channels for a number of samples. The MI data is fed to the CNN as a 2D array with the channels as rows and time-samples as columns. The split convolution favors this representation. The first convolution across time-samples can learn temporal features, and the second convolution across channels is better adept to learn spatial features.

Overfitting on small training datasets can be prevented through pretraining. HGD is a large MI dataset created under controlled recording conditions and therefore contains minimum noise. HGD is recorded with 128 electrodes from 20 healthy subjects and consists of 880 trials in the training set and 160 trials in the test set. Given that the training data available are larger than the BCID dataset, HGD is an excellent resource for pretraining deep learning models.

5.3 Training

Two techniques are often used for training systems on EEG datasets. EEG data is usually recorded in multiple sessions. Hence, one session is placed in the test set, and all the rest are placed in the training set. In this way, the system is tested on sessions that it has not seen before but belongs to the same subject. This within-subject training is preferable as the EEG signal is dynamic, and testing across subjects provides poor accuracy. The other training technique involves subject-to-subject information transfer. One subject serves as the testing set, and all the rest act as a training set. This process is repeated for all users. This cross-subject training technique is more challenging, and the evaluation is more robust and generalized. We used both techniques to train and test our proposed deep learning method.

The EEG data is cropped using a 2 s sliding window and then fed to the CNNs. Cropped training forces the CNN to learn generic EEG features rather than learn features specific to a trial or subject [37].

Convolutions are followed by nonlinearity, max-pooling, and dense layer with softmax. Performance improves when batch normalization and dropout are used. Exponential linear units (ELU) are used as the activation function. The number and sizes of filters and strides for each CNN model are provided in Table 2. Minibatch stochastic gradient descent is used for optimizing CNN parameters. The softmax function produces probability scores for each class. Batch normalization technique contributes to performance enhancement.

Any increase in performance is determined by gradually increasing the convolution-pooling blocks. CNNs with one, two, three, and four blocks show improved learning capabilities for specific filter sizes and frequency bands. The filter size and numbers are varied across models until the best combination is obtained for each CNN.

Using more than four convolution-pooling blocks results in continuous performance degradation, and thus CNNs with more than five blocks are not used in this fusion method. This observation is aligned with other studies that use CNN architectures with few layers for EEG decoding [28–30]. Deeper CNNs and residual networks with very deep architecture are not suitable, as no research has achieved good EEG decoding accuracy with them [37].

CNN with one convolution-pooling block (CNN-shallow) and four convolution-pooling blocks (CNN-deep) show reasonable performance with particular filter sizes. An initial filter size of 30×1 is used for CNN-shallow and 10×1 for CNN-deep. Shallow CNNs using larger filter size may be effective at learning specific temporal and spatial features, such as FBCSP, whereas the deep CNNs may be suitable for extracting generic EEG features. This study investigated whether fusing the features from these different CNNs improves classification accuracy.

6   Multilayer CNN Feature Fusion

In this study, a fusion method is proposed to combine CNNs for EEG classification. One-layer CNN [37] has been used and have achieved similar results as reported by the FBCSP method. CNN with more number of layers has been proposed to achieve good decoding accuracy [37]. In this study, a fusion method using MLP and autoencoders is used to fuse CNNs. Different CNN architectures may be effective in extracting different types of EEG features. Hence, their fusion can help build generic features for EEG decoding. Feature fusion for CNNs has not been evaluated for EEG classification. EEG data is time-series recording that has multiple channel sources, low SNR, and a nonstationary nature, and thus extracting relevant features is a challenging task. Using multi-CNN feature fusion, this study aims to uncover generic and robust features to improve EEG classification accuracy.

Feature fusion is conducted using two different architecture autoencoders. These networks have been utilized for fusion and feature extraction [37]. The CNNs are pretrained on the HGD dataset, and then fused by removing their final softmax classification layer and concatenating the features with a linear layer. This architecture

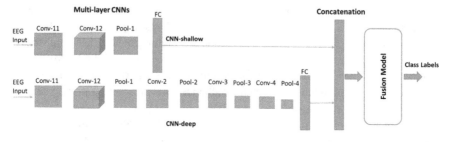

Fig. 5 Multilayer CNNs fusion

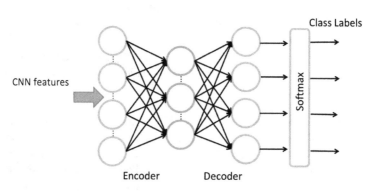

Fig. 6 Feature fusion model

of a multilayer CNN method is shown in Fig. 5. The multilayer CNNs method is now trained on the BCID dataset through the within-subject and cross-subject training approaches. A ninefold cross-validation scheme is used as a cross-subject scheme, data from eight subjects are trained, and the remaining one subject is validated. The resulting multilayer CNN features from the concatenation layer are fed to the autoencoder. The network is then trained and fine-tuned on the combined feature vector, and the output is sent to the softmax layer for the acquisition of the probability score for the MI classes. The overall fusion architecture is provided in Fig. 6.

7   Cross-Encoding with Autoencoders

An autoencoder is used as a fusion model. The CNN feature set is fed to the input layer of the autoencoder and then passed through the fully connected hidden layer for the reconstruction of the same input feature set at the output layer. The hidden layer has a lower number of neurons, as depicted in Fig. 6 [23], and the output layer has the same number of nodes as the input layer in order to reconstruct its own inputs. The hidden layer acts as a bottleneck that removes redundancy and learns the most important features required to reconstruct the input. The autoencoders act as an unsupervised learning technique. During training, input x is mapped to the hidden layer during the encoding stage, and the hidden layer z output is mapped to the output layer to reconstruct the input during the decoding stage. After an unsupervised autoencoder training, supervised fine-tuning is conducted for the simultaneous training and optimization of network parameters with the backpropagation algorithm [21].

In this study, we aim to learn discriminative features that can be used by a classifier to distinguish between the different motor imagery tasks for EEG data. Individual differences always exist between subjects and between recording sessions even when the EEG is recorded in controlled environments and optimal settings. These differences increase the difficulty of combining recordings from different subjects for the identification of general patterns in EEG signals. This problem can be addressed by taking the average over many very short trials so that the differences cancel each other out. However, EEG recording is a tiring and time-consuming activity. Therefore, this strategy is infeasible. Hence, we devise an alternative strategy to determine signal patterns from the raw EEG data that are stable across subjects and represent generic EEG characteristics.

Many studies utilized autoencoders for learning CNN features [34] and achieved improvements over CNN classification. In the present study, autoencoders are used for fusion and learning of the combined feature vector. The concatenated feature is fed to the autoencoder to learn generic EEG features. The autoencoders model has 100 hidden nodes, which show good learning capability. The cross-trial encoding scheme is used according to previous autoencoder training approaches [42]. Autoencoders are trained for within-subject and cross-subject features. In within-subject training, the autoencoder is forced to reconstruct another trial belonging to another session from the same subject and class instead of simply trying to reconstruct same input trial when fed with a combined CNN feature set from a particular session and class for a subject. If there are n_C trials for a particular class C, then n_C^2 pairs of input and target trials can be constructed for the autoencoder training. In this manner, the autoencoder increases the training samples and learns robust and generic underlying characteristics for the EEG data. In the cross-subject training, the autoencoders are given features belonging to one subject and are forced to reconstruct features belonging to any other subject for the same class. Subsequently, a softmax layer is used for the identification of class labels for the reconstructed output features. In this manner, the autoencoder provides better performance for within-subject and cross-subject testing. Cross-encoding autoencoders in this way leads to adaptations that reflect individual differences between subjects and provides common representation across subjects. Similar to an autoencoder, the training objective here is to minimize a reconstruction error. Therefore, this is an unsupervised training with the only difference is that we have paired trials based on their class labels. The distance used is based on the dot product for reconstruction error. In cross-subject training, the trials are paired within subjects and then trained with trial pairs across subjects. In

Fig. 7 Cross-encoding with
autoencoders

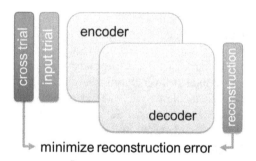

minimize reconstruction error

this process, the autoencoder is enabled to adapt to differences between the subjects
by conducting the training across all pairs of trials across subjects and using the best
weight for each subject. This cross-encoding scheme is depicted in Fig. 7.

By using the multilayer CNNs feature fusion approach, we are able to utilize
CNNs that vary in filter size and number of layers. This approach can extract
different convolutional features at different levels. CNNs have achieved good EEG
decoding accuracy [37, 43] with different depths of convolution layers and filter
sizes. Therefore, in this work, not only CNNs with different depths and different
filter sizes but also fused features from these CNNs are used in the construction of
a comprehensive feature vector.

8 Experiments and Results

Deep CNN model [37] is selected as a baseline for the evaluation of our proposed
multilayer CNNs fusion methods. This CNN method shows best results for EEG
classification [34, 44]. The deep CNN model [30] is implemented in PyTorch,
and the model is tested on the BCID dataset. The comparison between the overall
accuracy of our proposed methods with that of other methods is shown in Table
3. The proposed MCNN method outperforms other methods on BCID and HGD.
Our method achieved 74.1% accuracy for subject-specific training and testing on
the BCID dataset. Individual pretrained CNNs are tested, and the results show that
the fusion methods improve performance, as shown in Table 4.

Table 3 Subject-specific classification results obtained for the BCID and HGD datasets

Methods	Description	Accuracy (BCID)	Accuracy (HGD)
Ang et al. [40]	Filter Bank CSP	68.0%	91.2%
Tabar et al. [34]	1D CNN with SAE	70.0%	–
Lawhern et al. [44]	CNN with depth and separable convolutions	69.0%	–
Schirrmeister et al. [37]	CNN with cropped training	72.0%	92.5%
Proposed method	**CNN-A**	**74.1%**	**94.0%**

Table 4 Classification results for CNNs with different number of Convolution-Pooling Blocks layers with a corresponding convolution filter size

Models	Conv-filter size	Accuracy (BCID)	Accuracy (HGD)
CNN-shallow	30×1	73.7%	89.1%
CNN-deep	10×1	72.8%	92.8%

Table 5 Cross-subject classification results for the BCID and HGC datasets

Methods	Description	Accuracy (BCID)	Accuracy (HGD)
Ang et al. [40]	Filter Bank CSP	38.0%	65.2%
Lawhern et al. [44]	CNN with depth and separable convolutions	40.0%	–
Schirrmeister et al. [37]	CNN with cropped training	41.0%	69.5%
Sakhavi et al. [45]	Temporal features with FBCSP and CNN	44.4%	–
Proposed method	**CNN-A**	**53.2%**	**77.7%**

One of the major contributions of this paper is cross-subject classification improvement. The CCNN method with cross-encoding technique provides cross-subject EEG classification results that are better than those reported in literature. This study is the first to investigate the effects of cross-trial autoencoder training, which showed state-of-the-art performance, as shown in Table 5. Cross-trial auto encoding not only helped us increase the training set manifolds but also helped autoencoders learn generic EEG features that are not subject specific. The proposed method achieved over 10% accuracy improvement for cross-subject classification in contrast to state-of-the-art deep learning models.

9 Conclusion

This study proposed a novel method for deep feature learning from MI EEG recordings that address issues and challenges for this domain. Multilayer CNN feature fusion method for fusing features from different CNN layers and architectures were proposed. Then, we used a cross-encoding technique to determine the difference between individual subjects and trials and to apply the network to stable and common patterns across subjects. The results obtained by the proposed methods prove that CNNs with different architectures, depths, and filter sizes have overwhelming effect on accuracy and can extract different feature representations that can be fused to improve classification accuracy. Using pretrained CNNs can help improve feature learning and training on small-sized datasets. The cross-encoding approach used for autoencoders can help improve cross-subject classification. The proposed methods can learn a general representation of EEG signals that aid cross-subject classification. Experimental results conducted on different challenging datasets confirm the superiority of the proposed fusion methods as compared with state-of-the-art machine learning and deep learning methods for EEG classification. The proposed method has been evaluated for both subject-specific and cross-subject classification on challenging public dataset.

This method can be used as a cognitive system in a smart city environment to help stakeholders communicate and control devices using motor imagery signals.

For future work, we aim to further refine CNN models and fusion methods to improve within-subject and cross-subject classification accuracy. We intend to determine robust features that allow our methods to be used as part of advanced BCI systems.

Acknowledgments The authors extend their appreciation to the International Scientific Partnership Program ISPP at King Saud University for funding this research work through ISPP-121.

References

1. Z. Emami, T. Chau, Investigating the effects of visual distractors on the performance of a motor imagery brain-computer interface. Clin. Neurophysiol. **129**(6), 1268–1275 (2018)
2. F. Lotte et al., A review of classification algorithms for EEG-based brain–computer interfaces: a 10 year update. J. Neural Eng. **15**(3), 031005 (2018)
3. A.M. Chiarelli, P. Croce, A. Merla, F. Zappasodi, Deep learning for hybrid EEG-fNIRS brain–computer interface: application to motor imagery classification. J. Neural Eng. **15**(3), 036028 (2018)
4. M.-P. Hosseini, D. Pompili, K. Elisevich, H. Soltanian-Zadeh, Optimized deep learning for EEG big data and seizure prediction BCI via internet of things. IEEE Transactions on Big Data **3**(4), 392–404 (2017)
5. J.R. Wolpaw, N. Birbaumer, D.J. McFarland, G. Pfurtscheller, T.M. Vaughan, Brain–computer interfaces for communication and control. Clin. Neurophysiol. **113**(6), 767–791 (2002)
6. T.M. Vaughan et al., Brain-computer interface technology: a review of the Second International Meeting. IEEE Trans. Neural Syst. Rehabil. Eng. **11**(2), 94–109 (2003)
7. M.S. Hossain et al., Applying Deep Learning for Epilepsy Seizure Detection and Brain Mapping Visualization. ACM Trans. Multimedia Comput. Commun. Appl. (ACM TOMM) **14**(5), 10 (2018). 16 pages
8. M. Alhussein et al., Cognitive IoT-cloud integration for smart healthcare: case study for epileptic seizure detection and monitoring. Mobile Netw. Appl., 1–12 (2018)
9. S.U. Amin et al., Cognitive smart healthcare for pathology detection and monitoring. IEEE Access **7**, 10745–10753 (2019). https://doi.org/10.1109/ACCESS.2019.2891390
10. L.J. Greenfield, J.D. Geyer, P.R. Carney, *Reading EEGs: A practical approach* (Lippincott Williams & Wilkins, Philadelphia, PA, 2012)
11. G. Pfurtscheller, F.L. Da Silva, Event-related EEG/MEG synchronization and desynchronization: basic principles. Clin. Neurophysiol. **110**(11), 1842–1857 (1999)
12. K.K. Ang, Z.Y. Chin, C. Wang, C. Guan, H. Zhang, Filter bank common spatial pattern algorithm on BCI competition IV datasets 2a and 2b. Front. Neurosci. **6**, 39 (2012)
13. L. Tonin, T. Carlson, R. Leeb, J. d. R. Millán, Brain-controlled telepresence robot by motor-disabled people, in *2011 Annual International Conference of the IEEE Engineering in Medicine and Biology Society* (IEEE, Honolulu, HI, 2011), pp. 4227–4230
14. A. Ramos-Murguialday et al., Brain–machine interface in chronic stroke rehabilitation: a controlled study. Ann. Neurol. **74**(1), 100–108 (2013)
15. G. Muhammad et al., Automatic Seizure Detection in a Mobile Multimedia Framework. IEEE Access **6**, 45372–45383 (2018)

16. F. Nijboer et al., A P300-based brain–computer interface for people with amyotrophic lateral sclerosis. Clin. Neurophysiol. **119**(8), 1909–1916 (2008)
17. A. Krizhevsky, I. Sutskever, G.E. Hinton, Imagenet classification with deep convolutional neural networks. Adv. Neural Inf. Proces. Syst., 1097–1105 (2012)
18. Y. LeCun and Y. Bengio, Convolutional networks for images, speech, and time series, in MA Arbib The Handbook of Brain Theory and Neural Networks, MIT PressCambridge, MA 3361, 10, p. 1995, 1995
19. H.-C. Shin et al., Deep convolutional neural networks for computer-aided detection: CNN architectures, dataset characteristics and transfer learning. IEEE Trans. Med. Imaging **35**(5), 1285–1298 (2016)
20. A. Ghoneim et al., Medical Image Forgery Detection for Smart Healthcare. IEEE Commun. Mag. **56**(4), 33–37 (2018). https://doi.org/10.1109/MCOM.2018.1700817
21. Y. Bengio, P. Lamblin, D. Popovici, H. Larochelle, Greedy layer-wise training of deep networks. Adv. Neural Inf. Proces. Syst., 153–160 (2007)
22. M.S. Hossain et al., Improving consumer satisfaction in smart cities using edge computing and caching: A case study of date fruits classification. Futur. Gener. Comput. Syst. **88**, 333–341 (2018)
23. A. Antoniades et al., Detection of interictal discharges with convolutional neural networks using discrete ordered multichannel intracranial EEG. IEEE Trans. Neural Syst. Rehabil. Eng. **25**(12), 2285–2294 (2017)
24. M. Rawashdeh et al., Reliable service delivery in Tele-health care systems. J. Netw. Comput. Appl. **115**, 86–93 (2018)
25. X. Zhang, L. Yao, Q.Z. Sheng, S.S. Kanhere, T. Gu, D. Zhang, Converting your thoughts to texts: Enabling brain typing via deep feature learning of eeg signals, in *2018 IEEE International Conference on Pervasive Computing and Communications (PerCom)*, (IEEE, 2018), pp. 1–10
26. P. Mirowski, D. Madhavan, Y. LeCun, R. Kuzniecky, Classification of patterns of EEG synchronization for seizure prediction. Clin. Neurophysiol. **120**(11), 1927–1940 (2009)
27. X. Xie, Z.L. Yu, H. Lu, Z. Gu, Y. Li, Motor imagery classification based on bilinear sub-manifold learning of symmetric positive-definite matrices. IEEE Trans. Neural Syst. Rehabil. Eng. **25**(6), 504–516 (2017)
28. J. Decety, D.H. Ingvar, Brain structures participating in mental simulation of motor behavior: A neuropsychological interpretation. Acta Psychol. **73**(1), 13–34 (1990)
29. K.K. Ang et al., A randomized controlled trial of EEG-based motor imagery brain-computer interface robotic rehabilitation for stroke. Clin. EEG Neurosci. **46**(4), 310–320 (2015)
30. F. Lotte, A tutorial on EEG signal-processing techniques for mental-state recognition in brain–computer interfaces, in *Guide to Brain-Computer Music Interfacing*, ed. by E. R. Miranda, J. Castet, (Springer, Heidelberg, 2014), pp. 133–161
31. H. Ramoser, J. Muller-Gerking, G. Pfurtscheller, Optimal spatial filtering of single trial EEG during imagined hand movement. IEEE Trans. Rehabil. Eng. **8**(4), 441–446 (2000)
32. F. Lotte, C. Guan, Regularizing common spatial patterns to improve BCI designs: unified theory and new algorithms. IEEE Trans. Biomed. Eng. **58**(2), 355–362 (2011)
33. P. Bashivan, I. Rish, M. Yeasin, and N. Codella, Learning representations from EEG with deep recurrent-convolutional neural networks, in *CoRR*, vol. abs/1511.06448, 2015
34. Y.R. Tabar, U. Halici, A novel deep learning approach for classification of EEG motor imagery signals. J. Neural Eng. **14**(1), 016003 (2016)
35. H. Cecotti, A. Graser, Convolutional neural networks for P300 detection with application to brain-computer interfaces. IEEE Trans. Pattern Anal. Mach. Intell. **33**(3), 433–445 (2011)
36. S. Stober, Learning discriminative features from electroencephalography recordings by encoding similarity constraints, in *2017 IEEE International Conference on Acoustics, Speech and Signal Processing (ICASSP)*, (IEEE, 2017), pp. 6175–6179
37. R.T. Schirrmeister et al., Deep learning with convolutional neural networks for EEG decoding and visualization. Hum. Brain Mapp. **38**(11), 5391–5420 (2017)

38. P. Thodoroff, J. Pineau, and A. Lim, Learning robust features using deep learning for automatic seizure detection, in *Machine Learning for Healthcare Conference*, 2016, pp. 178–190

39. R.T. Canolty et al., High gamma power is phase-locked to theta oscillations in human neocortex. Science **313**(5793), 1626–1628 (2006)

40. K.K. Ang, Z.Y. Chin, H. Zhang, C. Guan, Filter bank common spatial pattern (FBCSP) in brain-computer interface, in *2008 IEEE international joint conference on neural networks (IEEE world congress on computational intelligence)*, (IEEE, 2008), pp. 2390–2397

41. C. Brunner, R. Leeb, G. Müller-Putz, A. Schlögl, G. Pfurtscheller, *BCI Competition 2008– Graz data set A*, vol 16 (Institute for Knowledge Discovery (Laboratory of Brain-Computer Interfaces), Graz University of Technology, 2008)

42. W. Wang, Y. Huang, Y. Wang, L. Wang, Generalized autoencoder: A neural network framework for dimensionality reduction. in *Proceedings of the IEEE Conference on Computer Vision and Pattern Recognition Workshops*, 490–497 (2014)

43. S.U. Amin, M. Alsulaiman, G. Muhammad, M.A. Bencherif, M.S. Hossain, Multilevel weighted feature fusion using convolutional neural networks for EEG motor imagery classification. IEEE Access **7**, 18940–18950 (2019). https://doi.org/10.1109/ACCESS.2019.2895688

44. V.J. Lawhern, A.J. Solon, N.R. Waytowich, S.M. Gordon, C.P. Hung, B.J. Lance, EEGNet: a compact convolutional neural network for EEG-based brain–computer interfaces. J. Neural Eng. **15**(5), 056013 (2018)

45. S. Sakhavi, C. Guan, S. Yan, Learning temporal information for brain-computer interface using convolutional neural networks. IEEE Transactions on Neural Networks and Learning Systems (99), 1–11 (2018)

CPSIA information can be obtained
at www.ICGtesting.com
Printed in the USA
LVHW061124271220
675113LV00011B/1901

9 783030 278465